Y

3

2

Cambridge History of Medicine

EDITORS: CHARLES WEBSTER AND CHARLES ROSENBERG

Bilharzia

Bilharzia

A HISTORY OF IMPERIAL TROPICAL MEDICINE

JOHN FARLEY

Dalhousie University, Halifax, Nova Scotia

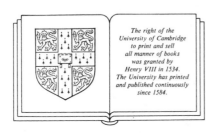

The right of the
University of Cambridge
to print and sell
all manner of books
was granted by
Henry VIII in 1534.
The University has printed
and published continuously
since 1584.

CAMBRIDGE UNIVERSITY PRESS

CAMBRIDGE

NEW YORK   PORT CHESTER   MELBOURNE   SYDNEY

Published by the Press Syndicate of the University of Cambridge
The Pitt Building, Trumpington Street, Cambridge CB2 1RP
40 West 20th Street, New York, NY 10011, USA
10 Stamford Road, Oakleigh, Melbourne 3166, Australia

© Cambridge University Press 1991

First published 1991

Printed in the United States of America

Library of Congress Cataloging-in-Publication Data
Farley, John, 1936–
Bilharzia : a history of imperial tropical medicine / John Farley.
p.   cm. – (Cambridge history of medicine)
Includes index.
ISBN 0-521-40086-4 (hardcover)
1. Schistosomiasis – Developing countries – History.   2. Medicine –
Great Britain – History.   I. Title.   II. Series.
[DNLM: 1. Schistosomiasis – history.   WC 11.1 F231b]
RA644.S3F37   1991
614.5′53 – dc20
DNLM/DLC
for Library of Congress   90-2430
                                                                              CIP

British Library Cataloguing in Publication Data
Farley, John *1936–*
Bilharzia : a history of imperial tropical medicine.
1. Tropical medicine, history
I. Title
616.9883009

ISBN 0-521-40086-4 hardback

CONTENTS

TABLES AND FIGURES

ACKNOWLEDGMENTS

This book has been a labor of love, bringing together many things that have long interested me: a professional fascination with parasites, a love of history, and a longtime interest in imperialism, whether of the Roman variety (I grew up in Britain in what was once an important Roman town), or of the more recent British vintage, which was already decaying when I became conscious of it.

Curiously, however, this study began and ended in the United States. It started one afternoon in the Harvard University office of Barbara Rosenkrantz, who told me that the period of procrastination was over; I had to start. The first notes were taken in the magnificent archives of the Rockefeller Foundation situated, I am glad to say, some miles away from New York, and the final chapters were tied together while I was a Scholar in Residence in that idyllic Italian enclave of the Rockefeller Foundation on the Bellagio promontory overlooking Lake Como. To Barbara, the archivists in Tarrytown, and the staff of the Villa Serbelloni I extend my sincere thanks.

My mecca, however, had to be in London, which even the Rockefellers admitted was the seat of empire and whose benevolence helped build what has been for many years the center of my world – the library of the London School of Hygiene and Tropical Medicine and particularly its vertiginous mezzanine balcony. I would like to thank Ms. Gibson and her staff for their help over the years, and David Bradley for providing space in the Ross Institute that I was able to call my own. I wish also to thank Bill Bynum, in whose department at University College I spent part of a sabbatical, and Shula Marks who made me realize how important South Africa was to my story and allowed me to attend one of her seminars in South African history at the Institute for Commonwealth Studies. I would also like to thank Sheila Willmott and the staff at Winches Farm field station in St. Albans, the very helpful staff at the Public Record Office, and the unknown gentleman in the British Foreign Office who took pity on me and allowed me access to some very recent medical documents. But my work on the British scene would have been impossible without the initial help of John Flint, my colleague in

Dalhousie University's History Department. Under his guidance, I took the first serious steps into British imperialism, discovering not only where to start but, more significantly, where to find it and how to find it.

Finding information about a London-centered empire was child's play in comparison to such activity in the United States, where the search provided an excuse to indulge my love of train rides. (Like Paul Theroux, I have never heard the whistle of a train without wishing I was on it.) In particular, I would like to thank Linda Brink at the Harvard Medical School, who manages the records of the American Society of Tropical Medicine; the staff at the Tulane University Library and Archives in New Orleans; the archivists at the Chesney Archives at Johns Hopkins University Medical School; Mary Pritchard at the Harold Manter Laboratory at the University of Nebraska, where American parasitology began and where, today, the records of the American Society of Parasitology are housed; the archivists at the University of Illinois at Urbana, where the H. B. Ward Papers are located; librarians at the Walter Reed Army Institute of Research in Washington, D.C., and at the Naval Medical Research Institute in Bethesda; and, closer to home, the archivists at McGill University, where one could, until recently, earn a Diploma in Tropical Medicine (fieldwork in the Caribbean!).

My very warmest thanks go to "Chip" Burkhardt at the University of Illinois not only for arranging access to its magnificent library (a feat that took him only seconds to arrange) and providing much needed comfort on the statistical probability of being struck by tornadoes (which always seemed to occur when I was there) but, more especially, for beating down the forces of athletic law-and-order to gain access to the swimming pool – a feat that took much, much longer! I would also like to thank Gert Brieger for his hospitality during my numerous visits to the Johns Hopkins Institute of the History of Medicine, and neither shall I forget the welcome I always received in Baltimore from the late Lloyd Stevenson and his wife; he continued over the years to take a fatherly interest in what I was about. Thanks go also to J. Allen Scott and John Weir, whom I interviewed and who read over those parts of the text relevant to their involvement in the bilharzia story; and Elizabeth Fee, who read over my material on the Johns Hopkins School of Hygiene and Public Health. I would also like to thank Sheila Penney and Elizabeth Haigh, who read over early drafts of the manuscript; Joe Harvey and David Patriguin, for helpful advice; and Kenneth Mott and Paulette Duchesne, for their great help during a wonderful couple of weeks rummaging around the library of the Parasitic Diseases Programme at the WHO in Geneva.

But I owe my greatest debt to three very special people: Sheila Zurbrigg, from the perspective of her experiences in working in India and her present historical interest in malarial epidemiology, prodded me to move in new directions and reminded me constantly that there was much more to bilharzia than worms and snails. Robert Joy, of the Uniformed Services University of the Health Sciences in Bethesda, always gave a helping hand when asked, always seemed to know where American documents were located, and took considerable pains to read over the almost-final draft of the manuscript. And finally, Peter Jordan, now retired but still active after a lifetime of medical service in British Africa and after directing the famous St. Lucia Project, also read over the draft manuscript and, over pub lunches in St. Albans, told me his likes and dislikes and made many helpful suggestions and comments about the disease.

I am naturally very grateful to those who have provided funds for travel and research. CUSO took me to Africa many years ago, the Rockefeller Foundation provided numerous summer grants that enabled me to spend time at their archives, and the Toronto-based Hannah Institute for the History of Medicine kindly provided a small grant for that all-important final visit to the WHO library in Geneva. Finally, and most important of all, I would like to acknowledge the Social Sciences and Humanities Research Council of Canada which, with much appreciated civility, has supported this project from its inception far too many years ago.

J. F.

Halifax, Nova Scotia

1

Introduction

Tropical medicine is unique among medical specialties in being defined by reference to the part of the world where it is practiced and where its diseases are endemic.[1] This occurred because the discipline arose as part of Western imperialism when explorers, military personnel, colonial administrators, businessmen, and finally settlers came face to face with a new set of diseases – tropical diseases, for which they had no answer and which were, at times, particularly virulent. To combat these problems, schools of tropical medicine were launched where physicians and parasitologists learned what was known about the tropical pathogens, their life cycles, the diseases they cause, and how to cure and prevent them.

There is, however, more to tropical medicine and its history than the discovery of pathogens, the unraveling of life cycles, and attempts to eradicate them. These and other medical and scientific events were and are influenced by political and social events beyond the narrowly defined sphere of medicine and parasitology. Founded as one aspect of European and American imperialism (defined simply as the domination of one society over another), imperial policies and attitudes largely determined the nature of tropical medicine.[2]

Until very recently, however, this sociopolitical component to tropical medicine has been largely ignored by those writing about its history. These narrative histories described when, where, and by whom significant discoveries were made. Some of these, such as Harold Scott's two-volume *A History of Tropical Medicine*, have become classics. Published in 1939, it dealt with the work that had been done up to that time on virtually every important tropical disease.[3] Although there are a few introductory chapters on the army, the navy, and the colonies, the main text gives an account of scientific discoveries made on each of many specific tropical diseases (although not bilharzia). The implication from the story that Scott and others tell is one of triumph over disease; the picture they portray is of "diseased natives" made well by white man's medicine. Others who served in the colonies, put on the defensive by a tide of anti-imperialist sentiments, were only too willing to advance this story of victory over disease, and the triumphs of tropical medicine have almost become the last justification for imperialism.[4] Most people would, I suspect, agree with the two historians who wrote: "Whatever political disadvantages colonialism might possess, from the biological standpoint its record is one of the greatest success stories of modern history."[5]

In more recent years a few historians have been more analytical and critical in their studies.[6] Indeed one of the earliest of such studies goes so far as to challenge what everyone seems to have accepted as a truth of empire. "With the apparent partial exception of West Africa," the authors wrote in contrast to what most believed hitherto, "the unhealthiest period in all African history was undoubtedly between 1890 and 1930," and "colonial rule . . . has largely created the continent's present disease environment." Thus, as these same authors assert, the story of tropical medicine becomes not simply the triumph of enlightened medicine over the useless and often harmful practices of "ignorant savages," but an attempt to control diseases that they themselves helped to create. Goodyear, for example, has argued that epidemics of yellow fever in the Americas can be linked to the sugar industry.[7] But despite this historical activity, R. MacLeod is probably correct when he notes: "There is as yet little coherent perspective on the relations between medicine and empire."[8] Certainly nobody has been able to do for the late nineteenth and early twentieth centuries what Philip Curtin has done for the earlier years in his now classic *The Image of Africa*.[9]

But to write a comprehensive modern history of tropical medicine that covers both the imperial and the medical aspects of all tropical diseases has become, I think, an impossibility. The range of diseases is so large, the information sitting in various archives and libraries on such diseases as malaria and trypanosomiasis so vast, and the machinations of the imperial powers so complex, that no scientist or historian (who tends to specialize as much as does the scientist) could ever do the subject justice.

What I have attempted here is only "a" history of tropical medicine. To do so, I have restricted myself in various ways. Only two empires are discussed, the British and the American, and I deal only with some of the countries that were either part of these empires or heavily influenced by them. The time frame is restricted also. It begins in 1898, when the British Colonial Office set in motion a series of events that led to the founding of the Liverpool and London schools of tropical medicine, and when the American Army was decimated by tropical diseases in taking over Cuba, Puerto Rico, and the Philippines following its rather shallow victory in the Spanish-American War. I end less precisely in the 1970s. By then the British Empire had collapsed, the International Health Division of the Rockefeller Foundation had more or less retired from the scene, and the WHO was in full flower, lavishly housed in its modern quarters overlooking Geneva. More importantly, the book ends, as I shall suggest, when tropical medicine seems to have entered a new post-imperial stage of its history.

It would be wrong to repeat the errors of the past, however, by dealing with only one dimension of the issue. To talk only of empire and the socioeconomic background while, at the same time, ignoring the technical and scientific aspects of disease and disease control would be as unbalanced as those early histories that spoke only of scientific triumphs. But again necessity demands that one restrict the number of diseases with which to deal. I have chosen one disease, bilharzia or, as it is commonly called today, schistosomiasis.

Bilharzia is a disease caused by the eggs of small, threadlike parasitic worms that live inside the blood vessels of the gut, liver, and bladder. Today these parasites are said to infect over 200 million people in 74 tropical countries of Africa, the Middle East, Asia, Latin America, and a few Caribbean islands, and in 1976 was listed as one of the six diseases of most concern to the WHO.[10] There are many reasons for this choice, not least of which being my own long-standing interest in these parasitic worms. More significantly, however, focusing on bilharzia enabled me to examine some of the basic assumptions about tropical medicine that Westerners have long accepted. Because bilharzia is mainly a disease of rural poverty that has rarely threatened the health of white officials or colonizers to any great extent, the question of motivation and priorities can be addressed more fruitfully for bilharzia than for diseases like malaria, which have threatened the health of white and native inhabitants alike. Furthermore, bilharzia is one of the most obvious examples of a disease whose prevalence has increased over the years because of human activities; it is not a disease that has quietly succumbed to the technology of Western medicine.

In addition, the disease does not occur in India. My task was greatly simplified by being able to ignore India and the British India Office, thereby focusing exclusively on the Colonial Office, which never had charge of that most prized possession of Great Britain.

Thus, I have attempted to use bilharzia as a "case study" by which to examine the much broader issue of tropical medicine in the British and American empires from 1898 to the 1970s.

IMPERIAL MEDICINE

My basic theme is that tropical medicine from 1898 to the 1970s was fundamentally imperialistic in its basic assumptions, its methods, its goals, and its priorities; it was the age of imperial tropical medicine. Few, I suspect, will disagree with this interpretation of events before World War II, for quite clearly in those years tropical medicine was an important part of empire building and empire maintenance. As stated consistently at that time, the basic goal of tropical medicine was to render the tropical world fit for white habitation and white investment. Its practitioners were members of colonial services, armies of occupation, and mining and fruit companies. What, if anything, should be done about the health of the native inhabitants was determined by the policies of these Western agencies without reference to the needs of the indigenous communities. Not surprisingly their health needs became a priority only when their diseases were felt to threaten the health or profits of the white man, or when imperial policies demanded that the health needs of the indigenous populations be addressed. In addition, because Christian duty and the white man's burden always included medical and sanitary work, medical missionaries were also an important part of the picture although one that I shall ignore. It was an age of imperial medicine in that the imperial agencies defined what the major medical problems were, what were the causes of these problems, and what needed to be done to overcome them. This was an age of imperial medicine also in that the imperial agencies imposed their solutions on the population without involving them in any way.

I shall argue, however, that tropical medicine after World War II was also imperialistic in the sense that health policies continued to be imposed by outside agencies, whether they were the declining imperial powers or the increasingly influential professional classes and international organizations. Tropical medicine, as before, continued to be imported, technical, and scientific; and even when, as in the 1940s, a more socially oriented approach briefly appeared, it was only because Western medicine was at that time flirting with so-called social medicine. There was, however, in this postwar era a rising concern with what were perceived to be the health problems of the tropical or Third World communities, but both the nature of these problems and the solutions to them continued to be imposed and Western. Even if control slowly passed into the hands of Third World personnel, no fundamental changes took place, for they had been trained in Western ideas and shared the professional goals and beliefs of their Western colleagues.

I believe that a fundamental shift away from this imperial-styled medicine began to take place only in the 1980s. In 1979, the WHO finally endorsed the idea that all people have the right to participate in their own health care planning and implementation, to dictate priorities, and to utilize methods that they can use and afford. Community participation has become the new creed, and minimally trained health workers are becoming the major agents of this new primary health care delivery system.

The policies and attitudes of imperial medicine and the new primary health care approach, which succeeded it, are reflected in the story of bilharzia.

What follows is my attempt to superimpose the story of this one disease against the broad backcloth of imperial tropical medicine.

BILHARZIA: WHAT IT IS

Unfortunately the disease is generally known today by two names, bilharzia or schistosomiasis. The reason for this is to be found in the past. Theodor Bilharz, the discoverer of the parasitic worm responsible for the disease, placed the worm in the genus *Distoma*, a broad genus that was soon abandoned as more types of parasitic worms were discovered. Numerous generic names were thereafter invented to house Bilharz's worm, including *Schistosoma* Weinland, 1858 (the name that must stand today according to the rules of zoological nomenclature). However, in the past, in an understandable desire to honor the name of Bilharz, the disease was often called bilharziasis or bilharziosis. But in 1949, members of the WHO Study Group on Bilharziasis in Africa, ignorant of the tight rules of zoological nomenclature, recommended that the name *Bilharzia* be used for the worm genus and bilharziasis for the disease. A recommendation to this effect was made to the International Commission of Zoological Nomenclature which naturally ruled, in 1954, that the generic name *Schistosoma* must be retained, but that the disease could nevertheless be called bilharziasis.

This ruling makes little sense, and I have not followed it. Bilharziasis should be used to designate the disease only if the generic name of the worm were *Bilharzia*, just as trypanosomiasis is used to denote the disease caused by protozoans of the genus *Trypanosoma*. Thus, because the generic name *Schistosoma* must be retained, the disease can be called "schistosomiasis" as is commonly done today, but there is no justification for the term "bilharziasis."

On the other hand, just as malaria, and not "plasmodiasis," is used to denote the disease caused by organisms of the genus *Plasmodium*, the word "bilharzia" can be used for the disease caused by worms of the genus *Schistosoma*. Many still know the disease as bilharzia, and so I shall, with no apologies to anyone, use this word throughout the book. I prefer short historical names over unpleasant tongue-twisters (particularly because the ugly derivative "schisto" is now widely used).

Bilharzia, known also by many local names such as "red-water fever," "snail fever," "big-belly," and "Katayama disease," is caused by eggs of blood vessel-inhabiting worms of the class Trematoda and genus *Schistosoma*. These eggs induce an immunological response after they become trapped in the body organs, especially the liver, gut wall, and urinogenital tract. It is these immunological responses that constitute the disease.[11]

Bilharzia is, in reality, not a single disease but a complex of diseases induced by the eggs of five principal schistosome species, three of which – *Schistosoma haematobium*, *S. mansoni*, and *S. japonicum* – are particularly important. *Schistosoma haematobium* inhabits the veins of the bladder area, and the eggs that are not trapped in the body are discharged in the urine. The other two species inhabit the mesenteric veins of the gut, and their eggs are discharged in the feces. In every case, the worms may also be found in the liver and portal blood system.

Distribution and prevalence

The diseases caused by these three species have a worldwide tropical distribution but are mercifully absent from the Indian subcontinent. *Schistosoma haematobium* is highly endemic in the Nile Delta and Valley, and has an irregular distribution in the Middle East countries and North Africa. It occurs in most West and Central African countries, along the coastal countries of East Africa from Somalia to Natal, and in the islands off the east coast (Figure 1.1a). *Schistosoma mansoni* is also highly endemic in the Nile Delta and now seems to be spreading into the Nile Valley (Figure 1.1b). In sub-Sahara Africa its distribution is similar to, although more irregular than, that of *S. haematobium*, but unlike *S. haematobium*, *S. mansoni* occurs also in South America (Brazil, Surinam, and Venezuela), and in some islands in the Caribbean (Dominican Republic, Puerto Rico, St. Lucia, and others [see Figure 1.1c]). Oriental bilharzia, caused by *S. japonicum*, is endemic to the Yangtze Valley and many coastal provinces of mainland China. It occurs also in Central Sulawesi, and the Philippines (see Figure 1.1d). There are also a series of smaller foci in Thailand and Japan, and an *S. japonicum*-like form has been identified in Malaysia (Figure 1.1d). The other two species, *S. intercalatum* and *S. mekongi*, have a much more restricted distribution. The former occurs in Cameroun, Gabon, and Zaire; the latter in the Mekong River valley of Laos and Kampuchea.

Over 200 million people in 74 countries are said to be infected with the worms, although the data on which such figures are based are rather unreliable. There is little doubt, however, that in villages of the Nile Delta, and in other areas where there is constant contact of the human host with water, the prevalence can be almost as high as 100 percent.

Pathology

Most people who carry the parasite suffer only minor although unpleasant symptoms: blood in the urine, occasional diarrhea, and cramps. But as the trapped eggs increasingly induce inflammatory reactions in various body organs, the classic symptoms of chronic bilharzia can appear. The morbidity, or severity, of these reactions is very variable and generally related to the "worm load" – that is, the number of worms being carried in the body. There

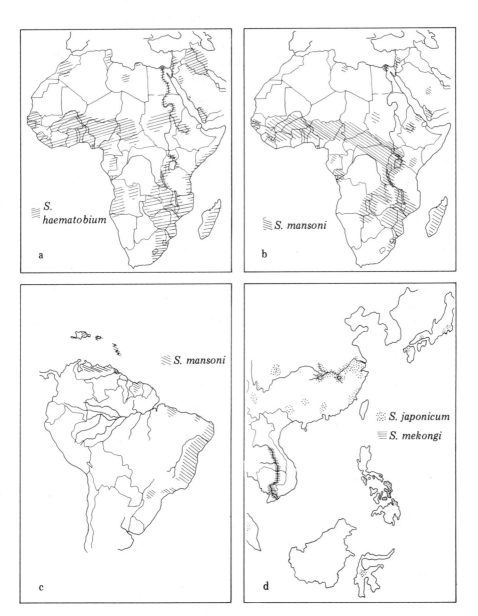

Figure 1.1. Distribution of the human schistosome species: (a) *S. haematobium* in Africa; (b) *S. mansoni* in Africa; (c) *S. mansoni* in South America; (d) *S. japonicum* and *S. mekongi* in the Orient.

are also pathological differences among each species and among strains of the same species.

In very general terms, an infection with *S. haematobium* can cause lesions to occur in the bladder and ureter around the entrapped and calcifying eggs. In addition to the discharge of blood in the urine, and painful and excessive urination, various malfunctions occur as urinary and kidney passages become blocked with these lesions. In the intestinal schistosomes, the lesions occur in the gut wall and liver. This can result in the venous drainage of the liver being blocked, which in turn can lead to a compensatory increased arterial flow to it. As a result of this, portal hypertension and the classic enlargement of the liver and spleen can occur. Eggs of all three species may also become trapped in the lungs, and in *S. japonicum*, nervous disorders or "cerebral schistosomiasis" can also occur if egg aggregates come to rest in the brain.

Life cycle

The worm eggs, whose shapes are highly diagnostic for each species, when shed in the urine or feces of the human host hatch to produce a minute, short-lived larval stage called a "miracidium" (see Figure 1.2). These miracidia bore into and invade the tissues of specific snail hosts, where they undergo asexual reproduction eventually to produce the final larval stage. This final stage, the "cercariae," are released daily in very large numbers from the snail, swim freely in the water, and then will bore directly into the skin of the human host. In the human, the parasite migrates to the liver via the heart and lungs eventually to mature in the veins of the liver, gut, or bladder. Eggs will appear in the urine or feces approximately 30–40 days after infection.

Epidemiology

The disease has a very complex epidemiology, resulting in part from a very intricate relationship between the parasite and the snail intermediate host. There are not only strains of each schistosome species but also a multiplicity of snail species and varieties that vary in their susceptibility to these strains. Also the taxonomy of these snails has long been a source of almost total confusion and seems always to be in a constant state of revision.[12] I shall, however, ignore the history of these controversies.

Both *S. haematobium* and *S. mansoni* are transmitted by species of freshwater pulmonate snails (the group to which most freshwater snails belong). Those of *S. haematobium* belong to various species complexes of the genus *Bulinus*, whereas species complexes of the genus *Biomphalaria* act as the snail host for *S. mansoni*. *Schistosoma japonicum*, on the other hand, is transmitted by amphibious prosobranch snails (a group to which most marine snails belong but which has also a few genera of amphibious freshwater forms) belonging to the

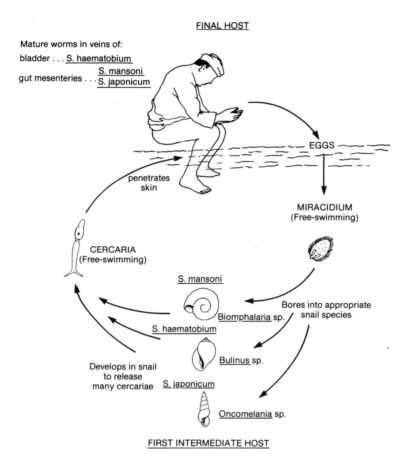

FINAL HOST

Mature worms in veins of:

bladder . . . S. haematobium

gut mesenteries . . . S. mansoni
S. japonicum

EGGS

penetrates
skin

MIRACIDIUM
(Free-swimming)

CERCARIA
(Free-swimming)

S. mansoni

Biomphalaria sp.

Bores into appropriate
snail species

S. haematobium

Bulinus sp.

Develops in snail
to release
many cercariae   S. japonicum

Oncomelania sp.

FIRST INTERMEDIATE HOST

Figure 1.2. Life cycle of the human schistosome worms

species *Oncomelania hupensis* of which there are six geographical subspecies. Another prosobranch snail, *Tricula aperta*, endemic to the Mekong River, acts as the intermediate host of *S. mekongi*.

Bilharzia is a chronic disease of economic poverty of mainly rural areas, where children and adults, because of recreational, domestic, religious, and occupational reasons, come regularly into contact with freshwater contaminated with the schistosome cercariae. In cases of *S. haematobium* infection, the prevalence of the disease and the intensity of infection peak in the teenage years; this is less true for other species, however.

Reservoir hosts play an important role in Oriental bilharzia, where the parasite is naturally transmitted between humans and other vertebrates, including many domesticated animals such as cattle, pigs, and dogs. Although animals are believed to play little if any role in the transmission of the other two schistosome species in Africa, rodents are believed to act as important reservoirs of *S. mansoni* in South America.

But very little was known about bilharzia in 1898 when our story begins. Then, Queen Victoria was on the throne, the British Empire was at its zenith, and the Americans first set about acquiring their own.

PART I

The imperial approach (1898–World War II)

2

1898: A declaration of war

So long as London remains the focus of the world's commerce and
the nerve centre of a great tropical Empire, it is an imperial
necessity that there should be in the metropolis an institution
where the study and treatment of tropical diseases can adequately
be carried out. Upon nothing so much as upon bodily vigour does
tropical colonisation depend for its success: it is the basis of pioneer
work in the exploration of uncharted regions in search of oil and
other minerals and in the transformation of jungle land into rubber
plantations and tea gardens and the cultivation of other tropical
commodities: it is indispensable alike to the missionary, to the
soldier and to the official who in isolated regions executes the
functions of British government.   F. A. Lyon[1]

In 1898, nearly three centuries after the British had first settled among the
malarial swamps of semitropical Virginia and had opened their first factory on
the coast of pestiferous India, and over two hundred years after the Royal
Africa Company had gained a monopoly in the West African slave trade, the
British declared war on tropical diseases. In the year 1898, Colonial Secretary
Joseph Chamberlain set in motion a chain of events that led to the founding of
the London and Liverpool schools of tropical medicine, headquarters of a new
army that set out to rid the Empire of disease.

Such a long delay may seem peculiar; for two centuries and more, staying
alive had been the most urgent problem faced by British settlers, troops, and
government officials alike. In the early nineteenth century, for instance, the
annual death rate per thousand for British troops in the West Indies was
approximately eight times that in Britain, and in the Cape Coast of West
Africa the death rate had reached the astronomical number of 668, almost fifty
times as high as the death rate at home.[2] But two important events of the late
nineteenth century had provided a new impetus toward this declaration of
war: the emergence of the germ theory of disease and British expansion into
new tropical territories.

GERM THEORY AND EMPIRE

The germ theory of disease and the discovery that these disease agents could be carried by intermediate and vector hosts had generated a more optimistic attitude toward the tropics. By 1898, Patrick Manson had implicated the mosquito in the transmission of nematode filarial larvae, and he and Ronald Ross had uncovered the role of the mosquito in the passage of the malarial parasite. Likewise, in the Americas, Carlos Finley had postulated that yellow fever was transmitted by the mosquito, and Theobold Smith had shown that ticks transmitted the agents of Texas cattle fever.[3] These discoveries led to the realization that many of the white man's problems in the tropics could be attributed to disease germs and their vectors rather than to the climate per se, and to the belief that the tropics were now potentially safer for Europeans. As an article in the *British Medical Journal* noted in 1897: "Get rid of or avoid these disease germs and we get rid of a principal obstacle to the colonization of the tropics by Europeans."[4] On the surface, at least, it now seemed relatively simple.

In earlier years, many of these diseases were assumed to result from the tropical climate itself. Although smallpox and others were believed to be contagious, the great majority of "infectious" fevers were thought to arise, basically, from poisons in the tropical air. These poisons, expelled perhaps by decaying organic matter, initiated changes in the body that had been rendered susceptible by such "predisposing causes" as high heat and humidity as well as by excessive eating, drinking, and sexual passions. The problems could certainly be addressed by following a series of rules and regulations that years of painstaking observations had shown to ameliorate the situation; but, fundamentally, because the tropical climate itself was the major cause of the infectious fevers, the Europeans were limited in what they could do.

Nevertheless, after midcentury, the threat posed by tropical diseases was no longer what it had been earlier. In 1854, for example, the *Pleiad* expedition to the Niger and Benue rivers had returned with no European fatalities, whereas only 13 years before, 55 of 159 Europeans had died during the notorious Niger expedition. According to Philip Curtin, increased use of quinine therapy, better precautionary measures such as netting to keep out dangerous effluvia, and the abolition of heroic therapy had combined to make a real difference. Thus, even before the germ theory, African exploration was no longer, as Livingstone expressed it, "quasi-suicidal."[5]

But Africa in particular was still a dangerous place, and the possibilities of colonizing such disease-ridden lands remained as remote as ever. But with the germ theory in place, the future looked brighter. Acute tropical fevers that debilitated so many colonial officials were no longer assumed to have a climatic cause and thus to be basically unavoidable. As Patrick Manson explained in his *Tropical Diseases*, published in 1898, "Acute disease, with active tissue changes, is not so caused. In the tropics, as in temperate climates, in the European and in the native alike, nearly all disease is of specific origin."[6] Similar views were expressed by Luigi Sambon. "It is not the mere influence of climate which opposes colonization in tropical lands," he noted, "but the competition of other living organisms – from man, wild beasts, and snakes to protozoa and bacteria – with which we have to struggle for existence."[7] In theory at least, the outcome of that struggle seemed no longer in doubt; white people could escape from the acute diseases of the tropics as they were at that time escaping from diseases of temperate climates. They declared war on tropical diseases believing, at last, that they could win.

But the germ theory did not in any way alter the opinion that a tropical climate exerted a pernicious long-term effect on Europeans, especially the women and children. To avoid physical and moral degeneration, British children were still sent home to the "more bracing and healthy atmosphere of Europe." Dr. A. Davidson, in his text of 1893, was quite explicit on this problem:

The child must be sent to England, or it will deteriorate physically and morally, – physically, because it will grow up slight, weedy, and delicate, over-precocious it may be, and with a general feebleness. . . . Morally, because he learns from his surroundings much that is undesirable, and has a tendency to become deceitful and vain, indisposed to study, and to a great extent unfitted to do so.[8]

EXPANSION OF THE BRITISH EMPIRE

The declaration of war against tropical diseases coincided also with the acquisition of new tropical territories by the British (Figure 2.1). By the 1890s, the British Empire – which only a few decades earlier had consisted of India; a group of white, temperate-zone colonies that seemed destined to follow the path of the American colonies; and a hodge-podge of trading centers, strategic outposts, and coaling stations – had been transformed, almost overnight, into a vast empire, including much of Africa. This acquisition of African territories acted as the major stimulus for the Colonial Office's war against tropical disease. British tropical medicine was thus "colonial medicine." It dealt with the diseases of those parts of the Empire administered by the Colonial Office: Africa, the West Indies, and Southeast Asia. The medical problems of India were not their concern; they were handled by the lofty India Office and the India Medical Service.

By the end of the nineteenth century, the British had added the foreign-office protectorates of Northern Nigeria, Southern Nigeria, and the Northern Territories of the Gold Coast to their older small coastal crown colonies of

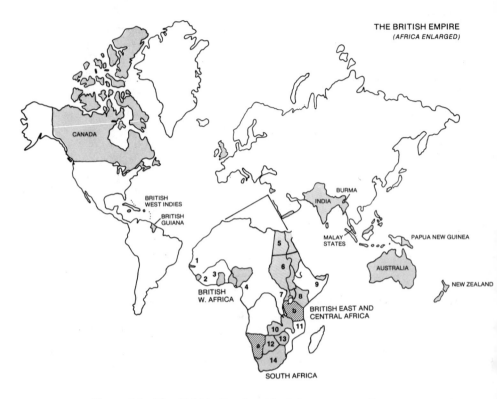

Figure 2.1. The British Empire (shaded area: 11 million square miles; population: 370 million): 1, Gambia; 2, Sierra Leone; 3, Gold Coast; 4, Nigeria; 5, Egypt; 6, Anglo-Egyptian Sudan; 7, Uganda; 8, Kenya; 9, British Somaliland; 10, Northern Rhodesia; 11, Nyasaland; 12, Bechuanaland; 13, Southern Rhodesia; 14, South Africa. Acquired after World War I (hatched areas): a, German South West Africa; b, Tanganyika.

Lagos, Gold Coast, Sierra Leone, and Gambia. During the same period, Cecil Rhodes expanded the territories administered by his British South African Company to include Mashonaland and Matebeleland (Zimbabwe). North of the Zambezi River this company also controlled what later became Northern Rhodesia (Zambia), while the British Foreign Office took over the British Central Africa Protectorate (Malawi) of the Lake Nyasa watershed and the beautiful Shire Highlands. In 1882, the British had also occupied Egypt and, by the end of the century, had expanded control over the Sudan and two protectorates covering the headwaters of the Nile: Buganda and British East Africa (Uganda and Kenya). Only German East Africa (Tanzania) prevented the Union Jack from flying on every mast on a line between Cairo and Capetown.

With the birth of this new tropical empire came a corresponding surge in imperial enthusiasm and the idea of a "racial duty" owed by Britons to their subject peoples. Much of this enthusiasm was directed toward the white settler colonies of British stock, "a great homogeneous people, one in blood, language, religion and laws, but dispersed over a boundless space."[9] But Britain also had a Christian duty to govern India, and now the "white man's burden" had been increased by peoples of the savage and mysterious Dark Continent. Such views of duty and empire were fervently championed by Joseph Chamberlain, who took up the reins of the Colonial Office in 1895 and gave to it a status never enjoyed before. Until then, the Colonial Office, unlike the India Office, had never been considered an important branch of the Government, and had reached its nadir in midcentury when 11 colonial secretaries held office in the 13 years between 1852 and 1865. Under Chamberlain's leadership, however, the Colonial Office began to acquire many of the African territories administered initially by the Foreign Office. By 1914, to all intents and purposes, all of the British possessions in Africa had become colonies, whereas the older white colonies of Australia, New Zealand, Canada, and South Africa had been transferred to the Dominion Division of the Colonial Office.

The British attack against tropical diseases was largely motivated by the desire to protect the health of officials working in tropical climates administered by the Colonial Office. To achieve this end, the British sought primarily to improve the level of medical service offered to these officials, and to investigate the diseases which threatened their lives. "You send out soldiers and sailors, and you think you are bound to send medical men to look after them," Joseph Chamberlain was reported to have said. "Do you think of the large staff of able civil servants you send out, and what is being done for them in the event of failing health?"[10]

But saving lives was also a matter of simple economics. The diplomatic maneuvers in European capitals by which Africa was dismembered in the 1880s and 1890s were effective only because the European powers recognized one another's zones of "effective occupation." To "effectively occupy" a protectorate in Africa required government officials to be posted there so as to ensure the effective cooperation of the other European powers. Economy alone – always a prime concern for the British – dictated that these officials complete their tours of duty without being incapacitated by tropical illnesses. "The all important element in the success of commercial operations," Lord Brassey remarked in an address to the London School of Tropical Medicine, "is that those who conduct them should not be compelled very frequently to absent themselves from their posts of responsibility."[11]

But there was also the matter of Christian duty. Protecting colonial officials from the scourges of tropical diseases would, in the words of Patrick Manson, enable "our countrymen to carry out some of the duties imposed by circumstances of our race."[12] But, although concerns were continually expressed toward the "welfare and progress of the races we govern," the Colonial Office was content to leave African health in the hands of the missionary societies, who, realizing that modern scientific medicine could be used as a powerful evangelical tool, began to specifically recruit medical missionaries in the 1890s.[13] While hospitals and trained physicians were to be provided for the benefit of the colonial administrators, native hospitals also would be built for the benefit of those Africans aware of the advantages of "white man's medicine." But there would be no massive campaign to drive African patients into these hospitals, no great strategic plan to clean up Africa and to turn Africans into sanitized Englishmen. The British, as the Empire evolved in the twentieth century, were not converters.

By the end of the nineteenth century, the British no longer believed, as they had earlier, that the "natives" were convertible and capable of civilization. Following the Indian mutiny, racial disdain and distrust toward all non-Europeans had slowly enveloped the Empire. Indeed, the germ theory provided a powerful new thrust toward this racially segregated Empire. The "natives" themselves had replaced the tropical climate as the major threat; they were the source of disease germs. Thus, to protect the health of white officials, separate white communities had to be built, set apart by a *cordon sanitaire* from the "diseased natives," all of whom had to be excluded during the hours of darkness when the mosquitoes were biting. As Swanson remarked, "'The sanitation syndrome,' equating black urban settlement, labour and living conditions with threats to public health and security, became fixed in the official mind, buttressed a desire to achieve positive social controls, and confirmed or rationalized white race prejudice with a popular imagery of a medical menace."[14]

The menace of tropical diseases, therefore, provided one justification for successive British governments to develop a new imperial policy toward their African territories. The old nineteenth-century empire of "civilization, Christianity, and commerce," of self-interest and a civilizing obligation, had given way, by the 1920s, to an empire of almost permanent wardship. Africans, West Indians, and others were drawn into an empire of "trusteeship," in which civilization had become an almost unattainable goal.[15]

The idea of a trusteeship grew out of the First World War concern about the future of the German colonies, and the desire to prevent colonial rivalries from triggering hostilities in the future. The theoretical solution to these concerns involved an open-door trade policy, in which all powers would have equal access to colonial markets, and a protectionist policy toward the colonial people to prevent future exploitation by the colonial powers. If the allies decided to keep the German colonies, the *New Statesman* of 1916 argued, they might and ought to give a solemn undertaking to hold these territories in trust for civilization, to treat the interests of the natives therein as paramount, and to preserve in perpetuity the principle of the Open Door. . . . If at the same time France and Great Britain consented to make their own tropical dependencies in Africa subject to the same trust, the moral effect of the understanding as a demonstration of our good faith would obviously be enormously enhanced.[16]

Such a policy, of course, would be a denial of the validity of the old notion that colonies existed to serve the commercial interests of the colonizing power. A new colonial ideology would be needed for the postwar world. The British found theirs in the so-called dual mandate, first laid down by Frederick Lugard, Governor of Nigeria from 1912 to 1919, whose *The Dual Mandate in British Tropical Africa*, published in 1922, came to be viewed as the bible of British colonial policy.

The dual mandate, or the idea that British and colonial interests must be made reciprocal, was, in many ways, merely the old Empire in new clothes. The concepts of the old mercantile Empire were retained in the new Empire which still needed European brains, capital, and knowledge to make the colonies productive for the benefit of the civilized world. The old idea of a civilizing mission was also retained; the British genius for governing would bring law, liberty, responsibility, justice, and many other advantages to Africans. As Lugard himself expressed the concept of reciprocity:

Europe benefited by the wonderful increase in the amenities of life for the mass of her people which followed the opening up of Africa . . . Africa benefited by the influx of manufactured goods, and the substitution of law and order for the methods of barbarism.[17]

The British Empire gradually evolved into an empire of economic exploitation, coupled with a civilizing and a protective trusteeship policy toward Africans.

The British tried to execute these policies indirectly. Basically, they rejected both classical models of colonial government: "direct rule," whereby the colony was totally ruled by the European power; and "indirect rule," whereby Europeans merely supervised a colony in which local rulers, rules, and customs continued unchanged. The British opted for a modified indirect rule "by native chiefs, unfettered in their control of their people as regards all those matters which are to him most important," while, at the same time, being "subordinate to the control of the protecting Power." In this process, according to Lugard, there were not two sets of rulers, "but a single government in which the native chiefs have well defined duties and an acknowledged status equally with British officials." By these means the British aimed both to "civilize" Africans and to preserve African society as a bulwark against some of the evil effects of European civilization – an idea that appealed strongly to the aristocratic *noblesse oblige* traditions of the British colonial officer. It was also a means of exercising control in a morally defensible manner.

Above all, however, indirect rule was inexpensive; everything was done on the cheap. Under this system, each colony was to be financially self-sufficient, involving minimal government and minimal cost to the British taxpayer. Preservation of the status quo took priority over change, and any change that did occur was necessarily of the gradual variety so as not to undermine traditional African ways, or involve any unnecessary expenditure. It was an Empire with no goal in mind other than being there; an Empire, in the words of the historian D. K. Fieldhouse, on an "indefinite holding operation"; an Empire over which the sun never set, in space or in time.[18]

THE FIRST SCHOOLS OF TROPICAL MEDICINE

On October 4, 1897, Dr. Gage Brown, who had recently been replaced by Patrick Manson as Medical Advisor to the Colonial Office, wrote to Joseph Chamberlain suggesting that, before proceeding to their postings, medical officers be required to attend either Dr. Manson's lectures on tropical medicine given at St. George's Hospital in London, classes at the Royal Victoria Military Hospital at Netley, or a short course of instruction in their host country. He had reached this conclusion, he explained, after reading Manson's address to St. George's, given three days earlier, entitled "Necessity for special education in tropical medicine."[19]

Manson (Figure 2.2) had returned from China and Hong Kong in 1889 with every intention of retiring to a quiet life in Scotland. But financial problems brought him back to London where he opened a consulting practice near Harley Street. In 1892, he was appointed Physician to the Seamen's Hospital Society in Greenwich, and two years later began to give public lectures on tropical medicine at Charing Cross and St. George's hospitals. In the lecture of October 1, which had so impressed Gage Brown, Manson spoke of the "very grave disease in our educational system," of modern medical graduates being "utterly inadequate to qualify for tropical medicine," and of the inertia of a narrow-minded medical establishment who failed to understand the problems faced by medical graduates, one-fifth of whom served in the tropics.[20]

As a result of this lecture and the urgings of Gage Brown, the Colonial Office forwarded a memo to the War Office, the Foreign Office, the India Office, the General Medical Council, the Seamen's Hospital Society, and all 26 British medical schools. Mr. Chamberlain was, according to this memo, "anxious to do anything in his power to extend the benefits of medical science to the natives of tropical colonies and protectorates, and to diminish the risk to the lives and health of those Europeans who . . . are called upon to serve in unhealthy climates." He requested, therefore, that British medical schools

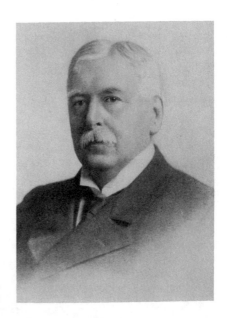

Figure 2.2. Patrick Manson (Reproduced
by permission of P. E. C. Manson-Bahr)

provide instruction in tropical medicine for colonial medical officers, similar
to that provided by the Army Medical School at Netley to medical officers of
the army and India service.[21] With this memorandum dated March 11, 1898,
the British declared their war on tropical diseases.

The reaction to this memo was predictable; most of the medical schools
rather smugly supported the status quo. Similarly, both the War Office and
India Office expressed satisfaction with the existing four-month training
program received by their medical officers at Netley, suggesting that Netley
itself could well become the training center for all colonial medical officers,
both military and civil.[22]

The Netley program was the successor to the Army Medical School which
had been opened at Fort Pitt in Chatham, following the medical horrors of the
Crimean War. Not only did the Indian Government provide half of the
funding for this school, but also a retired Indian service officer was tradition-
ally allotted the Chair of Military Medicine, with responsibility for diseases of
the tropics. In 1863, it moved to the imposing Royal Victoria Military Hospital
at Netley (Figure 2.3), built overlooking Southampton Water to receive sick
and wounded troops disembarking at Southampton.[23] Netley was, therefore,
the most obvious center from which the British attack against tropical diseases
could have been initiated and directed. But, because of Netley's close ties with
the India Office, that was not to be. Since the Colonial Office, not the India
Office, was to become the main instigator of the war against tropical diseases,
neither Netley nor the Royal Army Medical College at Millbank, where the

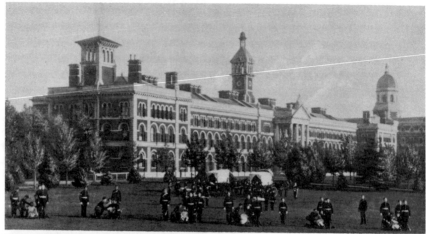

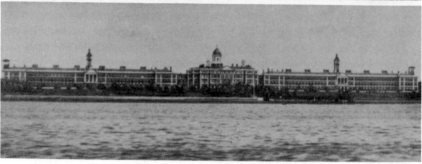

Figure 2.3. The Royal Victoria Military Hospital and Army Medical School at Netley. *Top,* Ambulance and stretcher bearer's drill. *Bottom,* The 480-yard frontage overlooking Southampton Water (Courtesy of Royal Army Medical Corps Archives, Aldershot)

School was relocated after the Boer War, came to play the major role in the history of British tropical medicine.

Not all respondents to the Colonial Office memorandum were so complacent, and so willing to accept the status quo, however. Liverpool and Edinburgh, for example, unlike the other British medical schools, promised limited action. But the Seamen's Hospital Society, no doubt under Manson's coaching, realized that the Colonial Office memorandum presented a golden opportunity. The Society set out immediately to gain the prize as the *only* school of tropical medicine in the country.

The Seamen's Hospital Society had its beginnings in the aftermath of the Napoleonic Wars, when a fund was established for the relief of distressed mariners. The Society, formed in 1821 to administer this fund, received the gunship *Grampus* on loan, converted it to a hospital ship, and moored it at Greenwich, downstream from the City of London. Eleven years later, the Admiralty replaced the ship with the considerably larger *Dreadnought*, which had earlier seen service as Vice-Admiral Collingwood's flagship. In 1870, the hospital came ashore when the Society rented wards in the Greenwich Infirmary, and in 1890 the Albert Dock Branch Hospital opened its wards.[24] These hospitals provided unique clinical material, as the Society noted in their reply to the Colonial Office's memo, with an average of 190 tropical-disease cases being treated each year. But before a school could be located at Greenwich, they explained, it would be necessary to build a new wing for the hospital, and to erect a new building to house laboratory and lecture rooms. Showing considerable speed and initiative, they even forwarded a budget: £10,000 for a new wing to the Albert Hospital, £3,550 for lecture and laboratory space; and a £3,100 annual maintenance allowance.[25]

Manson, far from wanting every medical school in Britain to teach classes in tropical medicine, had hoped for a single school all along. By June, Chamberlain seemed to have acquiesced to Manson's view. He now felt that only one school was necessary. What is more, he now favored the Seamen's Hospital at Greenwich; Manson was to have his way. In a detailed memo to the notoriously tight-fisted British Treasury, the Colonial Office put forward the case for a single school of tropical medicine at Greenwich and requested a contribution of between £1,500 and £2000 toward the cost of new lecture and laboratory space. The major request for a new hospital wing was ignored, while, following the dictates of British colonial policy, the colonies themselves were expected to meet the remaining costs. "As the scheme is mainly intended for the benefit of Africa," Chamberlain explained, "so upon Africa the bulk of the expense will fall."[26] The Treasury split the difference and promised, four days later, to invite Parliament to grant £1775. By July 1898, the foundations of the new school were being laid at Greenwich. From initial memo to building had taken only four months (Figure 2.4).

To the total surprise of the Colonial Office, the initial Chamberlain memo also led to the founding of a second school of tropical medicine, at Liverpool. Alfred Jones (Figure 2.5), senior partner in the Elder Dempster Company which dominated the West African shipping business, announced at a dinner of the Royal Southern Hospital that he would give £350 per year to promote the study of tropical diseases. Toward the end of 1898, a committee was formed to plan a new school, and representatives of the Liverpool Chamber of Commerce, steamship and sailingship owners, the Royal Southern Hospital, and University College Liverpool formed a management committee to run the school under the chairmanship of Jones. The school opened on April 22, 1899, six months before the opening of its rival school in Greenwich. From the beginning, considerable friction existed between London and Liverpool,

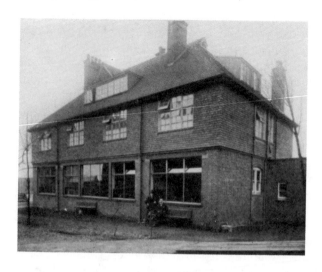

Figure 2.4. London School of Tropical Medicine, Royal Albert Docks, Greenwich (Reproduced by permission of P. E. C. Manson-Bahr)

brought on by the decision that all future colonial medical officers, whether graduates of Liverpool or not, must attend the course at London. This decision implied an inferior status for Liverpool, and even though the decision was to be reversed in 1900, friction continued because of the unequal grants given to the two schools. But, with fewer than 30 students per year, this grant

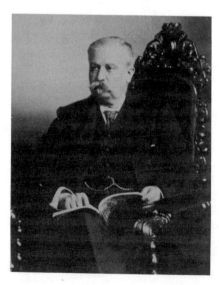

Figure 2.5. Alfred Jones (Reproduced by permission of Dr. P. N. Davies, the University of Liverpool)

difference was understandable. Liverpool always remained small in comparison to London.[27]

At Greenwich, 96 qualified physicians, including nine women, attended one of the three 12-week sessions given in the first year of operation. Of these 96, there were 42 from the colonial service, 27 from railway and trading companies, 16 missionary doctors, and seven from the military. They were run through a series of lectures, laboratory sessions, and clinical examinations dealing with specific tropical diseases. In teaching and research, the school emphasized protozoology and helminthology (parasitic worms); there was very little emphasis on bacterial diseases such as cholera, and only the briefest exposure to "hygiene in the tropics."[28] Liverpool was almost the same.[29] Basically, before the 1930s, there were three departments: tropical medicine, entomology, and parasitology, with the latter heavily emphasizing protozoology. No bacteriology or hygiene was offered until 1913, when Ronald Ross was bumped from the Alfred Jones Chair of Tropical Medicine to become Professor of Tropical Sanitation for five years.

Tropical medicine became the main impetus for the emergence of parasitology as a discipline in Britain.[30] The serious study of parasites had begun many years before in the early nineteenth-century German universities, but for most of the nineteenth century the only parasites known belonged to a single group of organisms, the parasitic worms or helminths, and their study was usually termed "helminthology" rather than parasitology. With the discovery of parasitic protozoa by Rudolf Leuckart (Figure 2.6) in the late 1870s, however, and the realization that helminths were not the only animals found in the body, the term "parasitology" gradually came into more general use. Parasitism was recognized as a way of life shared by many animal groups, although in practice those who studied it concentrated on the helminths, the parasitic protozoa, and often, by the end of the century, that aspect of entomology concerned with insect and other arthropod vectors.[31]

Many factors lay behind this emphasis on protozoa and helminths, although the Liverpool situation needs little explanation. The Liverpool School was financed by those with financial interests in West Africa. Its eyes were, therefore, focused firmly on West Africa, where they recognized malaria to be the major health problem undermining the "conditions of life" in which Europeans were forced to live. On the first of many expeditions sent out by the Liverpool school to West Africa, they had discovered the malarial mosquito, and, with Ronald Ross as holder of the first Alfred Jones Chair of Tropical Medicine, protozoology and particularly malariology became the major focus.

But London had no such limited geographical focus, although it, too, made the decision to ignore bacteriology and hygiene. This decision can be ascribed partly to Manson, whose indifference to these topics is well known. Yellow fever and typhoid, for example, take up only 30 pages of his famous text,

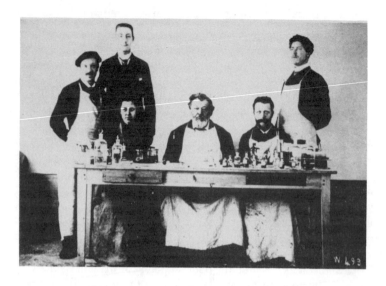

Figure 2.6. Rudolf Leuckart and assistants, the world's first parasitological laboratory, University of Leipzig (Courtesy of the University of Illinois Archives)

published in 1898. This indifference can be explained, partly at least, by his earlier experiences in China.[32] Basically he had little faith in changing the unsanitary habits of the Chinese or indeed the African. "In retrospect," his biographer noted, "one is struck by the scarcity of reference either to pharmacology or to sanitation" in his China journals, and quoted Manson's own words on the issue:

Unless you get people willing to receive them, there is very little use offering sanitary privileges or trying to carry out sanitary measures. I recollect that an elaborate system of drainage and of model municipal sanitation was supplied to the Chinese. Water-taps, traps, drains, ventilators, and all the rest of it were placed at their disposal. The Chinese turned on the water-taps, but they were too lazy to shut them; and naturally, the supply calculated to last a year was exhausted before the year was half over. The traps had gratings which had been placed over them to prevent them being choked; gratings and traps were ruthlessly removed to facilitate the escape of domestic rubbish. To give these things to Chinamen unappreciative of their purpose and ignorant of their use, was like giving a monkey a fiddle; they did not understand them and they broke them.[33]

Manson's feelings aside, the main cause for London's emphasis on protozoa and helminths appears to have been interuniversity jealousies. In November 1898, two weeks after the medical schools had been informed of the decision to build a single school at Greenwich, King's College Medical School forwarded its belated reply to the original Colonial Office memorandum. Basically the letter extolled the virtues of its bacteriological laboratory, and supported the idea of special training in tropical medicine, which must, they noted, "of necessity include thorough practical training in bacteriological methods." After pointing out that over a thousand graduates, many of whom worked in the tropics, had already passed through their Department of Bacteriology, and that all of these "had been especially instructed in the bacteriology of cholera, plague, malaria [sic] and other tropical diseases," the authorities of King's College Medical School came to the crux of their argument: "The council trust that the Government would be willing, in any arrangements they may eventually make, to recognize instruction given in the bacteriological laboratory of King's College as a qualifying course in Tropical Medicine."[34]

A month later, the Principal of King's College and its Professor of Bacteriology, Dr. E. Crookshank, met at the Colonial Office to argue that in ascertaining whether a candidate had a complete training in tropical medicine, "provision should be made for the full recognition of a course of bacteriological training in any laboratory of public standing and established reputation." However, they were quick to add, King's had the best equipped laboratory in London, and to open other such laboratories would lead to unnecessary competition and the undermining of King's. Their final suggestions to the Colonial Office were not made without self-interest in mind. Rather than a single course at Greenwich, they suggested a six-week course in a bacteriological laboratory (presumably King's); a course of lectures on tropical medicine and hygiene at Greenwich, or "any other medical school"; and a clinical course at Greenwich in conjunction with the London hospitals.[35] Clearly, if such a scheme had been allowed to go through it would have resulted in the complete emasculation of the Greenwich school.

To add to this threat from King's, Manson must also have been aware of Netley as a potential rival. The military school had long enjoyed a strong reputation in military hygiene and was rapidly gaining equal renown in bacteriology following the appointment of Almroth Wright in 1892.[36] More ominously, the school had plans to move into London; in 1902, it began offering some classes, including hygiene, in the Medical Staff College on the Victorian Embankment.

Bacteriology now became a thorny issue. To agree to the King's proposal, Manson told Chamberlain, would mean that "every medical school or bacteriological laboratory in London and throughout the country would have an equal claim to be regarded as affording a qualifying course of study."[37] To justify the existence of a single special school, through which all medical officers had to pass, it was clearly necessary to avoid duplication with King's, Netley, and other medical schools. What better way than to omit bacteriology and hygiene from the curriculum of the new school? By 1900, training in bacteriology was available at most British medical schools; indeed, it was the most obvious sign that a school was progressive and entering the spirit of modern medical science. Michael Worboys expressed it best, when he wrote: "In an important sense tropical medicine was defined initially by what an orthodox medical degree left out."[38] It had left out parasitology.

Although the link between parasitology and tropical medicine seems somewhat fortuitous, the split between parasitology and bacteriology was not. It reflected the growth and delineation of two scientific disciplines in the 1880s, parasitology and bacteriology, whose practitioners believed there to be a scientific rationale for the division. Basically, diseases caused by bacteria were thought to differ fundamentally from diseases caused by the nonbacterial parasites. The latter were never contagious; their life cycles always involved passage through an intermediate or vector host in which obligatory stages of development took place. Bacterial diseases, on the other hand, were usually contagious, although they might also be transmitted mechanically and accidentally by arthropods.[39]

Manson himself made these important distinctions in his address at the opening of the London School of Tropical Medicine on October 2, 1899. Why, he asked his audience, is tropical medicine so special as to warrant special training in distinct institutes? Why, he asked, may a physician "be competent to deal with disease in England but sadly incompetent to deal with disease in Africa?" By 1899, the answer to both these questions seemed obvious: Unless trained for the tropics, European doctors would have difficulties in the face of specific diseases that occur only in the tropics and which they would not have seen before. Why, he then asked, should one meet different diseases and pathogens in the tropics, given that the "climate" of these pathogens is the human body, all of which are chemically the same? "Viewed as a culture media for pathogenic organisms," he said, "the negro and the Esquimaux are identical, just as the king and the beggar." Obviously, Manson continued, it is the tropical external climate that influences the distribution of pathogens; this climate limits many pathogens to the tropics and brings about diseases with "a limited climatic range." But, he added, coming to the crux of this argument, such climatic rules do not affect bacterial pathogens. They are cosmopolitan precisely because they live in the human body and rarely come under the influence of the external climate. Instead, "transmitted directly from host to host, they can be acquired in any climate when suitable social conditions occur." Thus, strictly speaking, plague, leprosy, cholera, typhoid, and even yellow fever (then considered to have a bacterial cause) were cosmopolitan and not specifically tropical diseases. On the other hand, diseases caused by protozoa and parasitic worms could be strictly tropical. They were often so limited because they usually involved passage through intermediate or vector hosts (mosquitoes, flies, snails, etc.) that were endemic to the tropics, not to temperate zones. Thus, Manson concluded, students of tropical medicine must be exposed chiefly to these diseases of limited climatic range, not to diseases of the ubiquitous bacteria.[40]

But, although bacteriology was never a major component in the teaching of British tropical medicine, there were small diagnostic and research bacteriological laboratories scattered throughout the Empire: By 1910, Kuala Lumpur, Ceylon, Hong Kong, Mauritius, Lagos, British Guiana, Uganda, and Townsville in Queensland had such facilities with an annual cost to the British taxpayer of a little in excess of £12,000, most of it in salaries.[41]

I have made much of this link between tropical medicine and parasitology because it has had serious implications. It gave added credence to the assumption that because of the climate, inhabitants of the tropics appeared to suffer from a different set of diseases than did the British. Africans suffered from "tropical diseases" such as sleeping sickness, malaria, and bilharzia perhaps, whereas the British, at home, had to endure "nontropical" measles, pneumonia, and tuberculosis. Thus, the British colonial medical officer, who needed to be able to diagnose and treat those special tropical diseases that he and his British colleagues were likely to acquire, naturally was specially trained to diagnose and treat diseases caused by protozoa and parasitic worms. But it was only too easy, however, to slip into the totally false assumption that these "nontropical" bacterial and viral diseases, which we know today are among the primary causes of death among African children, were Western diseases of no particular importance in the tropics.[42] Thus tropical medicine, by concentrating on helminths and protozoa, became a discipline that ignored some of the basic public health problems of the tropical colonies.

The link between parasitology and tropical medicine also led to the belief that these parasitic diseases could be prevented without the involvement of the people with the diseases. The reason, the argument went, was that these parasites spent part of their life cycles as larval stages within intermediate hosts; therefore, the parasites could be destroyed very easily by killing these hosts. This technical view of prevention was as attractive to the British medical officer in the 1920s as it was to officials of the WHO in the 1960s. For success it merely required suitable chemicals to kill mosquitoes and snails, and scientifically trained experts to administer them. The population at risk could be ignored.

Nevertheless, British medical officers of the early twentieth century were obviously better trained than their predecessors. Opting for a life of adventure, danger, and considerable satisfaction, they set out into the Dark Continent where untold diseases lay in wait to cripple them and the duty-bound British colonial officers. To a society whose emotions had been torn between memories of past cholera epidemics and the romantic sufferings of the consumptive, it offered glimpses into the exotic. "Black shapes," in the words of Joseph Conrad, whose *Heart of Darkness* appeared in 1902, "crouched, lay, sat between the trees leaning against the trunks, clinging to the earth, half coming out, half effaced within the dim light, in all the attitudes of pain, abandonment and despair. . . . black shadows of disease and starvation."

There was clearly work to be done – a Queen's Empire to be made safe.

3

1898: Another war, another continent

Empire was the thread that linked Britain and the United States in their wars against tropical diseases. But if the British war began with a silent memo from the bureaucrats in the Colonial Office, the Americans began their war with a blaze of guns and the cries of the sick and wounded. In February 1898, after the U.S. battleship *Maine* had been blown up in Havana harbor with much loss of life, the United States blockaded Cuban ports, demanded the withdrawal of Spain from Cuba, and declared war. By July, U.S. troops had landed in Cuba, occupied Santiago, destroyed the Spanish squadron, and also occupied Puerto Rico. Meanwhile in the Philippines the Spanish Pacific Fleet had been destroyed in Manila Bay, and by August a land force had occupied Manila. As a result of the Treaty of Paris, signed in December 1898, the United States found itself in control of the remnants of the once powerful Spanish Empire, including the tropical islands of the Philippines, Cuba, and Puerto Rico. The United States had taken on a role that many of its citizens regarded as a perversion of their own history; they, too, had become an imperial power.

THE AMERICAN "EMPIRE"

The American empire differed significantly from the British. It was administered by the Bureau of Insular Affairs within the War Department, not by a Colonial Office. There were no colonial officers; the empire was run by the officers and men of the U.S. Army. In contrast to the new British possessions in Africa, which were acquired after a series of diplomatic maneuvers in European capitals, the American empire was taken by direct military assault, not only against the Spanish, but also against those who were being "liberated." The American war against the Philippine *insurrectos*, who had themselves fought against the Spaniards and declared themselves a republic, lasted three years, cost the U.S. Army 7,000 killed or wounded, and left over 200,000 Filipinos dead from action, disease, and famine.

The American and British empires also followed different political guidelines. Rather than preserving indigenous societies, which was what the British tried to do with their twentieth-century empire, the Americans were "converters." The United States "attempted to fit her colonies into a republican framework; to treat them either as protostates of the Union and ultimately to absorb them completely, or as sovereign states with whom she was allied and who would finally throw off her tutelage."[1] To reach either of these desired ends, independence or statehood, the colonies had to be utterly transformed or converted into an American-like society. No other route was possible. As Elihu Root, Secretary of War during the Spanish campaigns observed, "people who have not yet been educated in the art of self-government," need "a course of tuition under a strong and guiding hand. With that tuition for a time their natural capacity will, it is hoped, make them a self-governing people."[2]

This process of tutelage was often seen to be equivalent to nation building on the North American mainland. There, territories were acquired and subjected to a short period of tutelage before being admitted to the Union. As Senator Perkins naively noted in 1900, "Porto Rico and the Philippines are ours to have and to hold and to dispose of as Congress in its wisdom may see fit. If we retain them, a period of pupilage – a time for education – must be theirs, so that they may be fitted to understand and have the capacity to enjoy the rights of American citizenship."[3] But, as everyone realized at the time, Filipinos and Puerto Ricans were not Anglo-Saxons, prepared for self-government "by centuries of discipline under the supremacy of law." They were looked upon as members of an inferior race, who, like the Indians and the blacks in the Jim Crow South, were not thought fit, now or ever, to acquire the full benefits of American citizenship or to acquire political equality.[4] Members of the anti-imperialist leagues and the Republican administrations under Theodore Roosevelt and William Taft were in full agreement over that thorny issue. But whereas the anti-imperialists wished to grant immediate full autonomy to these newly acquired islands, the Government chose to hold the islands under subjugation, fully conscious that many regarded this policy as "a radical and mischievous change in our system of government . . . wholly inconsistent with the spirit and genius as well as the words of the Constitution."[5]

Under the Republican administrations that held power until the election of President Wilson in 1912, American tutelage became an end in itself, not a process toward full independence on one hand or U.S. statehood and citizenship on the other. It was meant "to instill into the minds of their pupils the belief that it is the destiny of the Filipino people to remain forever under the control of the United States."[6] King George III must have turned in his grave when, less than 150 years after the Americans had gained their independence from Britain, President Taft asked of the Philippines:

Is it impracticable, is it wild to suppose that the people of the islands will understand the benefit that they derive from such association with the United States and will prefer to maintain some sort of bond so that they may be within the tariff wall and enjoy the markets, rather than separate themselves and become independent and lose the valuable business which our guardianship of them and our obligation to look after them has brought to them.[7]

In this process of tutelage and Americanization, tropical medicine was to play a crucial role.

There were other differences between British and American experiences which impinged on their approaches to tropical medicine. To the British, secure in their northern island home, tropical diseases were, by the twentieth century, the afflictions of exotic peoples in far-away lands. Not so to the Americans; these tropical diseases could constitute a domestic threat. As anyone can testify who has spent the excruciating summer months in the American South, along the Mississippi Valley, or even on the Eastern seaboard, much of the United States is humid and semitropical. Many tropical diseases, such as hookworm and malaria were, and sometimes still are, endemic to certain areas of the country, particularly, of course, in the economically deprived South. "In the South," noted Creighton Wellman, who was to become a major figure in American tropical medicine, "the great handicap of disease has been felt the most painfully because, in addition to all the sickness rife in the north, we have various tropical and subtropical scourges which add to the already too heavy burdens which have been laid upon a long suffering humanity."[8]

During the nineteenth century, physicians in the South, aware of these diseases, had long demanded special training in distinct Southern medical schools. John Warner has argued recently that although this medical movement paralleled political movements in favor of cultural and political separation from the North, it cannot be ascribed simply to political moves by physicians motivated by their Southern identity. Rather, he argues, it became a means of enhancing the much maligned professional status of Southern physicians "by carving out an important realm of medical knowledge in which they were uniquely able to excel." Rather than follow the authoritative directives of Northern and European physicians, Warner points out, Southern physicians were urged to "observe their region's diseases, formulate their own theories, and publish their pathological and therapeutic discoveries." As a corollary to these views, it was naturally considered "the greatest piece of folly" for Southern medical students to learn their trade in the North or in Europe.[9]

The New Orleans School of Medicine, founded in 1856, was generally regarded by Southern physicians as the institute best fitting Southern needs. In the era of proprietary medical schools with their rock-bottom standards, the

New Orleans School set new standards by lengthening the term and empha-sizing clinical work on the Paris model, using the resources of the huge Charity Hospital.[10] "This institution," one of its founders noted, "is of special importance to the Southern Medical Student, on account of its presenting the very types and varieties of disease he will meet with when he goes into practice." The first Chair of Tropical Medicine in the United States was actually established in New Orleans, long before the departments and schools of tropical medicine were established later in the twentieth century. Edouard Dupaquier, a native of New Orleans, returned from Paris in 1885 and eventually was appointed to the Chair of Clinical Therapeutics at the New Orleans Polyclinic. In 1902, the title of the Chair was changed to Clinical Therapeutics and Tropical Medicine.[11] But, with the South's defeat, a distinc-tive Southern medical school was no longer a viable proposition. But many of these Southern physicians gained an expertise in tropical medicine, and the majority of Americans who pioneered the study of tropical diseases were Southerners.

But not only was the South home to some tropical diseases, it also could be threatened by many more diseases imported from the tropics. The Spanish-American War, indeed any war, added to this threat. At such times concerns were constantly expressed that new tropical diseases could be introduced into the country by troops returning from the tropics and that these new diseases could become endemic to the American mainland. Indeed, the Spanish-American War itself was in some small way a reaction to these threats. "Robbed of all superfluities," the Army surgeon John van Hoff wrote, "the real reason why we are in the Antilles today is because our people had determined to abate a nuisance constantly threatening their health, lives and prosperity." Spain was, he continued, "maintaining a pesthole at our front door and we could no longer endure it."[12] Thus, the U.S. Army Medical Corps became a major force in the war and in the Americanization that followed.

THE U.S. ARMY MEDICAL CORPS

The training received by members of the regular U.S. Army Medical Corps, who led the initial fight against tropical diseases, had been considerably upgraded in the 1890s with the opening of the Army Medical School in Washington, D.C. The curriculum of this school differed fundamentally from that at London and Liverpool. Since it was a school of military hygiene, its emphasis was naturally on preventive medicine, bacteriology, and hygiene, not helminthology and protozoology. American army doctors, practicing their trade among large groups of men in camps periodically visited by devastating epidemics, obviously needed to be trained in methods of hygiene and sanitation, and needed expertise in contagious bacterial diseases. As

Colonel Craig, one of America's foremost experts in tropical medicine noted, "The first and most important of the duties of the Medical Corps is the prevention of disease. Unlike the civil practitioners, the army surgeon is preeminently a sanitarian, and furthermore, a specialized sanitarian, in that he has to apply the science of hygiene to conditions not ordinarily encountered in civil life."[13] The Army Medical School, established by General Order on June 24, 1893, was indeed the first scientific school of hygiene and public health established in the United States. In its early years, a medical graduate took a four-month course, which included a large quota of lectures and laboratory sessions in military hygiene, bacteriology, general and sanitary chemistry, and pathology. Exposure to parasitology, the core of the London and Liverpool curricula, was limited to two lectures and five laboratory demonstration sessions given by Charles Stiles.[14]

Military necessity obviously dictated the nature of this curriculum. In addition, the emphasis on bacteriology and sanitation indicated that, unlike the situation in London, the military school was not seen as a threat by other medical schools. Indeed, the quality of these civilian schools was so abysmal in the 1890s, that few of them even presented classes in bacteriology. Furthermore, Surgeon-General George Sternberg, the founder of the military school, had had very different experiences from those of Patrick Manson. Sternberg had enlisted as an Assistant Surgeon in the Army of the Potomac, and in his long military career, both during and after the American Civil War, gained considerable experience dealing with yellow fever and typhoid epidemics which regularly devastated garrisons of the U.S. Army. In the 1870s, he began publishing research articles on bacteriology and yellow fever, a disease whose etiology remained a mystery, even though he and many others believed it to have a bacterial cause. In 1879, for example, he had been part of the unsuccessful National Institute of Health's Commission to study yellow fever in Cuba, and thereafter played a major role in the bitterly contested debates over the nature of the yellow fever "germ."[15] By the 1880s, he was widely regarded as one of the country's leading bacteriologists, a view that was further substantiated by the publication of his *Manual of Bacteriology* in 1892 and his appointment as Surgeon-General one year later.[16] Thus, in many ways, the differences between the London School of Tropical Medicine and the Army Medical School were a reflection of the two men who controlled them.

The political, geographical, and personnel differences between the American and British empires had a major impact on the manner in which each country fought its war against tropical diseases. The British, in these early years, focused primarily on the training of medical officers so as to improve the medical care given to British colonial officials. They did this by rounding out their medical education, and by familiarizing the physician with those diseases not covered in British medical schools. But the American war against tropical diseases was seen in a wider context. Not only were the lives of troops garrisoned in the new tropical possessions to be protected, but also it became politically necessary to show that to be civilized *and* American was also to be clean, sanitary, and healthy. Thus the war against tropical diseases became part of the political weapon of tutelage, displaying, by its success, one of the great advantages that could be bestowed by American civilization. "The glory and merit" of this war, one enthusiast noted in 1900, "justly belongs and of right should accrue to the American army of occupation," by whose efforts Cuba "will eventually be transformed into a paradise of health, wealth and beauty."[17] The twin necessity of protecting the lives of troops and displaying the values of American civilization dictated the weapons: active hygienic and sanitation campaigns supported by a network of bacteriological laboratories. By such means the Medical Corps became a major force in support of American imperialism.

The Medical Corps received a black eye in the war. Although the military victory was achieved with few battle casualties, the medical costs were high as thousands were struck down by disease. But this was hardly the fault of the Corps. Following the Civil War, the U.S. Army had passed through its "dark ages," reduced to little over 27,000 men. With the Spanish-American War, however, the size of the army increased very rapidly to 274,000 men of whom approximately 215,000 were volunteers. Finding men for the army was not difficult; keeping them healthy was. To assist in that process, the Medical Corps also increased its strength with the addition of 113 volunteer surgeons, many of whom were incompetent and poorly trained. Also, the Corps carried little prestige or authority. Its budgetary and manpower requests were consistently ignored, and its sanitary recommendations went unheeded. The results were predictable.

On July 17, 1898, the Vth Corps of 16,500 men occupied Santiago in Cuba, encamping on the surrounding hills. By the end of the month, yellow fever was killing 15 troops every day, and malaria and dysentery had reduced the Corps to an "army of convalescents." As Graham Cosmas vividly described the situation: The Corps "degenerated into a mob of shambling scarecrows. Men stumbled glassy-eyed through their duties until they collapsed and stretcher-bearers, themselves sick, carried them away." The Corps was forced to beat a hasty retreat to a quarantine station at the east end of Long Island, leaving all their supplies and equipment behind in Cuba; an American Dunkirk had taken place without a shot being fired. Meanwhile, 150,000 filthy, undisciplined volunteers sat out the war in large Southern army camps. At Chickamauga, one officer reported, "It is impossible to walk through woods . . . without soiling one's feet with fecal matter"; 21,000 of those in the volunteer camps came down with typhoid, 1,500 of whom died, and, in a war that lasted only a few weeks, 2,500 Americans died from disease, and only 363 from battle. "For the Army," Graham Cosmas wrote, "the war ended in sickness, confusion, and complaint."[18] But the Medical Corps recovered quickly, drawing considerable credit from their sanitary campaigns and research activities in the Philippines, Cuba, and Puerto Rico.

The United States had encouraged Filipinos in their struggle for independence from Spanish domination, but in 1898, after the Spanish-American War, the Philippines were transferred from Spanish to American rule. The Filipinos, under Emilio Aguinaldo, revolted against this U.S. subjugation and so began a long period of guerrilla warfare. The Americans sought to pacify the people and build a new nation by what they called "actual deeds." These "deeds" involved the wholesale Americanization of Philippine society, from reforms in government and education to such mundane matters as road building. But, there was also a medical component to the war, and the Medical Corps played a major role in quelling the Philippine insurrection. The Americans should, the Chief Surgeon in the Philippines believed, instruct the Filipinos in personal hygiene. By doing so, he noted, America had shown "humanity in war, and [such instruction] has made a deep impression on the Filipinos and has been an important factor in winning their allegiance to our Government."[19] W. Cameron Forbes, Governor-General of the Philippines from 1909 to 1913, was even more enthusiastic. The Americans, he wrote, were "doing God's work here."[20] A recent account of this period was equally positive: "Because of the widespread distributions of doctors and the immediate statistical evidence of their effectiveness, the army's public health work was an important force for pacification, bringing to the Filipinos vivid evidence of the humanitarian and benevolent intentions of the United States."[21]

But there was always the reverse side of the coin. As two historians have recently argued, the medical and sanitary changes brought to these islands were part of a ruthless program of Americanization in which the war against disease and the war against the Filipino *insurrectos* were, basically, part of the same event. The sanitary war was joined not only because ill health and unsanitary conditions among the Filipinos often became a threat to the health of the Americans, but also because by doing so Philippine society could be reconstructed on an American model. This sanitary reconstruction would then boost commercial activity by rendering the islands more appealing to American investors, and, at the same time, result in a more healthy and efficient workforce.[22]

In 1902, a cholera epidemic in which up to 200,000 people are estimated to have died, began to slice its way through the Philippines. The American Army immediately unleashed a "cholera war" in which they carried out extensive search operations to locate infected villages. These villages were then cordoned off or razed to the ground, and their inhabitants placed in detention camps, or, as the Chief Surgeon preferred to call them, "detention pavillions." There, often by force, they were administered viscious drugs such as benzozone (a powerful oxidizing agent and germicide, which can cause severe burns). Furthermore, wartime destruction of local rice crops and the implementation of strict quarantine regulations against the cholera bacillus brought about widespread famine in the cordoned villages that were left standing, and this in turn increased the mortality from cholera and other diseases. Bodies were then forceably expropriated and cremated. No attempt was made to enlist the support of the local populations, and thus, to many Filipinos, it seemed that cholera had become an excuse to continue the war against them.

Similarly, an outbreak of plague was kept in check by a military operation against filth and the ubiquitous rat, which had recently been implicated in the spread of the disease. Houses found to contain infected rats were often torn down, and the wretched inhabitants transferred to "detention camps" for "the temporary residence of homeless people." Other houses were disinfected with carbonic acid, and all clothing and articles burned. Their occupants were then forced to take disinfectant baths, and exposed persons were also moved to the detention camps. This was certainly war on a grand scale.

A system of depopulation is being actively carried on; infected houses and unsanitary hovels in their neighborhood are attacked and cubicles and partitions are removed, outhouses and structures built in yards and unfit for human habitation are destroyed, letting in the sun and air; sewers and drains are flushed by the fire department . . . ; all evicted people are given shelter in tents until they can find dwelling places.[23]

At the same time, William Gorgas was ordered to do battle with yellow fever in Havana. It was a simple matter of self-preservation. Yellow fever was endemic to the city, but because of the lifelong immunity acquired by those who survived an attack, the disease there seemed to strike only foreigners, including, of course, invading armies. "Had not Spain surrendered, indeed, it is almost certain that the United States would have been obliged to withdraw its troops," noted the biographers of Gorgas.[24] To make matters worse, Havana also acted as the seedbed for continual epidemics of yellow fever that struck at American cities as far removed as New Orleans and Boston. Believing the disease to be associated with filth, the U.S. Army ordered Gorgas to cleanse the city – something an occupying army was well qualified to do. Under Gorgas's direction, his biographers claim, Havana "now became as orderly, as clean, and as civilized in its appearance as Fifth Avenue. All the tin cans, vegetable heaps, and other extraneous matter had been removed."[25]

Medicine also played an important role in the Americanization of Puerto Rico. There, in July 1898, American troops under General Miles had landed at Guanica Bay and Ponce. They came not to make war, Miles pronounced, but to bestow "the advantages and blessings of enlightened civilization." According to Brigadier General Guy Henry, the second Military Governor, this would be done by affording the Puerto Ricans "kindergarten instruction in controlling themselves without allowing them too much liberty." Once again the American Government avoided the basic question of the end to which this tutelage was directed. The Foraker Act of 1900, which bestowed civilian government on the island, determined that Puerto Ricans were not American citizens, and that the island was a "dependency" or "possession," rather than a territory – a step away from statehood. Tutelage, as in the Philippines, became an end in itself, and the assumed results of this activity – better roads, higher standards of education, and better public health measures – were used by successive governors to justify American presence on the island.[26] "There is every reason to believe," reported Henry Carroll enthusiastically in 1899,

that sanitary conditions are abreast of, if not superior to, those in the British West Indies, with sanitary appliances of American manufacture far superior, and all at the end of a few months. When the American army established itself, intelligent officers of experience took up the "white man's burden" with an individual sense of obligation and a devotion worthy of the American citizen soldier.[27]

One of those medical officers to take up the "white man's burden" was a young army surgeon, named Bailey Ashford. A graduate of Georgetown University Medical School and the Army Medical School, he was put in command of the general hospital at Ponce. Ashford developed an understanding of and a sympathy with the problems of the island rarely found among conquerors, and later married the daughter of Don Ramon Lopez, founder of the island's first newspaper.[28]

Ashford was responsible for starting a campaign against hookworm. Following a devastating hurricane that hit the island in 1899, he not only discovered widespread anemia among its victims (Figure 3.1), but also found that the problem was not alleviated by the better food available in the hospital. Anemia, Ashford concluded, after noting the telltale signs of eosinophilia and discovering eggs in the stools of the *jibaros*, was due primarily to hookworm infections, not simply to malnutrition as usually presumed. Ashford also recognized, however, that although such a disease may well be due primarily to a parasitic infection, its seriousness was determined by the economic conditions of the victims. As he noted with specific reference to hookworm in Puerto Rico: "It seems to us that we have in the fact of poor and insufficient food, exposure, etc., a remarkable illustration of how, when resistance is lowered in the life of the whole population, an endemic disease becomes a veritable scourge."[29]

Although hookworm posed little threat to the health of American troops, it did pose an economic threat to the heavy American investment that was anticipated in order to develop sugar and coffee plantations on the island. Thus, Ashford was forced to use economic arguments in an attempt to convince the Government that a campaign against the worm should be initiated. Hookworm, he exhorted members of the American medical community, "is now the great scourge of the agricultural classes in Porto Rico, and what has come to be a most important economic question in the betterment of the islands."[30] After months of effort, Ashford finally achieved his goal: In

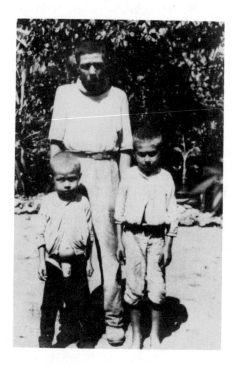

Figure 3.1. Hookworm victims, Puerto Rico, 1922 (Courtesy of the Rockefeller Archive Center)

1904, the Governor of the island finally approved the finances for a Puerto Rico Anemia Commission.

The campaign was essentially directed at mass treatment of the hookworm victims, with five doses of thymol, given a week apart, being considered sufficient to cure the patients.[31] Ashford did not believe that the disease could be eradicated by the implementation of sanitary campaigns. "I believe it not possible," he wrote, "that those degraded to the level of people whose life is bounded by a tropical plantation, enjoying little beyond the cutting of cane and the picking of coffee, can have a high standard of personal cleanliness."[32]

Medical research

Action against tropical diseases was taken also on the research front. Research into the etiology, prevention, and cure of tropical diseases became a major preoccupation of the U.S. Army Medical Corps. In 1898, Surgeon-General Sternberg commissioned the first of a series of commissions or boards set up to investigate diseases threatening the well-being of American troops and the success of their civilizing mission. This first one, commanded by Major Walter Reed, and including Victor Vaughan, future Dean of the University of

Michigan Medical School, dealt specifically with the typhoid outbreaks in the volunteer camps. Typhoid, they concluded, was passed via feces, filth, fingers, and flies and the epidemics in the volunteer camps had resulted from a breakdown in sanitation.

In the spring of 1899, Reed also took command of another board set up by Sternberg to investigate the perennial problem of yellow fever. The short period of complacency following the sanitation campaigns of General Gorgas had come to an end. The cleaning-up operation had not stamped out yellow fever as previously believed. Thousands of nonimmune immigrants arriving from Spain had created perfect conditions for a new outbreak of the disease, and once again many American personnel began to fall prey to the dreadful scourge. Those believing in the efficacy of cleanliness were shocked to learn that "Havana, the 'spotless town' of the Caribbean, was just as intensely ridden with yellow fever as was Havana 'the pesthole.'"[33] After another desperate attempt to improve sanitation, Sternberg appointed the board of Walter Reed, Aristides Agramonte, Jesse Lazear, and James Carroll, which immediately became embroiled in the ongoing debates over the cause and means of transmission of the disease.

By 1899, many believed yellow fever to be caused by a bacterium, *Bacillus icteroides*, which had been implicated two years previously by the Italian bacteriologist, Giuseppi Sanarelli. Many also assumed that the bacterium was transmitted directly by contaminated material or "fomites" in the bedding, vomit, blood, or feces of yellow fever victims. Sternberg disagreed with both of these assumptions, and so did Reed. Thus, in 1900, Reed met with Carlos Finley the Cuban physician who, many years previously, had provided evidence that the mosquito was the carrier of the yellow fever germ.

That insects could act as disease vectors had become apparent by 1900, although many physicians were still resistant to the idea. By then Manson had made public Ronald Ross's discovery that mosquitoes not only could remove the malarial parasite from human blood, but also, after the parasite had developed further within the insect's body, could inject the parasite back into a human.

With Reed back in the United States, the other members of the board began a series of experiments in which one mosquito, after feeding on the blood of a yellow fever patient, was allowed to bite James Carroll and another two volunteers. Although all of them came down with the disease, the experiments were not rigorous enough to prove the point; however, Reed did present a preliminary paper on the supposed etiology of yellow fever at the meeting of the American Public Health Association, held in the fall of 1900.

Later in 1900, Reed began a series of more adequately controlled experiments in which volunteers, after being offered up to $200 in gold for their pains, were either required to live with bedding, stained linen, and filth of previous yellow fever victims, or were subject to the bite of the *Aedes* mosquito. Only those exposed to the mosquitoes came down with the disease. As a result, Reed felt able to announce, at the Pan American Congress held in Havana, that "the spread of yellow fever can be most effectually controlled by measures directed to the destruction of mosquitoes." Sanitation was not the answer to the yellow fever.[34] The validity of this claim became clear a few years later when General Gorgas's antimosquito campaign during the digging of the Panama Canal prevented epidemics of yellow fever and allowed the canal to be completed.

Similar research boards were set up in the Philippines. There, after the insurrection had begun to take its bloody toll, President McKinley appointed the First Philippine Commission under the chairmanship of Jacob Schurman. The Commission received medical testimony from Simon Flexner and L. F. Barker of Johns Hopkins, who were both in the Philippines at that time investigating some of the medical problems. "We would like to know," the commissioners asked the two American physicians, "what effect the climate and maladies would have on Americans coming here, whether they could endure the climate or not, and what course of living perhaps they ought to adopt, and what maladies they would have to encounter." They were informed that many diseases seemed to be confined to the Filipino population, and that diarrhea and dysentery were the most prevalent disorders among whites. With this in mind, Dr. Barker advised the Commission that "if the government sent men out it would also be necessary to pay close attention to the public sanitation, water supply, drainage, removal of excrements, quarantine and to make a special study of the diseases, the same as the English, who have established a school of tropical diseases."[35] This was precisely what the commission recommended to the President in their report of 1900. Action quickly followed.

Four disease boards were set up in the Philippines. Each one consisted of a group of physicians working out of a pathological laboratory. While most of their time was spent on routine investigations, such as autopsies, and bacteriological analyses, each member worked independently on pieces of individual research.[36] The focus of this research was quite naturally aimed at those diseases that threatened the American population. The first, established in 1900 under the command of Richard Strong, future Chairman of Tropical Medicine at Harvard University, concerned itself with the vexing problems of diarrhea and dysentery. These, as Flexner and Baxter had already indicated, were major problems for the white population, second only to malaria and venereal disease in prevalence among American troops. Similarly, the second board, established in 1906, focused on beriberi, a serious problem among Filipino scouts attached to the U.S. Army, which had been linked to an improper diet by physicians of the Japanese navy.[37]

THE AMERICAN SOCIETY OF TROPICAL MEDICINE

These medical victories did not go unnoticed at home. On March 9, 1903, 19 local physicians from Philadelphia, sparked by the acquisition of the new tropical empire, attended the first meeting of the Society of Tropical Medicine of Philadelphia at the home of its founder and president, Dr. Thomas Fenton. Changing its name almost immediately to the American Society of Tropical Medicine, the initial council members agreed to restrict membership to a maximum of 200 "regular American physicians" interested in tropical diseases, and to admit to corresponding membership any foreign physician who had contributed to the field of tropical medicine.[38] They enhanced their prestige almost immediately by successfully inviting a host of eminent figures to become honorary members: Aristides Agramonte, James Carroll (who actually presented an address on yellow fever to 75 people at the Society's first public meeting in January 1904), William Gorgas, Charles Laveran, Patrick Manson, George Sternberg, Charles Stiles, William Welch, and even Robert Koch.

The society developed amazingly quickly from its modest provincial beginnings. By 1906, Gorgas, Agramonte, and Carlos Finley had all presented papers, and Creighton Wellman, then living in Angola, had the first of many papers read for him. A year later its potential membership was enlarged when scientists, as well as physicians, were allowed to become honorary members. In 1909, William Gorgas became the first president with international stature, and in 1910 the Society met for the first time outside the Washington–Philadelphia area. Under Gorgas's presidency, they began to press for an American civilian institute of research and teaching in tropical medicine and hygiene, commending this matter, as noted in a 1909 resolution, "to the consideration of the American capitalists."[39] A few years later, their endeavors were to be rewarded with the opening of the first School of Tropical Medicine in Tulane University, New Orleans.

The American war against tropical diseases, which had begun so disastrously among the human misery of Santiago and the Southern army camps, ended triumphantly with the discovery of the yellow fever vector, and the digging of the Panama Canal. The Medical Corps had played a major part in the double victory against the human enemy and tropical diseases, and in doing so had gained both scientific prestige and political influence; no longer could they be ignored. "Thank God," Walter Reed wrote in a letter to William Gorgas in the summer of 1901, "that the Medical Department of the U.S. Army, which got such a "black eye" during the Spanish-American War, has during the past year accomplished work that will always remain to its eternal credit."[40] Cuban independence in 1902, for example, was attained only with the Platt Amendment, which gave the United States the right to intervene again should yellow fever or other diseases again threaten Cuba or the United States. Indeed, between 1906 and 1909, Cuba was reoccupied and a sanitary regime was imposed that addressed the commercial and military priorities of the Americans, not the public health needs of the Cuban society. The policy addressed specific diseases and their control, while the problem of rising infant mortality, malnutrition, poor housing, and unclean water remained outside the scope of the American-constituted health system. For that to occur, Cubans had to wait another 70 years.[41]

And what of bilharzia, which is endemic to both the Philippines and Puerto Rico? Little was known about the worms in those early years, but to Dr. Gonzalez Martinez of the Puerto Rican Anemia Commission belongs the credit of discovering the worm for the first time in the Western Hemisphere. "Bilharziosis recti is particularly common," he wrote in 1904, speculating that the worms may have been introduced from Africa by the slave trade.[42] Two years later "distomiasis–bilharzia disease" was noted in the Philippines, and an accurate diagnosis of Oriental bilharzia made in 1908 following an examination of a Filipino scout. Captains Nichols and Phalen, who made the diagnosis, warned also that the highest prevalence of the disease was probably to be found on the islands of Samar and Leyte.[43] This statement was to haunt the Americans in 1944, when the American troops came ashore in the Leyte Valley.

By this time the British were already aware of bilharzia. By 1898, they had become masters of Egypt and the Suez Canal, the gateway to India.

Bilharzia (1850–1918): The Looss controversies

The sun is almost overhead beating down mercilessly from a cloudless sky; another excruciatingly hot day in the tropics. A group of children are playing around in the water of an irrigation canal, in Egypt perhaps, with their mothers gossiping together as they do the daily wash. A teenage boy urinates in the water. As long as he can remember his urine has been stained with blood; today is no different. His urine also contains small, oval, golden-brown eggs with a terminal spine. By urinating in the water and passing these eggs he was doing what millions of others had been doing for time immemorial – helping to disseminate the parasitic worm responsible for bilharzia.   [Author]

No other people on earth suffer the ravages of bilharzia to the extent of the Egyptian *fellaheen* (Figure 4.1). The figures are astonishing: 47 percent of the entire Egyptian population according to J. Allen Scott's estimate of 1937, 16– 20 million in the opinion of two Egyptian physicians in the 1970s. Villages in the Nile Delta with over 70 percent of their population carrying the worm are not uncommon; a recent survey of Luxor primary school children revealed 80 percent of them to be infected.[1] Indeed, so common is one of the species in Egypt and parts of the Middle East that in some areas one of the symptoms, hematuria – or bloody urine – is popularly regarded as the male equivalent of menstruation.

All this was unknown to the first wave of Europeans to arrive with the French invasion of 1798. In their three-year sojourn, many French troops contracted the disease, and there is even evidence to suggest that Napoleon himself can be counted among them.[2] Five years after the French departed, Muhammad Ali came to power and initiated a long period of European-styled reforms, many of which impinged directly on the bilharzia story.

South of Cairo, on both sides of the Nile, large dikes divided the land into a series of basins, some as large as 100,000 acres. Every August, floodwater of the Nile was diverted by short canals into these basins, where it stood two to three feet deep, depositing its rich silt into the soil. After ploughing, a rich winter crop was seeded, to be harvested in the spring. This "basin irrigation"

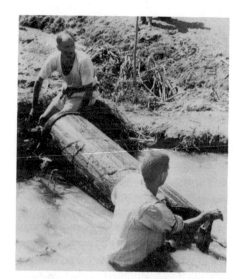

a

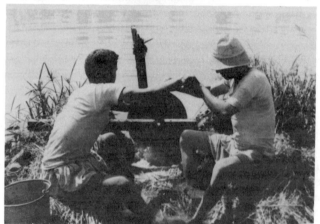

b

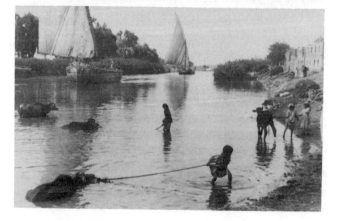

c

allowed only one crop per year, and left the fields empty and parched throughout the summer months.

Muhammad Ali left this system in place, but introduced significant changes north of Cairo in the Nile Delta. There, he not only oversaw the dredging of old canals and the digging of new ones, but introduced perennial irrigation. This was accomplished by digging deeper canals, or *Sayfi* canals, from which, even in periods when the Nile was low, water could be raised by screws and water wheels to irrigate summer crops. In particular, these deep canals were used to irrigate long-staple Jumel cotton, which was planted immediately after the harvesting of the winter crops and which quickly came to be Egypt's primary export crop.

Tremendous time and effort were required to keep the *Sayfi* canals open. To increase water flow in them, French engineers raised the level of the Nile by constructing regulating barrages on the river north of Cairo. The first of these, the so-called "Bridge of Blessings" 12 miles north of the city, was begun in 1847 and completed in 1861. But, as a Scottish engineer was to remark two decades later, the "barrage was a costly failure, of no more use than those useless old Pyramids a few miles off."[3]

Cotton brought only misery to the *fellaheen*. They were forced not only to dredge and dig new canals, but to clean out the *Sayfi* canals every year to prevent the accumulation of silt and weeds. But, in addition to these slavelike conditions, perennial irrigation provided an environment in which bilharzia flourished. We do not know by how much the disease increased at that time, but one study during the 1930s suggested that the changeover from basin to perennial irrigation increases the prevalence of the parasite at least ten-fold. Another study put the figure much higher: A 1–3 percent prevalence in a village under basin irrigation increased to 75–80 percent when perennial irrigation was introduced.[4]

A second series of reforms initiated by Muhammad Ali had a more positive impact on the disease: He opened military, technical, and medical schools under French and Italian directors. The first such medical school, opened in 1827 to train military surgeons, involved what historian Heyworth-Dunne called "a most curious situation." In the school, she wrote, "a hundred Egyptian students from al-Azhar who knew only Arabic and who had never

Figure 4.1. Bilharzia and the Egyptian *fellaheen*: (a) The installation of the Archimedian screw, an ancient water-lifting device consisting of a 10-foot-long cylinder with a wooden spiral inside. (b) The screw in operation. Prolonged exposure of hands and feet to water ensures infection with the schistosome worms. (c) Egyptian farmers take pride in keeping their cattle clean. Here, in the Mahmoudia Canal, the children carry out this enjoyable task and thereby expose themselves to bilharzia. (Courtesy of the Parasitic Diseases Programme, WHO)

received any training but in Arabic grammar, Koranic exegesis, Fikh, etc., gathered together in order to be trained in medical and scientific subjects of which they had not the slightest idea, by a number of European teachers who did not know the language of their students." These teachers (six Italians, four French, and one Bavarian) had their lessons translated into Arabic and dictated to the poor students.[5]

Also, in an attempt to replace the many foreign experts with their own nationals, the Egyptian Government sent students on educational missions to Europe. In 1882, for example, 12 of the best medical students were sent on a six-year mission to France, many of whom returned to take up positions in the medical school and hospital that had by then been transferred to the palace at Kasr al-Aini.

A series of economic crises and the death of Muhammad Ali in 1849 led to a breakdown in the educational system. The French director of the medical school resigned, and the new viceroy, Abbas I, unable to find an Egyptian or French replacement, turned to Germany. In 1850, Wilhelm Griesinger, Professor of Anatomy at Kiel, became Director, and the same year Theodor Bilharz (Figure 4.2) arrived to be his assistant. They were not strangers to each other; Griesinger had been an internist at Tübingen when Bilharz enrolled there in 1845.[6]

Both men were first and foremost research scholars, trained in the German system. Under Griesinger's direction, the Egyptian medical school continued to decline as a teaching institute and was actually closed for a short time in

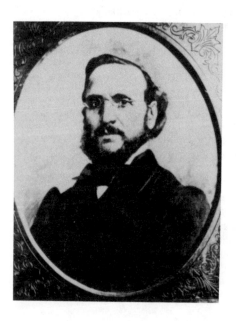

Figure 4.2. Theodor Bilharz (Reprinted with permission from M. Abdel-Wahab, *Schistosomiasis in Egypt*. Boca Raton, Fla.: CRC Press)

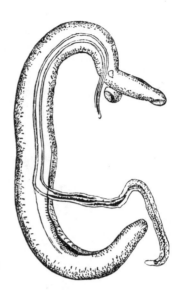

Figure 4.3. *Distomum haematobium*, from Cobbald's
Entozoa (1864)

1855. But, at the same time, these two men made the first crucial discoveries: finding and describing the schistosome worms and linking them to clinical and pathological symptoms.

In Tübingen, Karl Theodor von Siebold had recognized Bilharz's talents in anatomical studies, and it was to von Siebold that Bilharz addressed his first correspondence on May 1, 1851. He had discovered during an autopsy, he informed von Siebold, long white helminths in the portal vein with a flat body and a long spiral tail. This and subsequent letters were published by von Siebold in *Die Zeitschrift für wissenschaftliche Zoologie* of which he was editor. By the end of the month, Bilharz realized that these worms were unlike any other trematode. "Something more wonderful, a trematode with *divided* sex," he wrote, and went on to explain that the previously described worms with the flat body were males each of which was capable of grasping a single threadlike female worm in a fold of its body, giving the appearance of a tail. In a letter dated December 1, 1851, Bilharz named the new worm *Distomum haematobium* (Figure 4.3).

Distomum haematobium, distinct sexes
    Male: soft, white, filiform body, anterior "forebody" flattened, narrow, ventrally concave, dorsally convex, smooth surface. . . . "Hind body" behind the acetabulum with ventral surface rolled in to form a 'gynaecophoric canal' with rough exterior and smooth interior. The oral acetabulum subapical, triangular. The ventral acetabulum arises at the end of the forebody, diameter equal to oral acetabulum. Outside acetabulum surface finely granulated. The esophagus, with no pharynx, divides anterior to the ventral acetabulum and reunites again in the hind body. Genital pore behind ventral acetabulum and gynaecophoric canal.

Female: different shape, more delicate, thin, taeniform body. The anterior sensory organs are attenuated with a smooth surface, the tail ends in a narrow point. Acetabula and esophagus similar to male. The genital pore is present at the margin of the ventral acetabulum.

Length: 3–4 lines (i.e., 0.25 to 0.33 inch) but the length of female is greater.

Country: Egypt. In human portal vein before bifurcation. Female within male gynaecophoric canal always found in mesenteric veins, intestinal veins, hepatic veins, and splenic vein.[7]

By March 1852, Bilharz had discovered the characteristic eggs with the terminal spine or "pointed appendage," as he called it, and had watched as small active embryos emerged from the eggs. This organism, he wrote, "had a long, cylindrical cone-shaped form which was thicker anteriorly and more rounded posteriorly, with a proboscis-like protuberance anteriorly. It was covered completely with rather long cilia." He noted, too, the pear-shaped bodies which we know to be eyespots, but unfortunately, Bilharz was unable to observe any further transformations of these "infusorial-like embryos."[8]

Meanwhile, however, the medical school continued to decline. Griesinger returned to Germany in 1852, but Bilharz remained in Cairo, dying of typhus in 1862. During the 1860s, the French took over the school again, and although 31 Egyptian students had recently returned from study at Edinburgh and Munich, only two chairs at the medical school were held by them.[9] But, during the reign of Ismail Pasha (1863–79) Egyptians regained control of the school, and Bilharz's discoveries seemed to have been forgotten. As a result, when the worm was rediscovered in the 1870s by the Italian Prosper Sonzino, the physicians at Kasr-el-Aini believed a new discovery had been made. "Many of them," Sonzino wrote, "remember having seen or heard speak of Bilharz, but none of them remembered clearly. The memory had been preserved by tradition, but in time the tradition faded away."[10] Indeed the only Egyptians aware of the worm at that time were those who had studied in Germany; few Egyptians were able to read the scientific literature emanating from that country. From the European point of view, Egyptian medicine had reached a new low. And then the British came.

For the British, Egypt had tremendous strategic importance; it lay across the shortest route to India. To safeguard this route to the east, it seemed necessary to maintain a stable regime in the country and to block further attempts by the French to gain dominance. Seeing this stability threatened by mounting foreign debt and the Ahmed Arabi revolts, British troops occupied Cairo after defeating the Egyptian Army at the battle of Tel el-Kebir on September 13, 1882. The goal of the British "was to secure the stability and tranquility of Egypt so that it would not be torn by internal disturbances and thus threaten England's strategic route to the East."[11]

The necessary stability would be achieved, the British believed, only with the restoration of Khedival authority under the Ottoman Empire. With that achieved, they hoped, British troops could be rapidly withdrawn. But such proved to be impossible. The declining power of the Ottoman Empire threatened a power vacuum in the Middle East should the British withdraw. "Getting out of Egypt," the Consul General Evelyn Baring argued, "is a very different problem from getting out of Afghanistan."[12] The British were faced also with an unstable situation inside the country, where the Turkish-Armenian groups, favoring the rule of the Khedive, were opposed by Egyptian nationalists. Thus the "veiled protectorate" was maintained, and the British began to introduce a series of reforms, including, once again, reforms in education and agriculture.

As in the period of Muhammad Ali, these reforms had a considerable impact on the fate of bilharzia in Egypt. Irrigation engineers were brought over from India to improve the canal system and to rebuild the "Bridge of Blessings." This they achieved in 1884, but their greatest monument can be found many miles upriver, where their engineers selected Aswan as the most suitable site for a water-storage dam. The completion of the dam in 1902 brought huge tracts of land along the Nile Valley under perennial irrigation, while more acres were placed under summer irrigation in the Delta. By 1912, cotton accounted for 80 percent of Egyptian exports, and, during the 1890s, the highest cotton yields on record were realized. But a price had to be paid: The country lost its self-sufficiency in foodstuffs, and, one can only assume, the level of bilharzia rose to yet new heights.

Again, as in the time of Muhammad Ali, the medical school came under close scrutiny. A report highly critical of the school and the hospital appeared in the *British Medical Journal* of 1885. Its message was clear: Efficiency demanded European guidance. The medical school, the report noted, had 165 pupils in a six-year program, after which the superior ones were dispatched to France and Germany for further training. These better students, the report maintained, "are invariably found to be in an almost elementary stage of ignorance, and to have acquired only the most imperfect, inaccurate, and useless kind of knowledge." The Egyptian Medical School, the author concluded, is "in urgent need of reform."

The students are taught by rote from Arabic translations of old textbooks. There are no laboratories, physiological, anatomical, pathological, or histological. With trifling exception, the school may be said to be wholly destitute of materials for teaching. . . . The money spent is thus mainly wasted, and the school is a dangerous, because deceitful, sham.[13]

What were needed, according to the author, were anatomical and pathological collections, and modern laboratories. All entering students, the report further argued, should have knowledge of a European language, and, above all, someone from a London hospital medical school should be brought in to reorganize the school. In 1897, Dr. Cooper Perry of Guy's Hospital was sent

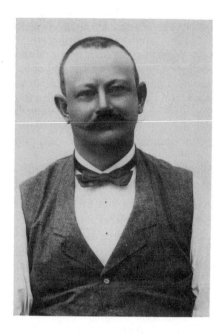

Figure 4.4. Arthur Looss (Courtesy of the University of Illinois Archives)

out to advise on the school's reorganization. As a result, in 1898, the language of instruction was changed again, this time from Arabic to English, and a considerable number of Europeans were added to the medical staff.

"There are now probably few countries in the world," stated the 1909 Annual Report of the Egyptian Public Health Department, "that offer so attractive and untouched a field of scientific investigation as does Egypt."[14] One to be so attracted was Arthur Looss (Figure 4.4) of the University of Leipzig, who arrived in Cairo during the British reorganization of the 1890s. He was to remain in Egypt and dominate the field of helminthology until the outbreak of World War I. In 1906, the young and inexperienced Robert Leiper arrived in Cairo to learn all he could from Looss. Leiper's name was to be ineradicably linked to bilharzia.

ROBERT LEIPER

At the first meeting of the advisory board set up in 1903 to oversee the distribution of the Tropical Disease Research Fund which had been set up to finance research activity at the London and Liverpool schools of tropical medicine, Patrick Manson, a member of the board by virtue of his office as Colonial Medical Advisor, proposed that money earmarked for the London School be used to hire two young lecturers in protozoology and helminthol-

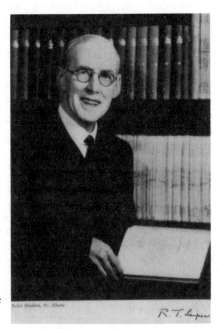

Figure 4.5. Robert Leiper (Courtesy of the Liverpool School of Tropical Medicine)

ogy. He proposed that each of them should be sent to Europe for six months training, thereby making "the Empire independent of Continental experts."[15]

On January 28, 1905, Robert Leiper (Figure 4.5) was hired as Lecturer in Helminthology at the London School. The "old man" as he is affectionately known today (he died in 1969), was an epitome of a "canny Scot" who, according to one anonymous source to whom I spoke, would have made a brilliant career selling real estate to the status-minded southern English. As Sheila Willmott wrote in her eulogy (and few people knew him better), "He expected, and received, love, respect and affection from many of his staff, students and co-workers, but he was not afraid of making enemies or of continuing feuds; indeed, at one time, he maintained that people worked better when there was friction."[16] He was clearly capable of exasperating anyone at anytime, but all those with whom I have spoken told me of his fascinating "Royal Tour" of the magnificent Roman remains of Verulamium and the equally inspiring St. Albans Cathedral close by.

Born in Kilmarnock in 1881, he gained his medical degree from Glasgow, but became more interested in parasitology, winning a Carnegie Research Scholarship in Glasgow examining helminths collected during the Scottish Antarctic Expedition. With this very limited background Leiper was appointed to the London position, and immediately began a process of self-education. Excused all teaching responsibilities, he spent the first six months acquiring a basic knowledge of tropical diseases by attending lectures and working on filarial larvae. Later in the year, he traveled to the Gold Coast, where he showed his mettle not only by discovering the elusive male Guinea worm, *Dracunculus medinensis*, but also by experimental proof of the method of infection. Finally, in January 1906, Leiper arrived in Cairo to work under Arthur Looss. He spent over 18 months in the Nile Valley before beginning his teaching duties at London during the 1907–8 session. During this long sojourn in Egypt, Leiper came into contact with bilharzia and began his investigations of the infamous worms.

BILHARZIA: 1906

By 1906, very little more was known about the disease than had been published 25 years earlier in August Hirsch's monumental *Handbook of Geographical and Historical Pathology*. "Endemic haematuria," as the disease was then known, was thought to be caused by a single species of worm, *Distomum haematobium*, found in the veins of the gut mesenteries and the bladder, and endemic to Egypt and Natal.[17] The worms were known to cause local lesions around the worm's egg masses trapped in the tissues, and to produce the telltale blood in the urine. The disease seemed to be associated with water. Thus humans were thought to become infected after drinking water that contained either the worm eggs themselves, or small organisms that carried the eggs or larvae of the worm. Others believed, however, that the worms entered the body directly through the skin or even through the urethra itself.[18]

By the time Leiper arrived in Egypt, a few more details had been uncovered. The disease was known to exist beyond the boundaries of Egypt and Natal and, if Patrick Manson could be believed, had even afflicted an Englishman who had visited islands in the West Indies. In addition, as mentioned in the preceding chapter, the disease had been reported from Puerto Rico during the Anemia Commission's survey. A few more details of disease pathology were known, but the life cycle still remained a mystery. At that time it was usual to believe that the active embryo or miracidium, which Bilharz had seen hatching from the egg, passed into an intermediate host (some freshwater mollusc, crustacean, or larval arthropod perhaps), where the cercariae were produced. Humans acquired the worms, Manson believed, by drinking water containing either the cercariae or these intermediate hosts.[19]

Once infected there was little one could do. A bland and nutritious diet was advised; spices, stimulants, and exercise were to be avoided. Manson prescribed male fern extract or methylene blue three times a day, and recommended washing out the bladder with a "weak boric acid lotion, and the internal administration of urotropine, uva ursi, buchu, perhaps small doses of cubebs, copaiba, or sandalwood oil, salol, benzoic acid, and so forth."

In addition, Manson noted, eggs passed with the urine had a terminally placed spine, whereas those released with the feces usually carried a lateral spine. Were there two species he wondered?

ONE SPECIES OR TWO?

While Leiper was in Egypt studying under Looss, Luigi Sambon, at the London School of Tropical Medicine, read a paper to the Zoological Society of London that was to fire a heated controversy between Sambon and Manson on one side and Looss on the other. This controversy centered around two scientific issues: the number of schistosome species and their life cycles.[20]

According to Sambon there were two African species of schistosome: *Schistosoma haematobium*, the old classic species with a terminally spined egg (Figure 4.6) described as *Distomum* by Bilharz; and another species described by Sambon as having an egg with "a large curved lateral spine" (Figure 4.6), that lived in the blood vessels of the gut, not the urinogenitals.[21] Such laterally spined eggs had been found before. In 1902, for example, Manson had described a patient from St. Kitts in the West Indies, with laterally spined eggs in the feces, "as so often happens in bilharzia ova from the alimentary canal."[22] But, in the past, such eggs had been assumed to be those of *Schistosoma haematobium*. Looss, for example, assumed them to be abnormal eggs produced only by immature females, whereas Griesinger and Bilharz had suggested that such laterally spined objects were pupalike capsules protecting the embryos that had freshly emerged from the terminally spined egg.[23] But, whatever these laterally spined objects were, they were assumed to be

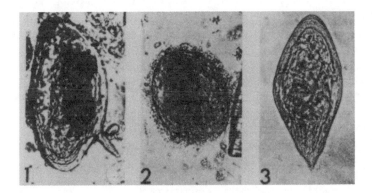

Figure 4.6. Eggs of the three human schistosome species: (1) the laterally spined egg of *Schistosoma mansoni*; (2) the egg of *S. japonicum* with a rudimentary spine; (3) the terminally spined egg of *S. haematobium*. (Reprinted from P. Jordan and G. Webbe, *Schistosomiasis: Epidemiology, Treatment and Control* [London: Heinemann, 1982], with permission of the authors)

produced by *S. haematobium*. Indeed, in 1864, the South African form of
S. haematobium was described as a new species, *Bilharzia capensis*, partly
because none of the eggs had lateral spines.[24]

But now Sambon, using a badly preserved adult worm and a few eggs from
the helminth collection at the London School, erected a new species,
Schistosoma mansoni, which differed from *S. haematobium* only by an egg with a
lateral rather than a terminal spine. In other words, according to Sambon,
S. haematobium was characterized by terminally spined eggs, and the new
species, *S. mansoni*, by laterally spined eggs. In a later address to the Society of
Tropical Medicine, Sambon admitted that he had used the egg as the main
criterion for speciation, but added the pious hope that careful study by others
"might disclose several peculiarities." However, he was quick to add, "for
zoologists the characters of the ovum should suffice for the determination of a
new species.[25]

To name the new worm after Manson was an astute move on the part of
Sambon; by its very name the worm received an authenticity it hardly
deserved. Manson himself gave it his blessing at the meeting. He felt strongly,
he said, that geography and pathology "were almost sufficient to make it clear
to logical minds that they were different species." F. Sandwich, author of *The
Medical Diseases of Egypt*, was more skeptical and unwilling to concede that the
Egyptian workers could have missed a second species if indeed one existed.
But even he had to pay court to political reality when he wrote: "If, however,
there was a new worm brought before the Society, or (before any members
of) an English-speaking race, he was quite sure it would be even more gladly
received if it were associated with the name of the President."[26]

But there was a second political reality overshadowing that meeting:
Arthur Looss. One of the world's foremost helminthologists and certainly the
greatest authority on bilharzia and hookworm, he had recently fallen out with
Manson over an alleged breach of scientific etiquette. Manson, according to
Looss, had used Looss's hookworm pictures without permission in his *Manual
of Tropical Diseases*. Manson's reference to "logical minds," Sandwich's respect
for Egyptian workers and indeed the whole idea that two species existed were
aimed in Looss's direction. Sambon, in his closing remarks, gave reality to the
shadow. There are, he exclaimed, "more and better reasons to separate
S. mansoni from *S. haematobium* than *Clinorchis endemicus* from *C. sinensis*" (a
direct reference to Looss's paper on *Clinorchis* in the *Journal of Tropical Medicine*),
and "the great German helminthologist at Cairo," Sambon assured his audience, "would soon give them a description of the adult form of *S. mansoni* in
his masterly way." Leiper, who was also in the audience, having recently
returned from Cairo, for once kept out of the dispute. But Looss did not.

In the next issue of the *Annals of Tropical Medicine and Parasitology*, published,
it should be noted, out of Liverpool not London, Looss fired a magnificent
broadside at Sambon, Manson, and indeed at the whole of British biological

science. It began ominously by reference to hurt pride and ego. "If Sambon's view were correct," Looss wrote, "all of us who have devoted attention to the subject would have indeed been wandering in the dark since the time of Bilharz himself, fifty-seven years ago. Since such a charge has practically been made I feel it necessary to take up the defence."[27]

Looss pointed out, with obvious reference to Sambon's concluding remark to the December meeting, that it was Sambon's job, not his, to prove whether or not the worm existed. "It is not customary among scientists," he wrote, "to assert something and call for help of others to establish it." One cannot, in other words, suggest that two species exist on the basis of egg spines and then demand that someone else provide the necessary descriptions. He could not accept this assignment, Looss snapped, Sambon himself must "take the trouble to prove it."[28]

In tone and substance, Looss's paper takes on the attributes of a lecture given by a German professor, fully conversant with the rules of scientific scholarship, to a group of Gymnasium students as yet uninitiated to the rules of the game. It can be seen also as an attack by a German professional on the sloppy and inadequate methodologies followed by the British in their biological laboratories. Looss was giving Sambon, and thus Manson, a dressing down. A German scientist with nearly a century of scholarly tradition behind him was speaking across a century of British neglect of laboratory science.

One could only distinguish new species, Looss lectured Sambon, by "constantly present and, if possible, easily recognizable zoological characters" that must be derived from the adult. No species of parasitic worm was distinguished *solely* by its eggs. "The fact is easily comprehensible. If I cannot tell whether two specimens I have before me are individuals of one species or individuals of two species, I cannot tell either whether slight differences I observe in their eggs are specific characters or not." Thus, Looss argued, until Sambon linked the egg characters with constant adult characters, "*Schistosoma mansoni* will find little approval with zoologists."[29] The egg shape, Looss continued, depended on the position of the egg in the ootype during its formation, and both shapes might occur in the same individual worm.[30] This observation, Looss noted, was reported by Bilharz – a fact that should have been known to Sambon, "when one takes the trouble to read it."

Looss took this opportunity to criticize the scientific training received by Sambon and, by implication, those in the London School. After claiming that laterally spined eggs were the abnormal produce of isolated or unimpregnated females, he argued that the production of abnormal eggs was well known to helminthologists. Ordinary medical men could not be expected to have such knowledge, he wrote, "but I strongly recommend studies of the sort to all those who indulge in 'formulating ideas' with reference to helminthological questions. Anyone would be laughed at if he tried to write a tale in a language of which he did not know the alphabet."[31] Finally, to make his criticisms crystal clear, he expressed his doubt that Sambon's ideas had the right to be classified as "rational inductive methods in advancing knowledge."[32]

Sambon reacted furiously to what he called this "violent and perhaps ill-considered" paper.[33] He pointed out, correctly, that much of the Egyptian data used by Looss was suspect because of the simultaneous existence of the two species. He denied, without any evidence, that a single female could ever produce both laterally and terminally spined eggs. "Until he can show me an actual specimen," he wrote, "I am bound to place the worm capable of producing the two kinds of eggs with the phoenix, the chimaera, and other mythical monsters." After accusing Looss of being blinded by theories that "often require a careful selection of facts," he fired his final shot in Looss's direction. "Though fully appreciating Professor Looss's vast erudition," he remarked sarcastically, "we must not forget that without the employment of good judgement it is quite easy to strain learning into absurdity."[34]

But a strong line of evidence that seemed to offer some support to Sambon's position had already been offered by the young Brazilian physician Piraja da Silva. In 1908, he had described a schistosome worm with laterally spined eggs, but had suggested that it was neither *S. haematobium* nor *S. mansoni*, but a new species entirely. His second paper on the subject, published the same year, was much more explicit: "We believe," he wrote, "that based on the shape of the egg, on its anatomy, its pathology, its geographical distribution and its measurements, the schistosomum we have observed in Bahia is not *Schistosomum mansoni*, but it is distinct from *S. haematobium*. Soon, perhaps, new findings will allow us to affirm the existence of a new American species: *Schistosomum americanum*."[35] Da Silva then visited Europe for two years and forwarded copies of his papers and specimens of the worm to Manson and Leiper.

Manson saw da Silva's findings as a triumph for his and Sambon's theory. "I think the large number of observations you have brought together," he wrote da Silva in his absolutely appalling handwriting, "finally dispose of any question there might have been about the specificity of the American *Schistosomum*. I do not think that Prof. Looss can refuse any longer to acknowledge this."[36]

A few years later Looss presented the "mythical monster": a female *haematobium* with two egg types. In addition, to counter Sambon's claim that laterally spined eggs occurred in the feces and terminal eggs in the urine, he quoted the work of an Egyptian student who found 10–12 percent of laterally spined eggs in the urine. "The females of *S. haematobium* can, and do, produce the two forms of eggs," he announced, "however much the impossibility of the process may be emphasized in order to save a theory."[37]

At this stage, Leiper agreed more with Looss than Sambon; he found it impossible to separate the two so-called species anatomically, and as he informed da Silva, "In *Egypt* everywhere you always find the females that are in the portal vein contain only one or two eggs and these are *almost invariably* lateral-spined even when the case is of terminal-spined eggs in the urine."[38] There was also the matter of competence. As Leiper mentioned in his letter to da Silva, "I studied for a year under Professor Looss and saw enough of his work to feel more reliance on his observations than those of Sambon."[39]

The evidence seemed clear. Whatever Sambon said and however correct he now appears to be, Looss had the better of the argument. He had the live material; Sambon only pickled specimens and eggs in jars. No wonder Leiper could at last announce his views on the issue. Looss, he wrote in 1911, had brought the lateral spine controversy to an end; there was only one schistosome species in Egypt.[40] In the words of Arthur Looss, "Egyptian bilharziasis is one entity."[41] Sambon was never to forget this slight to his reputation.

THE LIFE CYCLE CONTROVERSY

Looss's arguments with Sambon and Manson extended also into the intractable problem of the schistosome life cycle. By 1906, nothing new had been added to the observations of Bilharz: The egg hatched to release the embryo or miracidium that remained viable for only a few hours. What happened next remained a mystery. One was forced to draw analogies with better known species.

Manson drew his analogy with the sheep liver-fluke, *Fasciola hepatica*, whose life cycle had been partly elucidated in the 1880s by Algernon Thomas in Britain and, to a lesser extent, by Rudolf Leuckart in Germany. A miracidium, Thomas discovered, penetrated the tissues of lymnaeid snails eventually to produce many cercariae. In 1892, the missing piece of the puzzle fell into place with the discovery that sheep became infected by swallowing these cercariae that had become encysted on vegetation.[42] Thus, Manson reasoned, the miracidia of schistosomes also must pass into the body of a snail, a crustacean, or a larval arthropod to produce the cercariae. Then, either free, or in an encysted state, or even still in the body of the intermediate host, it must pass into humans with their drinking water.[43] Sambon, who not without cause had been castigated as "Manson's Boswell," naturally agreed. But others, often more familiar with the disease than either Manson or Sambon, felt that the worm was contracted by bathing in infected waters. By that time, considerable evidence had accumulated linking the disease with canal workers, or with young children who played in water.

But again the most authentic statement had come from Looss. In an 1894 paper he had assumed, like Manson, that the miracidia developed in a molluscan intermediate host. But his repeated attempts to infect the commonest snails and bivalves of the Nile Delta failed. Similarly, examinations of snails from the Nile Delta had apparently failed to locate a single type of cercariae that, in the opinion of Looss, could belong to the schistosomes (infected snails, when left overnight, will release clouds of cercariae, but at that time, the structure of schistosome cercariae was not known). Attempts also to infect crustacea, insect larvae, fish, and plants with miracidia had failed. Thus Looss denied the existence of intermediate hosts in the schistosome life cycle. Instead, according to Looss, the miracidia must penetrate directly into humans and form their larval stages in the human liver.[44] "I am thus forced to the conviction," Looss remarked 14 years later, "that man himself acts as intermediary host."[45]

However bizarre this theory may appear to us today, we should remember that Looss was the only one of those involved in the controversy to support his theory with experimental evidence. The evidence, of course, was entirely negative: Looss was unable to find snails with schistosome larvae in them, and unable to infect snails with schistosome miracidia in the laboratory. But even the weakness of this evidence was mitigated to a large degree by the assumed situation in Egypt. Given the extraordinarily high prevalence of infection in the *fellaheen*, it would have been natural to assume a similar level of infection in the snails, were they the intermediate hosts. But whereas 50–60 percent of the snails examined by Looss contained trematode larvae, not one was found with schistosome larvae in them. It is not clear how Looss came to that conclusion, given that the structure of schistosome cercariae was unknown at that time, but he can hardly have been expected to know that only an extraordinarily small number of infected snails is sufficient to maintain a high human prevalence of the disease. But there was a major flaw in Looss's argument. He claimed to have examined hundreds of specimens of *all* the molluscs common in the Nile Valley, whereas, in reality, he did no such thing.[46] But perhaps he can be excused; a laboratory-centered parasitologist would not have been aware of the rich mollusc fauna of the Nile Delta. German laboratory scientists were rarely naturalists.

There may, however, have been another reason why Looss should have proposed a direct life cycle for the bilharzia worm: If true, its life cycle would have closely resembled that of *Ancylostoma*, the hookworm. The Egyptian *fellaheen*, along with millions of others in the tropical and semitropical world, carry the hookworm nematode responsible for a disease marked by intestinal disorders and severe anemia. Discovered in 1838 by the Italian physician Angelo Dubini, it was again Bilharz and Griesinger who did much to link the presence of the nematode worm to specific clinical malfunctions of the body. And again, as in the case of bilharzia, Looss established its life cycle. But this time, his findings proved to be correct.

Looss described the young hookworm larva that emerged from the egg and then passed through one or two molts to reach the "mature larva" stage. But all attempts to feed experimental animals with these larvae failed, just as all attempts to infect snails with schistosome larvae had failed. This, and other peculiar findings, led Looss to conclude that the larvae of *Ancylostoma* can enter the human body directly by boring through the skin. Over the next few years, Looss not only showed this to be true, but described how the larvae, after boring through the skin, reached the lungs, crept up the tracheae to the esophagus, and then were swallowed. By this lengthy and quite bizarre migration they eventually reached the gut, where egg-laying began.[47]

This hookworm life cycle, disclosed by Looss between 1896 and 1901, resembled closely that described for the schistosome worm at much the same period. In both cases humans could infect each other directly through the agency of a free-living larval stage, found in feces-contaminated soil in the case of hookworm and feces or urine-contaminated puddles of water in the case of bilharzia. It may have seemed unusual that the life cycle of the schistosome trematode more closely resembled that of the hookworm nematode than that of other trematode species, but, as Looss remarked: "Our knowledge of the life-cycle of parasites has taught us enough never to be surprised that the parasites, perhaps more than any other animals, reject formulas and schemata set up by us when they are attempting to attain their special purposes and aims."[48]

Not surprisingly, given the well-deserved reputation of Looss, many lesser helminthologists accepted his "skin infection theory." F. Sandwich, in his *Medical Diseases of Egypt*, stressed that humans became infected with the parasite after bathing in water. But this took place, not by cercariae released from snails, but by miracidia hatched from eggs shed by infected humans. Frank Madden, Professor of Surgery at the Egyptian Medical School, likewise accepted Looss's theory in the first text devoted exclusively to bilharzia: "Any small puddle may become defiled with the urine or faeces of a patient suffering from bilharziosis; and, in a very short time, the water or mud is alive with miracidia, which may become applied to the bare feet, legs, or hands, penetrate the skin, and so lead to infection."[49]

Looss clung tenaciously to his theory. In 1909, for example, in answer to an article in the *British Medical Journal* that claimed infection was not due to bathing, Looss reiterated that his "skin infection theory" was in accordance with all the facts known at that time.[50] In that year, these supporting facts were to expand considerably when news from Japan percolated into Europe.

ORIENTAL SCHISTOSOMIASIS

In 1904, John Catto, a physician of the Indian Medical Service, while working in the London School of Tropical Medicine, described a new schistosome from some preserved material obtained from an autopsy of a Chinese man who had died from cholera in Singapore. The worm was clearly a new species; its structure differed from that of *Schistosoma haematobium*, and no spines were present on its eggs. This report of a new schistosome, named *S. cattoi* in honor of its founder, was the first indication that Europeans received of an Oriental schistosome.[51]

That same year, however, unbeknown to the Europeans, Fijiro Katsurada, Professor of Medicine at Okayama Medical School with an M.D. degree from the University of Freiburg, set out to investigate "*suishuchoman* disease," a serious affliction endemic to the district of Yamanashi, north of Tokyo. In April, he examined the stools of 12 patients with the disease and discovered schistosome-like eggs in five of them. A later autopsy of a scrawny cat with a distended abdomen located 32 schistosome worms with eggs identical to those found earlier in the humans. "For the time being," he wrote, "I want to call the parasite *Schistosoma haematobium japonicum*. Now there is no doubt that this very parasite is the cause of the dreadful endemic disease."[52] At the same time, other Japanese workers described the same worms and eggs from autopsies in the Katayama District, east of Hiroshima, where a local "Katayama disease" had been known for many years (Figure 4.7).

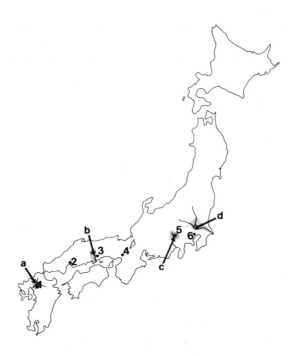

Figure 4.7. Endemic sites of *Schistosoma japonicum* in Japan: a, Chikugo River valley; b, Katayama in Takaya River valley; c, Kofu area in Yamanashi District; d, Tone River valley. Cities: 1, Kurume; 2, Hiroshima; 3, Okayama; 4, Kyoto; 5, Kofu; 6, Tokyo.

The Japanese, like the Europeans, could not agree whether the parasite entered the body through contaminated drinking water, or directly through the skin, or through an intermediate host. But they held one enormous advantage over those working in Egypt: *S. japonicum* occurred in domestic animals as well as in humans; field experiments were possible. In 1909, Kan Fujinami, Professor of Medicine at Kyoto University with postgraduate experience in Germany, and Hachitaro Nakamura, an Assistant Professor at the same institution, took 20 calves from a disease-free area into the Katayama District. The calves were divided into four groups. The first group, with mouths covered, were allowed to stand for several hours each day in irrigation ditches, in paddy fields, and in a local river. The second group were subjected to the same conditions but had their legs covered with waterproof boots. A third group was kept away from the experimental area but otherwise maintained in the same way, whereas the fourth group was allowed to drink the contaminated water and to stand exposed in it.

Autopsies revealed calves in groups one and four to be heavily infected, but a single worm was also found in one calf of group two. The authors were agonizingly honest in their summary of these results:

The entrance of the causative agent of this disease is definitely from outside of the body. In the case of calves, ordinarily, invasion is not through the gastrointestinal tract, but this route cannot definitely be rejected. It is not clear whether invasion is through the skin or the mucosa. There is only one case of a calf which was infected slightly through eating. Generally, the conditions for infection are very simple. It is sufficient to immerse a leg in the contaminated water for several hours a day in order to stimulate invasion of the disease-causing worm.

These experiments had established, if not absolutely, what Looss and others could only surmise. Their results could be and were interpreted as a confirmation of Looss's skin-infection theory.[53] The Japanese experiments had shown that at least one of the human schistosome species was acquired by skin contact with some waterborne stage of the parasite, and that stage was assumed by many to be the miracidium. Leiper was less convinced. In the 1910 report to the Advisory Committee of the Tropical Disease Research Fund, Leiper claimed that the Japanese believed that their experiments had confirmed Looss's hypothesis but, nevertheless, he still felt that the problem needed further investigation.[54]

But in reality, the two Japanese investigators took a more cautious view. They realized that the basic question had yet to be answered. What larval stage bored through the skin of those Japanese cattle? Was it the miracidium that hatched from the schistosome egg, as Looss believed, or was it the cercaria that had emerged from some intermediate host? The necessity of finding an answer to that question soon became apparent.

CONTROVERSIES RESOLVED

On October 24, 1913, at a meeting of the Advisory Committee of the Tropical Disease Research Fund, Ronald Ross, who was, by then, Professor of Tropical Sanitation at the Liverpool School of Tropical medicine, proposed that his colleague, Dr. J. W. Stephens, be sent to Cyprus to investigate bilharzia. J. W. Stephens had joined the staff of the Liverpool School in 1902 and had thereafter followed Ross's footsteps. When, in 1903, Ross had been appointed to the Alfred Jones Chair of Tropical Medicine, Stephens had replaced him as the Walter Myers Lecturer. Then, when Ross resigned from the Chair in 1913, Stephens had replaced him. Stephens was also the only member of the Liverpool School who had some experience with helminths; in 1909 he had taken an expedition to Egypt and worked in Looss's laboratory.

The disease was, Ross noted, a matter of great importance to the British garrison in Egypt.[55] This was hardly an overstatement. Not only had a recent study revealed that over 600 "Chelsea pensioners" had been disabled by bilharzia owing to infection during the Boer War, but now, if the "skin-contact theory" of Looss were true, then every puddle in every army camp was a potential source of the disease.[56] An artilleryman, returning home from Egypt, could be responsible for an epidemic of bilharzia in Woolwich Barracks! London could become another Cairo; the mind reeled. To make matters worse, the Looss theory seemed to have gained experimental support from the findings in Japan, although Leiper himself remained unconvinced. The problem had to be investigated, but if anyone were to do such investigating, it would have to be Leiper himself, the Lecturer in Helminthology at the London School. Whatever experience Stephens may have gained in Egypt, parasitic worms were the province of the London School, not Liverpool.

According to Ross and Stephens, the single endemic locus of *Schistosoma haematobium* in Cyprus provided an ideal experimental site. They could, for example, make comparisons with adjacent disease-free sites with relative ease – an impossibility in Egypt. Manson of the London School responded immediately to the Cyprus research proposal; he had a better idea. *Schistosoma japonicum*, the Oriental blood fluke, was an ideal experimental animal, he reminded his fellow committee members; unlike *S. haematobium* it could be transmitted very easily to lower animals. Leiper, he told the committee, was prepared to go to Shanghai to work on the life cycle of *S. japonicum* on a budget much lower than that proposed by Ross.

There were several factors to consider on both sides of the argument. *S. japonicum* was the better research tool, but Cyprus held many advantages over China. Locating the enigmatic snail host (if indeed there was one) in a quiet Cyprian village was one thing; finding it among the vast waterways of China was quite another matter. But reading the minutes of that October meeting leads one to suspect that no lengthy debate took place. The decision favoring

Manson's proposal seems, on the contrary, to represent another example of favoritism toward London at a time when considerable strains existed between the two cities, the two schools, and the two men, Ross and Manson.

The Liverpool School, of course, held a considerable grudge against the London establishment, since that first year when the London School had gained the sole right to train colonial medical officers. Their hostility toward London had not lessened over the years, even though, in 1900, Liverpool gained equal rights in this regard. Their suspicions were further aroused when the Advisory Committee of the Tropical Disease Research Fund continually granted less money to Liverpool than London, a quite understandable decision, given the much smaller size of the Liverpool School.[57] This festering sore was further exacerbated in 1907 when Ross wrote to the Colonial Office complaining of the pro-London bias displayed by the Advisory Committee.

The annual reports of the research fund, Ross complained, implied that only those at London did any work. Twenty pages of the previous year's report, he pointed out, detailed London's activities; only one page dealt with Liverpool. Such a difference bore absolutely no relationship to the quantity or quality of the work produced, Ross argued, but merely reflected the more verbose reports submitted to the Advisory Board by members of the London School. Leiper, in particular, was the recipient of some barbed comments: "Mr. Leiper's work is undoubtedly good," Ross sneered, "but the exceptional notice of it given by the Advisory Committee would appear to be chiefly due to the detailed nature of his report of it." What detail is required? Ross wanted to know, adding sarcastically that "under present arrangements hardship is likely to be inflicted on those institutions whose work by its very magnitude cannot easily be described in detail in the Report."[58]

The reaction to this letter was predictable. Both the Colonial Office and the Board of the Liverpool School expressed regret that the letter was ever written, and the letter was hastily withdrawn before ever reaching the eyes of the Advisory Board. Nevertheless, one has to assume that a person in Manson's position would have either read the letter or heard of its contents. He certainly read another letter from Ross, or rather Ross's lawyer, which he received ten months before the meeting at which the Cyprus plan was first broached.

Ross had resigned from the Liverpool School on September 23, 1912, giving only three months' notice. After some frenzied correspondence, he finally agreed to stay on as a special professor in tropical sanitation, with a salary of £400 per year. In return, Ross was expected to deliver a few lectures three times a year and to agree not to teach at the London School. Almost two months after these events, Manson forwarded a reference for Dr. W. T. Prout, who had applied for the position left vacant by Ross. This reference, following the normal custom, was printed and distributed to the selection committee. "I sincerely hope," wrote Manson in his reference, that his appointment may be successful, for it would, if I may use the expression, make good a defect in your system of teaching which I have long been anxious, in the interests of tropical medicine, to see remedied. A teacher of tropical medicine to be considered efficient should be not only a scientific man, but one having had extensive experience in tropical practice.[59]

Ross and the Liverpool faculty naturally objected to these insinuations of their teaching inadequacy, and Ross must have been particularly irked by reference to a scientific man of extensive practice. Ross met neither description; he held no medical or scientific degree beyond membership in the Society of Apothecaries (1881) and a Diploma in Public Health (1889), and thus was denied hospital facilities at the Liverpool Royal Southern Hospital. But Manson must have been amazed to receive a letter from Ross's lawyer threatening a libel suit unless he received a "full apology from [Manson] by return mail." "It is a very serious matter altogether," Ross informed his lawyer, "more especially that it opens up an old wound that everyone had hoped was healed years ago." Neither Manson nor the lawyer shared Ross's concern, and Ross was persuaded to drop the case after receiving a letter of apology from Manson. But only five months after Manson had agreed to pay four guineas of Ross's lawyer's fee, the Advisory Committee agreed to send Leiper to China, rather than Stephens to Cyprus, "to study the mode of spread of bilharziasis and to obtain, if possible, definite experimental evidence on this subject."[60]

Leiper arrived in Shanghai in March 1914, accompanied by Surgeon Lieutenant Atkinson, R.N., who had been seconded to the expedition by the British Admiralty concerned about the impact of the disease on their crews serving in the Yangtze River.[61] The Chinese expedition did not begin expeditiously. By June, the two men had fallen out. "I ought to give him a sound thrashing," Atkinson wrote his friend and fellow Antarctica explorer Apsley Cherry-Garrard; an act that could have been enacted with telling force on the frail Leiper by the ex-rugby player and boxer. Neither was their schistosome work progressing well. "Unfortunately," Leiper informed his wife, "we are completely boxed in re the schistosoma."[62] They had failed to find a Chinese infected with the parasites from whom a supply of eggs could have been obtained, and, when at last they were successful in obtaining eggs from an infected dog, none of the hatched miracidia successfully invaded any of the local snails tested. However, by that time Leiper no longer believed Looss's theory. "By experiment (on myself and others)," he noted in the letter to his wife, "it is already known that the miracidium cannot directly infect man." Because it dies after 24–36 hours, he explained, "it *must* therefore enter some intermediate host to survive." He was convinced that schistosome miracidia must penetrate a snail, where the parasite would pass through various larval stages before releasing the cercariae. He was also convinced that it was these cercariae that reentered the human host directly. He knew this much after receiving news of fresh findings in Japan.

In 1913, Keinosuka Miyairi and his assistant Masatsuga Suzuki made the all-important breakthroughs. They discovered that in their area of Japan miracidia penetrated local snails, developed into sporocysts in the tissues of the snail, and eventually liberated free-swimming cercariae. For the first time these schistosome cercariae were seen and described; they were forked-tailed (Figure 4.8):

A cercaria is provided with a powerful caudal tail and this is split, in its distal third, into two parts.[63]

Faced then with failure in China, and knowing of the important Japanese work, Leiper and Atkinson visited Katayama. There, guided by Fujinami, the instigator of the famous schistosome–cattle experiments, they collected specimens of the snail *Katayama* [= *Oncomelania*] *nosophora*, reported by Miyairi to be the intermediate host. On returning to Shanghai, the snail digestive glands were teased out, and the released cercariae allowed to come into contact with some laboratory mice.

The return trip to England, precipitated by the outbreak of war, became a scientific nightmare. A lady passenger in a neighboring cabin, Leiper related, "objected to my pied-piper companions," and forced him to leave the mice in the charge of an Indian butcher. All four infected mice died early in the trip, although a single male schistosome was recovered from the last to succumb. At Aden, Leiper sacrificed the last infected snail and allowed a single mouse to be exposed to the cercariae. Arriving at the London School in late October 1914, he was lucky enough, using his single surviving rodent, to locate male and female worms in its portal veins. The life cycle of *Schistosoma japonicum*, he reported, was similar to other trematodes in that its miracidia also invaded the tissues of snails to produce saclike sporocysts which in turn produced a multitude of cercariae. In *S. japonicum* these forked-tailed cercariae bored into the skin of Japanese workers in the paddy fields to complete the cycle. As such, Leiper wrote:

These experiments, carried out with the greatest precautions to avoid fallacy, convince me that the Looss hypothesis (which has so long dominated scientific opinion . . .) is entirely erroneous, and that the prophylactic measures based thereon would be wholly inefficient. It remains now to be demonstrated that *Schistosoma haematobium* . . . follows a similar course.[64]

Ross, meanwhile, continued to press for an investigation by Stephens into the disease in Cyprus or Egypt. At the end of 1913, they submitted a proposal on these lines to the Egyptian authorities and were greeted by an extremely hostile reply. They were well aware of the disease, the Egyptian Consul-General Lord Kitchener huffed, but in Looss they have "the greatest living

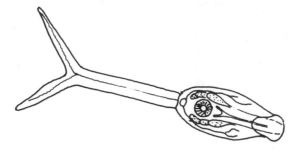

Figure 4.8. The forked-tail schistosome cercaria (slightly less than 1 mm long)

authority in bilharziasis and ankylostomiasis." In addition, he added, the Department of Public Health was about to address the problem. The point was made very clear: No outside interference would be tolerated.[65] A year later, however, Kitchener had returned to London as Secretary for War, Looss had been unceremoniously bundled back home to Germany and Leiper had arrived as War Office Consultant Parasitologist for the troops in Egypt with the honorary rank of Lieutenant Colonel R.A.M.C. (Royal Army Medical Corps). He was not welcomed and found himself the recipient of the type of hostility he often bestowed on others. But, as he told Victor Heiser of the Rockefeller Foundation later in the year, such circumstances "made it practically imperative for him to succeed in the mission which he had undertaken."[66] Leiper was never one to shirk a challenge.

The mission was clear. He was to investigate bilharzia in order to suggest preventive measures for the British troops garrisoned in Egypt and along the Suez Canal.[67] Leiper and his staff of J. G. Thomson and R. P. Cockin remained in Egypt until July 1915. Leiper then returned to the Military College at Millbank, where he worked until his position with the army expired in October of the same year. By November he was back in Egypt, this time alone, where he remained until February 1916.

No records remain of this important period in Leiper's life, beyond the formal reports published in the *Journal of the Royal Army Medical Corps*. Leiper, as far as I know, destroyed all his correspondence when he retired; it would have been totally out of character for him to have allowed some meddling historian to browse through his private papers. His report, published in six parts between July 1915 and March 1918, falls into two distinct sections. The first section, parts one to three, written while Leiper was attached to the Army, deals only with matters of prime interest to the military, such as means of transmission and methods of control. The final section, parts four to six, written after his discharge, deals with more theoretical questions, such as the number of human schistosome species in Egypt.

Leiper began his investigations in 1914 by collecting over 3,000 snails from a canal at El Marg, a small village northeast of Cairo. He soon found the forked-tailed cercariae in two common snail species, *Bulinus* sp. and *Planorbis boissyi*, and suggested, in his first report, that they might be the larval stages of *Schistosoma bovis*, from cattle, and *S. haematobium*.[68] Finding some laboratory animals susceptible to infection by these cercariae, Leiper carried back to England with him four mice, 26 rats, 16 desert rats, two guinea pigs, and four monkeys, all exposed to the cercariae. When examined, shortly after his arrival in England, those animals were found to be infected with large numbers of schistosomes. Thus, just as in Japan, the life cycle of the Egyptian schistosomes involved passage through a snail intermediate host and direct penetration of the cercariae into the final host.[69]

The practical implications of these findings to the British troops in Egypt were made abundantly clear in Leiper's first report. According to the Looss hypothesis, "all transient collections of water are dangerous if freshly contaminated. . . . Infected troops would be liable to reinfect themselves, to spread the disease among other troops, and to convey the disease to any part of the world." On the other hand, "large bodies of water, such as the Nile, canals, marshes, and birkets, are little liable to be infective." But with the discovery of snail intermediate hosts, "transient collections of water are quite safe. . . . Infected troops cannot reinfect themselves or spread the disease directly to others . . . and all permanent collections of water, such as the Nile, canals . . . are potentially dangerous, depending on the presence of the essential intermediary host."[70]

But how many human schistosome species existed in Egypt? Were Manson and Sambon correct in arguing for two species, *S. haematobium*, with terminally spined eggs, and *S. mansoni*, with laterally spined eggs? Or was Looss correct in believing the latter eggs to be the product of immature, unfertilized, or abnormal *haematobium* females?

Leiper addressed this problem only after discharge from his military duties. Before then, in his first three reports, he was content merely to state that "various bilharzia cercariae were found." The issue was not of military concern. The answer came suddenly in the fourth report: "*Planorbis* [*Biomphalaria*] *boissyi* is the intermediate host of *Bilharzia mansoni* in man in Egypt. . . . *Bulinus contortus* is one of the intermediate hosts of *Bilharzia haematobium* (*sens. strictu*) in man in Egypt."[71]

Only laterally spined eggs had been obtained from the rats, guinea pigs, and monkeys that Leiper had carried back to England after they were exposed to the cercariae from the planorbid snail. But it could still be argued that these laterally spined eggs were obtained from immature or isolated females; that the infections were of insufficient duration to allow the fully matured females to form and produce their terminally spined eggs. Thus Leiper returned to Egypt in 1915 in order to resolve the issue once and for all. He lightly infected a group of animals with enough cercariae from *Planorbis* [*Biomphalaria*] so that a supply of male and female worms would result in sufficiently low numbers to avoid early mortality of the host. In this way, he hoped, the host would live long enough to ensure infection with fully mature female worms. In addition, he also heavily infected animals with cercariae from *Bulinus*, so as to obtain enough worms and eggs for identification.[72]

These experiments proved so successful, that he was able to claim:

We have now established experimentally that the cercariae derived from *P. boissyi* gave rise to lateral-spined eggs, while those derived from *Bulinus* gave rise solely to terminal-spined eggs. . . . The young but sexually mature *B. haematobium*, derived from *Bulinus* infection, were well able to lay terminal-spined eggs . . . no evidence of a tendency to the formation of eggs with laterally-distorted spine was forthcoming.[73]

The conclusion was thus obvious: "The terminal-spined and lateral-spined eggs found in bilharzial infections are . . . the normal and characteristic products of two distinct species, *B. haematobium* and *B. mansoni*, and are spread by different intermediary hosts." Once again Looss had been found incorrect.

Leiper presented also a detailed report on control measures, for the way was now open for the application of Western biological technology.[74] Whereas, according to the Looss theory, eradication depended upon education and complete sanitary control throughout the country, now, with the discovery of intermediate hosts, eradication could be achieved by simply, or so it seemed, destroying the snail hosts without the cooperation of the Egyptians themselves.[75] Bilharzia had become a parasitic disease carried by a snail; thus the *fellaheen* could be safely ignored and allowed to continue in their time-hallowed ways. With the discovery of intermediate hosts, control seemed possible without any corresponding social action.

In rural areas the major remedy lay, according to Leiper, in finding some simple means of stamping out snails. Such methods, he argued, involved drying, clearing, piping, and chemicals. Basically, in the Egyptian agricultural system a "summer rotation" allowed sections of the canal system to become dry. Snails stranded in the drying mud could not survive, according to Leiper; only those stranded in residual pools were carried over into the following season. Thus, the snail population could be reduced either by reducing the number of such pools or by treating them with chemical manures, such as ammonium sulfate, in order to kill snails that otherwise might survive the drying season. In addition, Leiper explained, the canals were also closed in midwinter for silt and weed removal. If it were possible, Leiper argued, these canal clearance operations should be combined with the summer rotation, and the combination of clearing, drying, and chemicals should lead to the elimination of the snails. He also added, somewhat optimistically, that open drains should be replaced by underground pipes, as in England.

But the protection of British troops remained the prime concern. Any threat from cercariae in the camp water supply could now be eliminated by providing filtered water or water that had been rendered free of the larvae by standing for 48 hours, by heating the water to 50°C, or by treatment with chemicals lethal to cercariae. Thus the disease, Leiper concluded, "should now be treated as one of those diseases for which the individual is mainly, if not entirely, personally responsible."[76] Bilharzia was no longer a threat to a well-disciplined body of men where regulations to avoid snail-contaminated water could be rigorously enforced; bilharzia could not be passed directly from man to man: "We may foretell with reasonable safety, that the disease will never attain the terrible hold and produce the serious ravages which occur in heavily infected natives of Egypt."[77] More to the point, bilharzia should no longer impair military efficiency, and "the country may be saved the payment of large sums in compensation to men who need not have been infected."

The Colonial Office paid its respects to Leiper's work. "It constituted," they wrote to the Treasury, "not only a brilliant scientific discovery, but one of immediate practical benefit to the military authorities."[78] Looss's direct life cycle, in which the miracidia were believed to penetrate humans directly, had temporarily made bilharzia a "white man's disease." Not only was it a potential threat to his health in the tropics, but also it could be carried by him back into the temperate zones. But by discovering the indirect life cycle of the bilharzia-causing worms, Leiper had transferred the threat of disease from the British onto a people who had no choice but to wash, drink, work, and play in water contaminated with schistosome cercariae. The British military officer or colonial official did none of these things, and a well-disciplined body of men could be prevented from doing them. After Leiper's discoveries, bilharzia no longer constituted a major threat to British personnel in the tropics; with caution, they could ignore the disease.

Many years would pass before the British would again become interested in bilharzia. After the end of World War I, the cudgel was taken up by the Egyptian public health authorities and by the International Health Board of the Rockefeller Foundation.

5

The International Health Board

Between the two world wars, the International Health Board of the Rockefeller Foundation dominated the field of tropical medicine.[1] From its founding in 1914, when it was called the International Health Commission, until the closure of the International Health Division in 1951, the organization acted as an early version of the World Health Organization. What is more, the General Education Board, another branch of the Rockefeller philanthropies, funded the Johns Hopkins School of Hygiene and Public Health, which, arguably, became the single most important center for tropical medicine in North America. The Foundation also funded the formation of many foreign Johns Hopkins-like institutes such as those in Peking and London, both of which played a vital role in tropical medicine and the bilharzia story.

The beginning of the International Health Board illustrates again the strong link between American geography and the early history of tropical medicine. It grew out of the Rockefeller Sanitary Commission for the Eradication of Hookworm Disease, founded in 1909 as part of a Northern philanthropic and paternalistic concern with the South and its problems. By the turn of the century, hookworm disease was well known to Europeans. Associated with severe anemia and the curious symptom of dirt eating, hookworm, more than any other disease, had become associated with worker inefficiency. The problem had been clearly spelled out in a 1901 memorandum from the Governor of British Guiana:

Ancylostomiasis [hookworm] is an important disease from the standpoint of the employer of native labour. The invaliding and inefficiency which it causes among coolies, not to mention the deaths, are often financially a serious matter to the planter and mine owner. To them, any wisely directed expense or trouble undertaken for the treating and controlling of this helminthiasis will be abundantly repaid by the increased efficiency of the labourer.[2]

But before Bailey Ashford and Charles Stiles described the worms in Puerto Rico and the American South, respectively, hookworm was believed to be an Old World parasite.

Charles Stiles, a parasitologist, who had trained under Rudolf Leuckart in Leipzig, and had returned to the United States in 1891 to take a position with the Bureau of Animal Husbandry, discovered hookworm disease in South Carolina, Georgia, and Florida. There was no doubt, he reported in 1902, that hookworm "is one of the most important diseases of the South . . . and that much of the trouble popularly attributed to 'dirt eating' and even some of the proverbial laziness of the poorer classes of the white population are manifestations of uncinariasis (hookworm)." Six long years later, Stiles's message reached the ears of Frederick Gates, manager of the Rockefeller philanthropies, and the Sanitary Commission was created. With a $1 million grant from J. D. Rockefeller, Gates appointed Wickliffe Rose (Figure 5.1) Administrative Secretary to the Commission. The plan of campaign mapped out during the winter of 1909–10, after Rose had visited Bailey Ashford in Puerto Rico, involved a three-step process: survey, cure, and prevention.[3]

A large dose of thymol was assumed to act as the "cure." This property was discovered in the late 1890s, before which thymol was basically an external chemical used in wounds, as a substitute for carbonic acid, and in night commodes to deodorize the urine. It had been given internally as an antipyretic, the *United States Dispensatory* noted in 1896, but ringing in the ears, deafness, sweating, and "alarming collapse" often resulted. Furthermore, injecting thymol into the veins of dogs was reported to cause death by respiratory failure.[4] By the end of the century, however, it had become a powerful

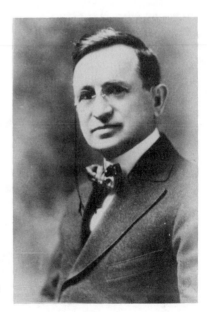

Figure 5.1. Wickliffe Rose (Courtesy of the Rockefeller Archive Center)

antihelminthic, but one that caused a "serious constitutional disturbance."[5] To prevent such disturbances, a saline purge was generally recommended, but by the time of the Sanitary Commission this had been replaced by Epsom salts. Epsom salts were required to sweep out the worms and, hopefully, to remove excess thymol before the side effects of nausea, weakness, and other malfunctions manifested themselves.

But after Looss had discovered that the larval stages of the hookworm required no intermediate host in which to develop, but, instead, matured in the soil, and then bored their way into the feet of their human host, the construction of sanitary privies came to be seen as a potentially powerful weapon in hookworm prevention. If used, these outhouses would prevent soil contamination by hookworm eggs in the feces.

Rose favored the use of thymol over the construction of privies. He felt, according to Ettling, that only when the Commission had demonstrated the power of modern medicine through dramatic cures, would the people of the rural South take any preventive measures. Stiles, on the other hand, had faith in the outhouse, and tried to design an efficient, cheap variety that people could afford. In this he failed; the Southern farmer could not afford Stiles's model, and the construction of privies became the least satisfactory aspect of the Commission's work.[6]

From the beginning of the campaign, Gates had a vision extending beyond the South. As early as 1910, he had asked Rose to survey the prevalence of hookworm around the world (Looss in Egypt received his copy of the Rose questionnaire in May 1911), the information from which was tabulated in *Hookworm Infection in Foreign Countries*, published by the Sanitary Commission. During the same period, J. D. Rockefeller granted 72,569 shares of Standard Oil ($50 million) to set up a philanthropic trust with the breathtaking goal of promoting "the well-being and to advance the civilization of the peoples of the United States and its territories and possessions and of foreign lands in the acquisition and dissemination of knowledge, in the prevention and relief of suffering, and in the promotion of any and all the elements of human progress."[7] After much controversy, this trust, the Rockefeller Foundation, was incorporated by the New York legislature in 1913.

By 1913, the Rockefeller organizations had gained considerable experience working in the South. Initially the problems there had been attributed to an inferior educational system, but, from the work of the General Education Board, founded in 1903, poverty had appeared as the basic problem. Now, however, disease had moved to center stage. At the very first meeting of the Rockefeller Foundation, the trustees had agreed that "advancement of public health through medical research and education, including the demonstration of known methods of treating and preventing disease," would constitute their most useful work.[8] But it was Gates who expressed this "Rockefeller creed" most succinctly when he wrote:

Disease is the supreme ill of human life, and it is the main source of almost all other human ills – poverty, crime, ignorance, vice, inefficiency, hereditary taints, and many other evils.[9]

On June 27, 1913, Gates and Rose presented a memorandum to the Board of the Rockefeller Foundation. "Whereas," they noted, the Sanitary Commission had found more than two million people infected with hookworm in the South, "involving vast suffering, partial arrest of physical, mental and moral growth, great loss of life, and noticeable decrease in economic efficiency over vast regions," and "whereas" the disease can be easily diagnosed, cured, and prevented with the result that "an intelligent public interest is awakened in hygiene and in modern scientific medicine and in practical measures for permanent public sanitation," and "whereas" over a thousand-million people are infected with the disease "in a belt of territory encircling the earth for thirty degrees each side of the equator," be it resolved "that this Foundation will extend the work of eradicating the hookworm disease to other countries and other nations, as opportunity offers," and will establish "agencies for the promotion of public sanitation and the spread of knowledge of scientific medicine."[10] On the last day of 1914, the Sanitary Commission was dissolved, and the International Health Commission was organized "for the prevention and cure of disease with the world as its field of operation" (Figure 5.2).

THE FIRST HOOKWORM CAMPAIGN

Initially, the activities of the International Health Commission, John Ferrell, assistant to Rose, noted in a letter to Looss, "will be limited to the continuation here and the extension to foreign countries of the work of the Rockefeller Sanitary Commission."[11] These foreign countries were organized into three geographical areas – Latin America, the West Indies, and the East. And, because most of these countries were colonies of Britain (Figure 5.3), the International Health Commission turned first to London.

In London, the color red was anathema, however much the British Colonial Office glorified in viewing atlases liberally reddened to show the extent of their Empire. Their Empire was run in the black and on the cheap, and colonial governors were expected to follow a policy of minimal government at little cost to the British taxpayer. Disease had always presented a threat to the economics of such an empire, and, in the first decade of the twentieth century, hookworm added its name to the lengthening list. Hookworm threatened not only the financial well-being of the mineowner and planter, but also menaced a system that could spend only locally derived public money to finance any health campaigns. Thus, much was written and little was done until American dollars were suddenly made available through the International Health Commission.

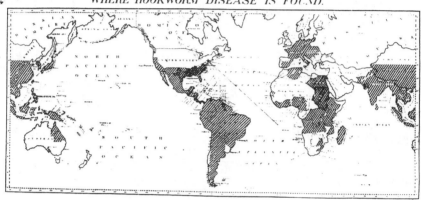

*Follow the RED lines to the dark areas in the Tropical Zone belting the Globe
WHERE HOOKWORM DISEASE IS FOUND.*

Figure 5.2. The International Health Commission's field of operations
(Courtesy of the Rockefeller Archive Center)

In July 1913, the American Ambassador in London, Walter Page, set up a meeting between the Colonial Office and Wickliffe Rose. Rose sailed for England in early August, but meanwhile, acting with some unusual alacrity, the Colonial Office set up a "hookworm committee" to prepare for the visit. The committee wanted one thing from the Americans: their money. The colonies possessed all the information they needed to combat hookworm, they noted; "the problem was largely one of money, as in the West Indies, or of treating large numbers of intractable savages, as in Tropical Africa, where conditions prevailed of which the American Commission could have no special experience."[12] Without money, they admitted, there had been "no general attempt to grapple with the problem in the Empire, as a whole."[13]

Rose spent 16 days in London, by which time he and the British had decided to launch hookworm campaigns in the British West Indies, Egypt, Ceylon, and Malaya, sites of important sugar, cotton, and rubber industries. Lewis Harcourt, the Colonial Secretary, immediately forwarded a memo to the West Indian colonies, the Foreign Office, India Office, and Egypt, asking them to cooperate with the International Health Commission, so as to secure for the Empire what had already been achieved in the American South.[14]

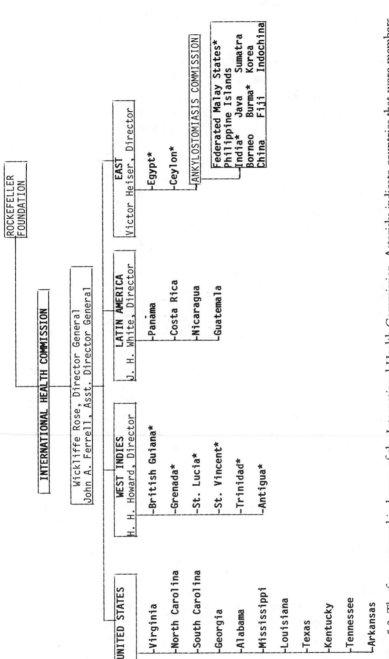

Figure 5.3. The four geographical areas of the International Health Commission. Asterisks indicate countries that were members of the British Empire. (Modified version of organization chart; courtesy of the Rockefeller Archive Center)

Rose arrived in Egypt in the spring of 1914, and immediately agreed to finance half the cost, and to expand an already operating, but limited, hookworm campaign, directed by Dr. A. F. MacCallan of the Egyptian Public Health Department.[15] MacCallan seems to have been yet another rather difficult character. According to Victor Heiser, the International Health Commission's wonderfully named "Director of the East," MacCallan was "dogmatic about everything," with an office of "one running mass of legs that loses its head when Dr. MacCallan's voice breaks the silence."[16] MacCallan was also somewhat ill-disposed to what he obviously viewed as American interference in a well-run British campaign. According to him, this American money was used to initiate a treatment-oriented campaign in Sharquia Province, utilizing five 50-bed traveling tent hospitals (Figure 5.4a). The full treatment (Figure 5.4b) took seven days: day 1, diagnosis, admittance, and laxatives; days 2, 3, 4, thymol (60 grains daily), a laxative, and a meal; days 5 and 6, rest and stool examination; and day 7, discharge or another bout with thymol.[17]

If it is hard to imagine poverty-stricken *fellaheen* being able to take such a seven-day "holiday," it is even harder to imagine them suffering through 180 grains of thymol. Indeed, the British were forced to hire six traveling "hookworm agents," who "beat up patients" to persuade them to attend. These actions were necessary, MacCallan explained, because "unfortunately the worms do not cause pain."[18] In such an environment, MacCallan's figures can scarcely be believed: Of 1,011 treated by June 1914, 628 had been cured and 383 relieved.[19] Perfect; but what happened to those who came and then fled in terror after their first dose of thymol, and were there no enterprising *fellaheen* who managed to avoid the "hookworm agents"? But the figures impressed Rose and the Colonial Office; nothing else really mattered.

But the campaign was short-lived. By the spring of 1915, all the hookworm hospitals had been taken over by the military; the war to end all wars had begun. In his final report on the campaign, MacCallan made his views known:

It should be understood . . . that the policy of surveying the country to obtain information as to the incidence of ankylostomiasis, and the inception of hospitals for the treatment of the disease, to the exclusion of sanitary reforms of the villages was dictated by the International Health Commission in consultation with the Director General, no practical method of effecting such reforms having been discovered.[20]

At this stage the International Health Commission seems to have lost whatever early faith they had in privies and sanitary reform. The difficulty of inducing Southerners to use privies and change their habits was one problem, but to attempt the same procedure with Egyptian peasants was quite another. Sanitation was impossible, given their filthy habits. "They have been driven as beasts of burden for so long," Rose noted, "that they are dumb animals."

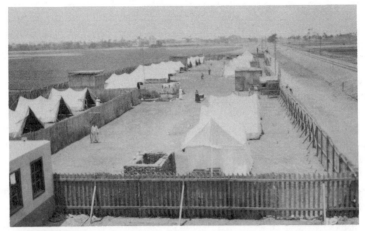

a

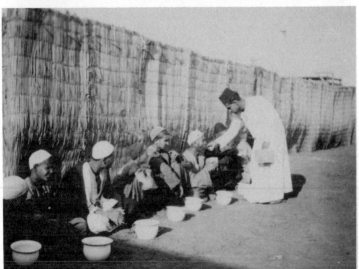

b

Figure 5.4. (a) Traveling tent hospital. (b) Patients taking thymol treatment for hookworm. From the First Annual Report of the International Health Commission, 1913–14. (Courtesy of the Rockefeller Archive Center)

Thus, "conservancy in the villages is absolutely impossible."[21] It was easier and cheaper to apply liberal doses of thymol.

Nevertheless, Rose regretted to see the campaign come to an end. Could the International Health Commission continue on alone, Rose cabled the Foreign Office? Not so, cabled Cairo, in turn: "The Department of Public Health consider [that the] proposal put forward cannot successfully be undertaken without assistance from the Egyptian Government, which assistance [the] latter are not able to give."[22] A few months later, however, the British, having unilaterally declared Egypt to be a British Protectorate and not a colony of Turkey, with whom it was now at war, had second thoughts: "It would be a great pity to do anything to stop the flow of American money."[23] But too late; Heiser found it impossible to visit Cairo in 1916 as promised, and the first contact between Egypt and the Rockefeller Foundation was broken.

Despite its short duration, however, this first hookworm campaign had an important bearing on the bilharzia story. It revealed to members of the Rockefeller Foundation the widespread occurrence and seriousness of the disease in Egypt. "I believe that probably 30% of the inhabitants have bilharzia," Dr. H. Finley from the American Mission Hospital informed Rose; the following year, Rose himself called bilharzia "one of the greatest scourges here."[24]

Hookworm occupies an important place in the bilharzia story. Hookworm, when discovered in the American South, first drew the Rockefeller fortunes into diseases of warm climates, and from thence to the world beyond. Hookworm thus attracted the Rockefeller organization into Egypt, where they discovered a concomitant disease, bilharzia. Hookworm is important, too, in revealing the motivations that led the Rockefeller Foundation into international health work. Quaker and liberal ideas of paternalism and "do-goodism" clearly played a role, but so did economics. In 1918, Rose asked George Cox to prepare a report on hookworm. Entitled "Economic value of the treatment of hookworm infection in Costa Rica," the report argued that success of any hookworm campaign must not only be judged by a reduction in morbidity, mortality, and suffering, but "must also show a monetary saving to the individual and the community." But, as the report showed, the real winners were the plantation owners. In one Costa Rican estate, where a two-year hookworm control program had taken place, there had been a 27 percent increase in earnings, a 47.8 percent increase in cultivation, and a 15 percent drop in costs. "The net result," Cox reported, is "happier, healthier, more permanent laborers producing more for themselves and for their employer." But it also meant increased unemployment. The savings to the employer could be passed on; "the increased efficiency of the laborers made it possible to reduce their number."[25] As Richard Brown has noted with some justification: To the International Health Commission "health is the capacity to work."[26]

A NEW CENTER OF TROPICAL MEDICINE

From their experiences in the South, and their campaigns in Egypt and other countries of the British Empire, those working for the Rockefeller philanthropies realized that a serious manpower problem existed: Outside the U.S. Army there were few Americans trained either in public health or in tropical medicine. Thus, the Rockefeller philanthropies set themselves the task of building a new profession of public health workers, which, because of the Foundation's involvement in international health, would impinge directly on tropical medicine. The task was passed to Abraham Flexner, Secretary of the General Education Board, who, after exploring the existing situation in the United States called together a General Education Board conference on October 16, 1914. As Elizabeth Fee has pointed out, of the three competing approaches to public health supported at that meeting – the social and political, the engineering or environmental, and the biomedical – the latter would carry the day.[27] Public health training, in other words, would be based primarily on the biological and medical sciences and oriented toward the medical profession. It would be concerned with a disease-oriented approach to public health, not with "congestion of population in cities, the condition of tenement houses, the elimination of slums, recreational centers, alcoholism, prostitution, and the standard of living," and similar problems, which, in the opinion of Edward Lewinski-Corwin, an economist at Columbia, "affect the public health as much as the sewerage system, food inspection, and the quarantine of measles."[28] Public health would focus on the prevention and elimination of individual diseases; it was a natural outcome of the widespread assumption that disease, to repeat the words of Frederick Gates, was "the supreme ill of human life."

This decision would have profound implications in the tropical world. Members of the International Health Board would address the problem of individual diseases but ignore the issues that many regarded as being of equal or even of more importance to health in the tropics. They viewed health simply as the absence of disease, which to the Western mind is often equated simply with the absence of pathogens. Thus health could be achieved only by the cure and elimination of each disease, one at a time, as it were. They chose to ignore the fact that the tropical world had not enjoyed the benefits of the social and sanitary movement that had taken place in the Western world during the late nineteenth century, and they therefore assumed that what can work in an affluent, sanitized, well-fed Western population must also work in the tropics. They assumed that diseases had only biological causes, which could be fixed; they ignored poverty, malnutrition, and other social causes, which could not.

In May 1915, as requested in the original October meeting, William Welch, Professor of Pathology at Johns Hopkins Medical School, presented his plan for the new school of public health. Entitled "Institute of Hygiene," he was quite specific on the basic goals of the institute:

The great need of the country today in the promotion of public health is the establishment of well equipped and adequately supported institutes or laboratories of hygiene, where the science of hygiene in its various branches is fruitfully cultivated and advanced and opportunities are afforded for thorough training in both the science and the art.[29]

As Fee has explained, the substitution of "institute" for "school," and "hygiene" for "public health," in the title of the document, implied that research, not teaching, should be the major emphasis, and that this research should be directed toward science, not practice. "A main function of the institute," Welch wrote, "should be the development of the spirit of investigation and the advancement of knowledge."[30] The institute, Welch further explained, should be an independent institution, housed in its own building, with its own laboratories, and its own full-time staff. It should be part of a university, closely related to a medical school, with access to "a good general teaching hospital." In addition, he noted, it should be organized into five major divisions. The Chemical, Biological, Engineering or Physical, and Statistical, should, he urged, take precedence over the Division of General Hygiene and Preventive Medicine, under which label Welch included "epidemiology, industrial hygiene, the principles of public health administration and other subjects."

Later that year, Rose, Greene, and Flexner began a series of site visits to choose the location of the new institute of hygiene. The outcome was in no doubt from the start; only Johns Hopkins University in Baltimore had a medical school and hospital suitable for an institute of hygiene of the type described by Welch. Indeed, only a few years earlier, J. D. Rockefeller had enthusiastically favored the Johns Hopkins Medical School with a $1,200,000 grant to build up its clinical departments. A document written by Gates in 1911, recommending this grant, leaves no doubt why, four years later, the Rockefeller Foundation would again favor Hopkins.

Most medical colleges, the document stated, were profit-motivated business ventures. This has led to "stagnation in the science of medicine," and lectures "that did and could do nothing more than to perpetuate from generation to generation a great body of false tradition."

In modern times, physics, chemistry, astronomy, botany have been reduced to sciences, because there has been money for apparatus, time for research and men ready to turn away from the allurements of money making to the higher walks of science. But while these glorious contributions to human knowledge, with their infinite promise to humanity, have been created, medicine until recently, say within the last generation, has scarcely advanced one step beyond medieval darkness. . . . Imagination cannot compass the torture that writhing humanity has needlessly endured because of it.[31]

Students' morals, Gates further maintained, were "contaminated by the known hollowness, shallowness and trickery of traditional medicine." But Johns Hopkins was different, Gates believed, "founded and organized in the spirit, not of commercialism, but of science and philanthropy." The first two years of study there, the report explained, covered the basic medical sciences. Such disciplines did not require the services of practicing physicians, he explained, but of those who "have given themselves up wholly to teaching and research on the comparatively meager salaries afforded them by the colleges. They have been content to exist on bread and butter, and they have lived, that is to say, their life has consisted in the enthusiasms of science and humanity." Clearly, as early as 1911, Johns Hopkins Medical School already possessed those characteristics now demanded of the new institute of hygiene.

In 1913, the General Education Board granted the Johns Hopkins Medical School an additional $1,500,000. In giving this grant, the *New York Tribune* noted that "the General Education Board recognized this institution as the greatest medical school in the country." Not to be outdone, the *Baltimore Evening Sun* headlined its report: "Hopkins Gift Makes School Without Peers."[32] Given this background, the site visits of 1915 were somewhat of a sham.

Visits were made to only four centers: Harvard, Columbia, Pennsylvania, and Johns Hopkins. In each interview, Rose, Director of the International Health Commission, asked about the availability of tropical disease cases. The new institute, in other words, was to provide professional manpower not only for the United States, but also for the International Health Commission as it set out to rid the world of disease. Although the answers to these inquiries probably had little impact on the final outcome, they show, once again, the favorable impression left by Johns Hopkins.

Pennsylvania and Columbia had little to offer in the field of tropical medicine, whereas Harvard tried to make a strong case for itself. But Hopkins had one overwhelming advantage in this regard: its Southern location. "We have a certain number of diseases which are more prevalent in the South," they told the Rockefeller visitors, mentioning in particular pellegra, amoebic dysentery, and hookworm, "which are practically never seen in New York." In addition, Dr. John Howland explained, "there is an enormous opportunity for the study of infectious diseases here in Baltimore on account of the Negro, because they have infectious diseases of all kinds all the time."[33]

A week after leaving Baltimore, the three participants presented their report to the General Education Board, recommending Johns Hopkins as the site of the new institute.[34] In June, the Rockefeller Foundation granted $267,000 and "agreed to co-operate with the University in the establishment of a School of Hygiene and Public Health for the advancement of knowledge and the training of investigators, teachers, officials, and other workers in these fields."[35] The School opened to students in the fall of 1918, using temporary facilities (Figure 5.5), and finally, in February 1922, received a $6 million endowment from the Rockefeller Foundation with which the new facilities were built on their present site at the corner of Wolfe and Monument Streets in Baltimore.

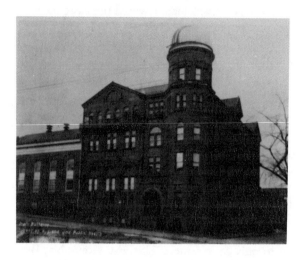

Figure 5.5. Temporary location of the Johns Hopkins School of Hygiene and Public Health from 1918 to 1925 (Courtesy of the Rockefeller Archive Center)

Curiously, despite becoming the most important source of expertise in tropical medicine in the United States, there was no department of tropical medicine in the School of Hygiene. But, as Welch was quick to point out, "The extension of the work of the International Health Board to tropical countries might be aided by the representation of tropical medicine in the School of Hygiene and Public Health."[36] As expected, their offerings were focused exclusively on the scientific and research aspects: A Doctorate in Public Health was offered only to physicians and senior medical students; medical and science graduates could obtain a thesis-requiring D.Sc. in Hygiene, which was essentially a Ph.D degree in the sciences; science graduates were offered a B.Sc. in hygiene (discontinued in 1923), whereas other medical students could obtain a Certificate in Public Health. Overall, the graduates of Hopkins went to the tropics armed with a research degree in the biological sciences.

Of the nine departments within the School, that of Medical Zoology, with its four divisions of protozoology, helminthology, medical entomology, and filterable viruses, came to have the most immediate link with tropical medicine. In many ways, the Department of Medical Zoology was the American equivalent to the London School of Tropical Medicine.

Medical zoology in the United States, like parasitology, helminthology, and protozoology in Britain, lay outside the mainstream of medicine. The practitioners of medical zoology were usually zoologically trained, interested in unraveling life cycles and means of infection rather than disease symptoms and pathology. Medical zoology was rarely if ever offered in American medical schools. It was one of those subjects that grew when the American medical schools moved into the universities, and the nonmedical faculties in turn saw the advantage in catering to the new breed of "premedical" students. In the United States, in contrast to Britain at this time, medical zoology became a premedical subject, offered to premedical students as part of their science training before entering medical school. Its position at Hopkins, however, was unusual. There, as in London and Liverpool, medical zoology became a postgraduate specialty.

Many members of the International Health Board honed their scientific skills in this department before moving overseas. The Department of Medical Zoology was headed by Dr. Robert Hegner, a graduate of Chicago with a Ph.D. degree from Wisconsin, who had won a research scholarship to Johns Hopkins in 1917 to work with the protozoologist Herbert Jennings. In 1919, Hegner recruited Dr. William W. Cort (Figure 5.6) to take charge of the Division of Helminthology. Both Cort and his division were to play vital roles in the bilharzia story.

Cort grew up in Colorado Springs, attended Colorado College, and, in 1909, moved to the University of Nebraska to study under H. B. Ward (Figure 5.7). Henry B. Ward was very much "the father of American parasitology." After three years of high school teaching in his hometown of Troy, New York, Ward traveled to Europe in 1888 to spend two years soaking up the

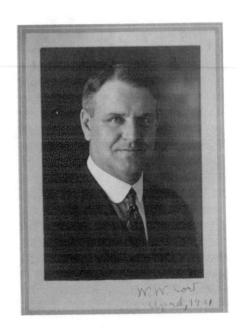

Figure 5.6. William W. Cort (Courtesy of the Alan Mason Chesney Archives of Johns Hopkins University Medical School)

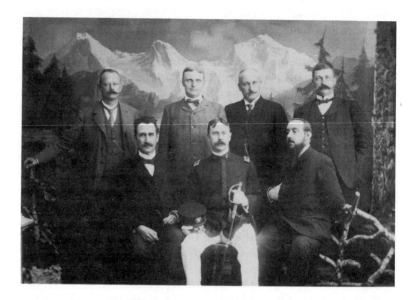

Figure 5.7. H. B. Ward (second from left, rear) at the International Zoological Congress, Bern, 1904, where A. Looss (rear, far left) announced his discovery of the hookworm life cycle. C. Stiles sits center front. (Courtesy of the University of Illinois Archives)

atmosphere of Göttingen, Freiburg, and Leipzig, where he studied under Rudolf Leuckart. He returned to gain his Doctorate at Harvard under E. L. Mark, and with these impressive credentials gained an appointment at the University of Nebraska in 1893, where he remained for 16 years. There, as medical zoology, parasitology steadily gained ground as an important class for all premedical students.

But parasitology developed in the United States for other nonmedical reasons. Land-grant colleges, which began opening at the end of the nineteenth century, were necessarily geared to practical needs, including animal husbandry and agriculture. They, therefore, had a place for the study of nonhuman parasites. Hiring faculty to teach both medical parasitology and veterinary parasitology became possible only after 1909 when Ward moved out of Nebraska to become Head of the Zoology Department at the land-grant University of Illinois. Here he opened the first graduate school in parasitology in the United States.[37]

William Cort moved to Illinois with Ward, obtained his Ph.D. degree in 1914, and, after two years at Macalester College in St. Paul, Minnesota, accepted a post at Berkeley. There he established a course in parasitology and helped investigate hookworm in Californian goldmines, an experience, he wrote, "that opened up the field of human parasitology to me." During these years, the summers were spent at the University of Michigan Biological Field Station on the shores of Douglas Lake, where Cort first met Hegner who led him to Hopkins. "I held the best position in my field in the world," Cort wrote later in life, "at the School of Hygiene and Public Health of Johns Hopkins University. All in all, from the director down, the School was a vigorous, inspiring place."[38]

Clearly, such a vigorous and inspiring place needed to be exported to other countries; only then would the benefits of scientific medical research be felt throughout the world and the dream of the Rockefeller Foundation fully realized.

THE LONDON SCHOOL OF HYGIENE AND TROPICAL MEDICINE

Plans to open schools of hygiene based on the Johns Hopkins model in Budapest, Prague, São Paulo, Toronto, and Warsaw were discussed after the close of World War I, and in May 1919, the International Health Board let it be known that they were interested in establishing such a school in London and "would be prepared to consider a definite proposition."[39]

London was crucial to the plans of the International Health Board. Nothing could be more urgent than establishing an agency that would spread the message of scientific medicine into the British Empire. "The proposed school of hygiene," noted the minutes of the International Health Board, "is to be imperial in scope and is to be open to qualified students from all countries."

The Board has in mind the importance of London as a strategic center for an institution of this kind; its incomparable wealth of experience in tropical medicine and practical public health administration; its commanding position in medicine and general science; the scope and distribution of the empire of which it is the political, economic and intellectual center; the part which the English speaking people have to play in the development of civilization.[40]

The British were prepared for such an offer of assistance. In 1919, the British Government had appointed its first Minister of Health, who, 18 months later, appointed a committee under the Earl of Athlone to investigate the needs of postgraduate medical training in London. Tropical medicine and public health received special attention in the report. Noting that the former was taken care of by the London School of Tropical Medicine, which had recently moved from Albert Docks to Endsleigh Gardens near University College, the report found the public health picture to be less rosy. To alleviate what they regarded as an "unnecessary and uneconomic" situation, they proposed to establish a single institute of public health in London – an institute of state medicine.[41] "We are hopeful," they concluded, with eyes turned toward New York, "that assistance towards its foundation and its endowment may be forthcoming from funds other than those of the State."

They were not to be disappointed. Following a memorandum from the Minister of Health,[42] the International Health Board pledged $2 million for the land, building, and equipment of a school of hygiene in London. The new school was planned not only "to cover broadly the field of preventive medicine," but also "to include courses offered by the London School of Tropical Medicine." Both the International Health Board and the Minister of Health stressed the necessity of close cooperation between the proposed school of hygiene and the London School of Tropical Medicine. Leiper was adamant on the matter. What is needed, he wrote in a private letter to George Vincent, President of the Rockefeller Foundation, was an institute of hygiene and parasitology, "in close proximity, or even contiguous with the School [of Tropical Medicine] and the College (i.e., University College)."[43] Whether he expected a total fusion of hygiene and tropical medicine is not clear, but he increased that likelihood by stressing the inadequate facilities of the new location in Endsleigh Gardens. In addition, Vincent was no doubt interested to learn, the School had proposed to open a department of tropical hygiene, but with insufficient funds no staff had been hired to run it. Thus, the old School of Tropical Medicine was amalgamated with the proposed new school of hygiene. In March 1922, the International Health Board authorized the purchase of the land on the corner of Gower, Keppel, and Malet Streets, and, in 1923, they agreed to provide $25,000 per year toward the operating expenses of what was to be called the London School of Hygiene and Tropical Medicine (Figure 5.8).[44]

"The building was to be a workshop where skilled labourers would pursue their tasks for the betterment of the human race," announced Sir Alfred Mond on July 7, 1926, at the laying of the foundation stone by Neville Chamberlain, the Minister of Health and Joseph Chamberlain's son. With music from *The Gondoliers, The Student Prince, The Mikado, and Rose Marie* (!) playing in the background, a cablegram passed to New York: "On the day of the laying of the foundation stone of the London School of Hygiene and Tropical Medicine, the American and British flags fly side by side at the dawn of a new era of preventive medicine."

The new school became a replica of Johns Hopkins, with virtually identical departmental organization. In both schools, the laboratory and scientific study of tropical medicine was located in the Department of Medical Zoology, made up of three subdepartments: protozoology, helminthology, and entomology. But in London, where tropical medicine enjoyed a more visible role than at Hopkins, both clinical and pathological studies of tropical diseases were covered by the Department of Tropical Medicine and Hygiene.[45]

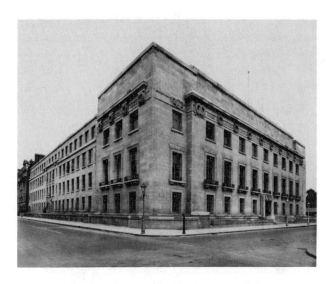

Figure 5.8. The London School of Hygiene and Tropical Medicine (Courtesy of the Rockefeller Archive Center)

Science dominated their studies. Whatever degree or diploma taken, whether for public health or tropical medicine, whether in London or Baltimore, the knowledge required was much the same. The student was required to know about the bacteria, helminths, protozoa, and viruses that caused disease; the insects that transmitted these agents; and the laboratory techniques required in studying them. The London School of Hygiene and Tropical Medicine had become the Johns Hopkins of the British Empire, carrying with it the mandate of the International Health Board to extend the benefits of scientific medicine to the British colonies.

THE PEKING UNION MEDICAL COLLEGE

London was not the only center to receive the gift of a Johns Hopkins. The Rockefeller Foundation, moving also into China, founded the Peking Union Medical College. There, two of the Foundation's employees discovered the snail host of *Schistosoma japonicum*, which had eluded Leiper and Atkinson a few years before.

With the acquisition of the Philippines, China had become a more significant factor in U.S. foreign policy. Following the Treaty of Tientsin in 1858, China had become an area of ferocious exploitation by the Japanese and Western powers. "Foreigners could go wherever they wanted, do as they pleased, independent of Chinese law, with foreign troops and gunboats never far behind."[46] By the 1890s, a chaotic, prostrate, and weak China seemed doomed for breakup and partition between the rival powers. But it was not to be; both Britain and the United States came to support the integrity of China and an "open door" policy for trade. But in general, American interest in China remained at a low ebb until the presidency of William Taft, who, following his election in 1909, sought to promote the economic interests of the United States by means of a massive expansion in foreign trade.

Nineteen nine was also the year in which Frederick Gates induced J. D. Rockefeller to fund an Oriental Education Commission, under the chairmanship of E. D. Burton, President of the University of Chicago.[47] The Commission, set up to investigate social, educational, and religious issues in China, argued, in their report, that new modern medical schools were desperately needed. In January 1914, the newly founded Rockefeller Foundation sponsored a China Conference to consider the educational and medical needs of China. As a result of this conference, the First China Medical Commission was sent to survey medical work and education in China and to select a site for "a large, well-equipped, well-conducted, and efficient medical school associated with a good hospital."[48]

By this time the reign of the Manchu Dynasty had ended, and a short-lived Republic of China was constituted. The revolutionary party, reorganized as the Kuomintang, won an overwhelming victory in the elections of 1912, but assassinations and power struggles once again led China into the chaos of civil war; by 1915, the age of warlords had begun. Undisturbed by such events, the Medical Commission spent four months of 1914 visiting 17 medical schools, finally recommending that the Union Medical College in Peking be the site of a new Western-style medical school.

The Union Medical College had its roots in the Peking Hospital of the London Missionary Society, set up in 1861 by William Lockhart, Senior Physician to the British Legation.[49] In 1906, however, in the aftermath of the Boxer Rebellion, which had destroyed the London Mission and its hospital, the various missionary bodies sought strength in unity and, with the financial help of the Dowager Empress Tz'u-hsi, opened the Union Medical College. It was not the first Western medical school in China, but, by all accounts, it was probably the best. With nine faculty in 1906, most with British degrees, 40 students enrolled for a five-year premedical and medical program.

On receiving the recommendations of the Medical Commission, the Rockefeller Foundation set up the China Medical Board, under the directorship of Wallace Buttrick. Flattered by the praise of the Rockefeller Foundation, tempted by hard cash, but worried about the future missionary direction of the school, the London Missionary Society agreed to sell the land and building to the China Medical Board for $200,000. With a board of 13 – seven from the

China Medical Board and six from the various missionary societies – the Peking Union Medical College was formed on July 1, 1915.

Earlier in that year, the China Medical Board invited William Welch and Simon Flexner to join with Gates and Buttrick on a Second China Medical Commission, to advise on future policy for the Medical College. Their report, of January 1916, set the tone for the college. It was to be the Johns Hopkins of the East, bringing scientific medicine to China just as Hopkins had brought it earlier to the United States. As at Hopkins, there would be stiff entrance requirements, a research-oriented faculty, and English, the scientific language, would be used as the language of instruction. "Medicine has so solved the problem of disease that it could almost be considered as an exact science," one of the participants remarked in an address following the laying of a corner-stone at one of the college's new buildings, and, in words that reflected the beliefs of the Rockefeller Foundation, went on to say that one "could almost say that medicine could command poverty and destitution, for disease was the maker of these things – the maker of the conditions that make for poverty, destitution, ignorance."[50]

The Peking Union Medical College actually opened in 1917 with eight students in the first year of a three-year premedical program. The first- and second-year students of the previous year, being unqualified to meet the new standards, were meanwhile transferred to other colleges. In 1919, the medical school proper, having "the potency of becoming one of the greatest centers of medical instruction in the world," opened its lecture halls to seven students, 11 faculty members, and 32 instructors.[51] Two years later, a new hospital opened its wards with a lavish dedication ceremony (Figure 5.9). John D. Rockefeller, Jr., and an entourage of scientists, secretaries, valets, and nurses attended the ceremony, after a voyage via private railcar across the continent to Vancouver, and luxury suites in the *Empress of Asia* ocean liner. Science pervaded those opening ceremonies like a Chinese mist. Papers such as "Biochemistry in retrospect and prospect," and "The origin of blood cells," shared the forum with the type of rhetoric one would expect from such occasions: "Scientific knowledge and technical skill must be dominated by idealistic loyalty to the highest and best influences of human life; and that idealism is an idealism based upon a deep and abiding religious conviction."[52]

The College was unashamably American, catering to students from wealthy Westernized families. The students were introduced to the delights of baseball and the inanity of American college football; they even had a school song!

Hurrah for PUMC
The College of our choice
'Tis here we learn such precepts
As makes our heart rejoice . . .

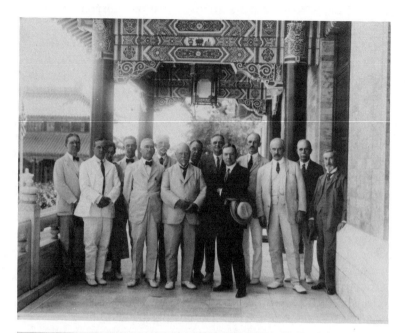

a

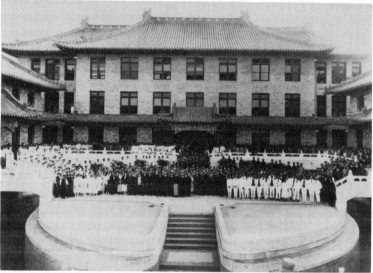

b

Figure 5.9. Peking Union Medical College: (a) J. D. Rockefeller, Jr., and others who attended the dedication ceremony, 1921; (b) staff of the college assembled at the hospital entrance, 1921. (Courtesy of the Rockefeller Archive Center)

She's taught us ills to lessen
And how disease to cure
By killing all bacilli
We heal the rich or poor.[53]

The song was not an accurate reflection of their future life in China, for it suggested that they must choose between healing the rich *or* the poor. In reality the choice had already been made; not for them the wretchedness of the Chinese peasant; they were carrying the torch of Western technological scientific medicine. Most of its graduates took up their medical careers in large urban centers, and were apathetic and unconcerned about the health problems of rural China.[54] In the words of John Bowers, the school became the pioneer medical center in Asia, "a self-contained island focused on scientific and educational accomplishments in a country beset by domestic and international disturbances."[55]

With chaos all around them, the College passed through what Bowers has called "the golden years." These were the years that witnessed the formation of the Chinese Communist Party; Chiang Kai-shek's seizure of the Kuomintang military and his northern expedition to drive out the war lords and gain control of the land; the establishment of the Nationalist Government in Nanking; the "white terror" that drove Chiang's old communist allies into the hills of Kiangsi; and the 1928 treaty that established the United States as the major ally of the Kuomintang Government. These were the golden years of quality, not quantity. Of the seven students admitted in 1919, only three graduated, and in 1924 only 64 students attended the College, eight in their final year. When, in 1925, the premedical program of the College was closed and students were admitted instead from premedical studies in other colleges, quality remained the priority. In a rigid adherence to rules, favored by American educators, students were required to have studied, for example, 12 hours of biology per week in which a three-hour laboratory session was considered equivalent to a single hour. Of these 12 hours, four were to be spent on each of general biology, invertebrates, and vertebrates. They even felt it necessary to detail the number of hours to be spent studying earthworms, echinoderms, turtles, and birds, among others. The British, never great admirers of American schooling, must have thought all these rules and regulations rather silly.[56]

The faculty were clearly the group that enjoyed the most benefits from these golden years. An interview in New York and a two-year appointment at the Peking Union Medical College quickly became the gateway to a successful career. An impressive group of American, British, Canadian, and Chinese, all with impeccable credentials from the best European and North American universities, combined ambition with adventure by joining its faculty. Among those to take advantage of the opportunity were Ernest Faust (Figure 5.10) and

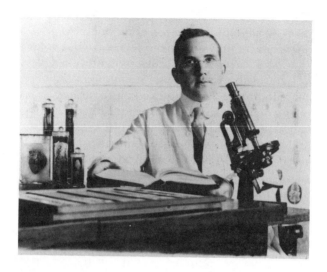

Figure 5.10. Ernest Faust (Courtesy of the Rockefeller Archive Center)

Henry Meleney, codiscoverers of the intermediate host of *Schistosoma japonicum* in China – perhaps the single most significant discovery pertaining to bilharzia in the decade.

BILHARZIA IN CHINA

Faust and Meleney both arrived in 1920. Henry Meleney joined the Department of Medicine after graduating from the College of Physicians and Surgeons at Columbia University. Faust, a native of Missouri, had not followed such a straight track to China. As a young man he had turned down a University of Missouri scholarship in 1907 in order to teach English and Latin in a rural Ozark school, and had then spent the summer of 1908 studying botany at the University of Michigan in order to teach science at the school the following year. Excited by this experience, however, he changed his plans and enrolled at Oberlin College, graduating in 1912. He then moved into H. B. Ward's laboratories at the University of Illinois, where he completed an M.Sc. degree in 1914, and a Ph.D. in 1917, working on the life histories of Montana trematodes. From there he began his long and illustrious career in parasitology and tropical medicine by moving directly to Peking, where he became an Associate Professor of Parasitology in the Department of Bacteriology, Parasitology, and Pharmacology.[57] Being so young and inexperienced, it was perhaps surprising that he got the job. But the letter of reference from Ward may have done the trick. "I am confident," Ward wrote, "that Faust will do more research than anyone else of whom I know."[58] Ward was correct in his assessment. John Grant, who occupied an office next to Faust in the College, remembered him as "an almost fictional type of a German scientific worker. He had little sense of humor, was a tremendous worker and given to meticulous detail."[59]

From the very start, Faust seems to have developed a special interest in bilharzia, known to be endemic in the Yangtze Valley and parts of southern China. At the opening of the Anatomical and Anthropological Association of China in 1920, for example, Faust presented a paper on "the present state of the schistosome problem," in which he pointed out that although much was known about the morphology of the adults and their larval stages, its life cycle in China remained a mystery.[60] The breakthrough came in Soochow, Kiangsu Province, during the summer months of 1922.

Meleney was having lunch in the cool of some trees, when some children and a 41-year-old man approached with the classical swollen belly of bilharzia. We "joked with them," Meleney wrote to Faust, "and finally persuaded the old man and two others to give us feces to examine. All three were positive." Meleney then visited their homes and found a small canal nearby, on the banks of which were several hundred snails that seemed different from the Japanese carrier of the schistosome parasite. They crushed 240 of them and found seven to be infected with cercariae that seemed similar to those of *S. japonicum*, and with which they infected two experimental mice. "On the whole I think this is quite promising," Meleney wrote, barely able to contain his excitement, "don't you?" But Meleney understood the caution of a parasitologist. "Dr. Snell [his companion] says you sent a terrible sceptic down here," he added in his letter. "[He] won't even believe a snail when he sees one. He thinks we've got what we're after. But I'm from Missouri. Anyway, we're having a good time and may bring home the bacon."[61] And bring home the bacon they did. In the 1923 issue of the *China Medical Journal*, they announced their findings: Cercariae released from snails along the canal shore, identified as *Oncomelania hupensis* by an American malacologist, produced mature worms of *S. japonicum* in experimentally infected mice. And, in addition, the miracidia hatching from the eggs of these worms successfully invaded experimental snails of the same species to produce cercariae again 72 days later. Also, they noted, these same "Chinese" miracidia successfully infected the Japanese snail host, *Blanfordia nosophora*, as it was called then, and the Chinese snail host was equally susceptible to miracidia of the Japanese *japonicum*; the Chinese and Japanese varieties of *S. japonicum* seemed to be identical.[62]

News of the discovery spread quickly. In 1923, an abstract appeared in the *Journal of Tropical Medicine and Hygiene*; a year later, both *Lancet* and the *Transactions of the Royal Society of Medicine* picked up the news. Then, in 1923, Faust returned to Johns Hopkins in a year's exchange with William Cort, and put together the important monograph *Studies on Schistosomiasis Japonica*, which appeared a year later as part of the monograph series of the *American*

Journal of Hygiene. This long and impressive work dealt with all aspects of the biology of the parasite: its structure and development in humans and snails; its distribution along the flood plain of the Yangtze Valley from the mouth of the river inland as far as Ichang; its compatibility with numerous reservoir hosts such as dogs, cats, oxen, and horses; and its intermediate host, *Oncomelania hupensis.*

Schistosomiasis japonica is not associated with the main current of the Yangtze River, but is found in the overflow areas and backwaters of the Yangtze basin, particularly in the region of lakes and canals adjacent to the River, where clear, quiet water is found. For this reason most of the endemic centers are found south of the River, particularly in the region of the three large lakes, the Great Lake, Poyang Lake and Tung Ting Lake, their tributaries, and intermediate lesser lakes, swamps and marshes.[63]

The authors presented also a rather pessimistic assessment of the control possibilities. Control of contaminated feces, elimination of reservoir hosts, public education, human treatment, and destruction of snails all presented difficulties, but none loomed larger than the Chinese themselves. "The cooperation of the native population in China cannot be expected at the present time," they noted. "With rare exceptions, neither the provincial nor the local authorities have any real interest in the welfare of the inhabitants," and, as they noted further, "it is not merely a public health problem; for within its scope are also included problems of economic and political life and general education."[64] Neither Faust nor Meleney, it is clear, carried any grand illusions about the possibility of controlling the disease in China. "I now agree with you," Meleney wrote to Faust "that the eradication of the intermediate host in China is a practical impossibility. Whether there is much more hope in other methods of eradicating the disease is also a doubt in my mind, when I think of the type of mind the Chinese have."[65]

Very little more was done about the disease between the period of Faust and Meleney's work and the wartime closing of the College in 1941. Clinicians in various parts of China reported new sites of the disease, and a few treatment campaigns with Fouadin and tartar emetic (to be discussed in the next chapter) were reported.[66] But quite clearly, with the discovery of the worm life cycle, a key scientific problem had been solved. This was not the time to deal with the disease in China; Faust was ready to continue his career in science. But it was not to be in China, where his request to head a separate department of parasitology was turned down by the Rockefeller Foundation. Thus, he returned to the United States in 1928 to take up a position at the newly reopened Department of Tropical Medicine at Tulane, America's first school of tropical medicine.

But elsewhere, the International Health Division had agreed to set up a program to eliminate not only hookworm, but also bilharzia. In 1927, the Division returned again to Egypt.

6

Bilharzia: Optimism in Egypt (1918–1939)

For the 21 years between the two world wars, a sense of optimism gripped the imaginations of those involved with the disease. In contrast to Manson's earlier statement that there was "no direct, or other, means by which the bilharzia can be destroyed," it now seemed that "bilharziosis need no longer be regarded as an incurable disease."[1]

Two chemicals, antimony tartrate (tartar emetic) and copper sulfate, were responsible for this brighter outlook. Both chemicals killed. The former, when injected into the bloodstream, was believed to destroy the adult parasites and their eggs; the latter killed snails. Together these chemicals could eradicate the disease by killing both the worm and its snail intermediate host. The successful use of tartar emetic for bilharzia was first announced in 1918 by Dr. J. B. Christopherson, Director of Civil Hospitals in Khartoum and Omdurman. Thirty grains of tartar emetic given over a 15- to 30-day period "is a definite cure for bilharziasis," he remarked, noting at the same time that care needed to be taken with the chemical that was, after all, a poison.[2] And it certainly was. As the 1899 American *Dispensatory* noted:

Symptoms of acute poisoning by the drug are an austere metallic taste; excessive nausea; copious vomiting; frequent hic-cough; burning pain in the stomach; colic; frequent stools and tenesmus; fainting . . . prostration, and death. Ten grains is the smallest dose reported to have proved fatal.[3]

Despite such side effects, however, antimony tartrate had long been used as an emetic at dosages up to 1 grain, and as a diaphoretic (agent that increases perspiration) at less dangerous levels. The *British Pharmacopoeia* of 1916 listed its medicinal properties as "diaphoretic, expectorant, alterative, emetic, circulatory and nervous depressant."[4] In 1915, it was used for the first time against a tropical parasite, *Leishmania*, and news of its subsequent success against bilharzia spread quickly into the British medical press. In 1921, for example, two physicians working in the Church Missionary Society's Hospital in Cairo reported the successful treatment of 1,000 cases.

The dosages given to bilharzia victims were severe. Progressively increasing doses of 1.0–2.5 grains were administered each day for the first four days. Two more dosages of 2.5 grains were given on days five and six, and finally, on alternate days, further dosages of 2.5 grains were given to a maximum of 20 grains. According to the two physicians in the Cairo hospital, 70 percent of those able to complete this arduous two-week treatment were freed from the worm.[5]

Antimony tartrate became the primary weapon in the Egyptian Public Health Department's attack on the disease, which commenced after the close of the 1914–18 war (Figure 6.1a,b). By 1921, an ankylostoma–bilharzia annex had been attached to each of five hospitals in Cairo and the Nile Delta, in which thymol (for hookworm) and tartar emetic were administered to literally thousands of Egyptian *fellaheen*. Each of these annexes occupied a fenced-off area of land adjacent to a general hospital. Each was supplied with a series of huts acting as laboratories, examination centers, treatment centers, and a doctor's office, while a duplicated series of tents was provided as posttreatment rest centers for members of each sex. The treatment was slightly less severe than that carried out earlier, with 2 rather than 2.5 grains being the maximum dose given. But to offset that advantage, the full treatment now took four weeks, not two.[6]

Although the annexes were built on the recommendations of the British-led Ankylostoma Committee which was reorganized after the war, the subsequent campaign was gradually taken over by Egyptian officials as the country painfully moved from British Protectorate status to virtual independence at the signing of the Anglo-Egyptian Treaty in 1936.[7]

The records of these treatment annexes, the hospitals, and parallel surveys of some Egyptian villages revealed for the first time the extent of the disease in Egypt. The small village of Saft el Enab, for example, showed that only 4.4 percent of the villagers were free from infection with parasitic worms; 83 percent of them carried a schistosome, and 74 percent were infected with *Schistosoma haematobium*.[8] Statistics from the treatment annexes are confusing and tell us very little about disease prevalence. But they do show that over 500,000 *fellaheen* attended the five treatment annexes between 1920 and 1923. Khalil was probably fairly accurate when he claimed that "about 70 to 80 percent of the total population of Egypt is infected with bilharziasis, i.e. 9 to 10 millions of a total population of about 13 millions."[9]

The rather irregular statistics produced by the staff of these annexes revealed also one of the major problems with the tartar emetic treatment: The majority of the patients failed to complete the four-week ordeal. At the Mansura annex in 1922, for example, 19 percent of the patients failed to complete the first week of treatment, 60 percent had dropped out by the end of the third week, and, in the end, slightly less than 20 percent completed the full course of injections. Other annexes reported similar results. Furthermore,

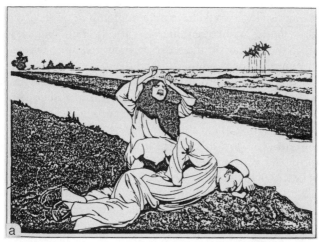

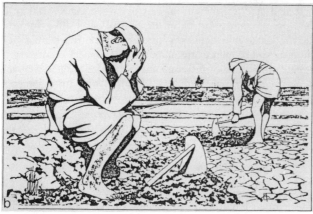

Figure 6.1. Egyptian propaganda posters showing victims of (a) bilharzia and (b) hookworm. From *Ankylostomiasis and Bilharziasis in Egypt* (Cairo: Public Health Laboratories, 1924)

completion of the ordeal did not guarantee a cure. Four weeks after completion of the 12 injections, reported the Tanta Annex in 1922, 51.9 percent of those examined still contained viable schistosome eggs in their urine, and, three months later, 38.2 percent still bore eggs.[10] But ineffective drugs were not the only problem. As Khalil so correctly noted, economic conditions were a major deterent in seeking treatment; a day in the annex was a day without wages.[11] Despite the manufacture of a new antimony drug by F. Bayer and Company in the late 1920s, named Fouadin (generic name, stibophen) after King Fuad,[12] which, according to Khalil, produced better results and which, given intramuscularly, was less dangerous than antimony tartrate, it was clear that these chemicals alone would have minimum impact on such an enormous problem unless joined with other lines of attack. But, luckily it seemed, another weapon did appear on the scene at about the same time: a beautiful green-blue chemical, copper sulfate.

A. C. Chandler, who first produced experimental data on the molluscicidal activity of the chemical, noted the attractive features of such agents in the treatment of disease. They offered, or so it seemed, a method of combating disease without involving the patient in any way, which appealed to the scientist and to the politician alike. The former could now deal with dilutions of chemicals rather than trying to understand the mentality of illiterate peasants; the latter could ignore the painful process of education or even more the politically explosive notion of upgrading and changing the lives of the masses, by opting instead for a simple mollusc-killing chemical. As Chandler noted:

If some efficient and practical method of destroying the snails could be found, this would furnish a logical point of attack in the control of all fluke diseases. . . . The fact, therefore, that fluke infections may possibly be controlled by attack upon an intermediate host instead of by reliance upon the enforcement of sanitary regulations makes the ultimate eradication of these infections, in spite of their relative incurability, a matter of brighter prospect than is the case with many other verminous parasites.[13]

Chandler, working in the gorgeous Willamette Valley of Oregon, as far away from the problems of Egypt as one could imagine, began testing with 18 chemicals, but soon narrowed them to the salts of copper, the cheapest of which was copper sulfate. He found that a minimum dilution of 1:500,000 killed all specimens of snails tested.

In 1926, Mohammed Khalil (Figure 6.2) directed the first Egyptian field test of the chemical at the Dakhla Oasis, far out in the western desert, where 65 percent of the population were estimated to harbor schistosome eggs.[14] Initially, Khalil accepted Leiper's advice that copper sulfate should be used only on the residual puddles left after the summer canal clearances, but when the testing time came the copper salt was added directly to a main spring-fed stream at a concentration of 5 ppm. After only four days, Khalil reported, all the bulinid snails were dead, and six months later there were still no snails to be found. Although 22 months later some living snails were found in the stream, the ever-optimistic Khalil reported that only 12 percent of the human population now passed ova. In 1929, having discovered a new stream containing living snails, the Oasis was treated again. Yet another survey, two years later, once again revealed no bulinid snails. Finally, in 1936, when the place was again reported to be snail-free and the population's health was said to be much improved, Khalil reported: "Out of 72 children born after 1930, the date

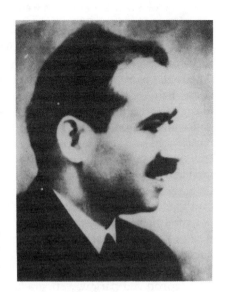

Figure 6.2. Mohammed Khalil (Reprinted with permission from M. Abdel-Wahab, *Schistosomiasis in Egypt*. Boca Raton, Fla.: CRC Press)

in which the preventive measures were taken, none showed any ova in the urine, although they frequented all the streams for bathing."[15] Such results, which were later to bear the brunt of much criticism, help to explain Khalil's future commitment to copper sulfate as the miracle drug in the control of bilharzia.

The euphoria generated by the apparent successes of tartar emetic, Fouadin, and copper sulfate was not shared by Leiper, who, in 1928, had been asked to advise the public health authorities in Egypt on control measures against the disease. Not surprisingly, given his background in the London School of Tropical Medicine, Leiper stressed the necessity for further research: "The simple formula of 'irrigating the veins with tartar emetic and the canals with copper sulphate' may express in an epigrammatic form our present views on bilharzia eradication but it holds out a promise of facile success which is not likely to be realized in our present state of ignorance."[16]

Thus, warned Leiper, Egypt needed to reorganize its scientific community to encourage research into such important matters as the habits and life histories of the susceptible snails. But because "it may be truly said that the modern concept of a civilized community is one in which zymotic diseases are under control and parasitic diseases are absent," Leiper also argued that the provision of pure water and the disposal of sewage were absolute necessities.[17] The Rockefeller Foundation could not have agreed more, for by this time they were thoroughly committed to removing hookworm and other diseases by sanitizing the world.

THE ROCKEFELLER CAMPAIGN IN EGYPT

Killing snails had little appeal to members of the International Health Division of the Rockefeller Foundation, who had gained their experience combating hookworms, which, unlike schistosomes, have no intermediate host to kill. Despite this basic difference, however, Victor Heiser, Rockefeller's "Director of the East," believed, "the fundamental problem even for the control of bilharzia is the prevention of soil pollution." Thus, in 1927, following an earlier invitation, the trustees of the Division agreed to provide funds and an experienced sanitary engineer to oversee the sanitization of Egyptian villages. This time, however, unlike their previous foray into Egypt, they were to provide their own scientific personnel. Such an engineer, Heiser noted, needed "initiative, industry, tact," and on a more basic level, "the willingness to bring about the complete installation of the right kind of latrines in a suitable village of several thousand population."[18] In addition, in order to appraise the effect of these latrines on the transmission of hookworm and bilharzia, the Division agreed also to enlarge their staff by the addition of two parasitologists, J. Allen Scott and Claude Barlow (Figures 6.3 and 6.4).[19]

Both Scott and Barlow were graduates of Johns Hopkins School of Hygiene and Public Health. In 1929, the year of their arrival in Egypt, Barlow, a medical graduate of Northwestern University, was already 53 years old, with 21 years of experience with the American Baptist Foreign Mission Society in China. The much younger Scott, after graduation from Wesleyan, had taught biology at the University of Vermont. In 1925, he entered the Division of Helminthology at Hopkins as a Rockefeller Research Assistant to work on hookworm under the direction of W. W. Cort, out of which came a D.Sc. in Hygiene two years later. The year 1925 was also when Barlow submitted his thesis on the life cycle of *Fasciolopsis buskii* for the same degree.

In 1921, Barlow had been given a Rockefeller grant to study the life cycle of this large intestinal trematode of man and pig in China. "Today is a red letter day for me," Barlow wrote to J. D. Rockefeller, Jr., on October 13, 1922, "because it is my birthday and on it I have found the infection method of the Fasciolopsis." Including in the letter a beautiful representation of the life cycle, he could not curtail his excitement – the excitement of discovery to which many aspire but few attain.

This may not be so exciting to you as it seems to me but it has been one of the greatest games I have ever played and now that I have tracked the dragon to his den, the most important part of the game is yet to be played, the killing of the dragon. . . . I have worked unusually hard and in the intense heat of the summer. The work on the open fields was almost unendurable and I lived alone. All the other foreigners were gone from the field to the mountains for the summer but I did not notice the heat, the absence of my family, or that of the other workers because of the intense interest and exacting nature of the work. I averaged eighteen hours a day at the microscope. I am

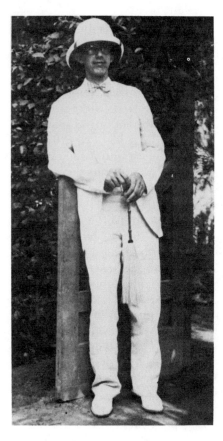

Figure 6.3. J. Allen Scott (Courtesy of J. Allen Scott)

happy in the outcome of the work and my greatest joy is to know that the disease can be easily controlled.[20]

Barlow ended his letter with this rather touching tribute:

In a really personal sense I feel that you have been my partner in this work and I want to thank you for that. . . . If I had but applied to an impersonal foundation, had dealings entirely by letter, and made reports to people whom I had not seen, I fear you would not have entered into the problem at all but I had your picture before me as I worked in the Lab and the partnership seemed very real. Had you not supplied me with what I did not have, I could not have supplied you with what you lacked.

"We are proud of the relationship," J. D. R., Jr., answered in a gracious reply, "but what we have done is insignificant in comparison to what you have done and are doing."[21]

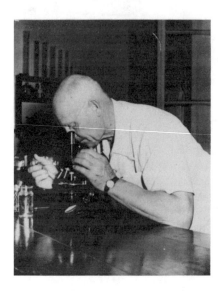

Figure 6.4. Claude Barlow (Courtesy of
the Rockefeller Archive Center)

Encouraged by friends in America, Barlow returned home to submit his
work as a thesis toward the Hopkins degree. This was accomplished, and the
work published as a monograph of the *American Journal of Hygiene*. But he did
not return alone. Having already become accustomed to self-experiment, he
attempted to bring back some living worms by swallowing 32 of them taken
from the body of a Chinese patient. An American newspaper reporter,
commenting on the monograph, was ecstatic: "Behind the technical terminol-
ogy and dispassionate scientific conclusions," he wrote, "there lies a human
and pulsating story. It is a story of patient and unremitting toil, of persever-
ance in the face of repeated discouragement, of seemingly unsuperable obstacles overcome, of personal heroism unsurpassed on any battlefield since the
first Egyptian pharaoh led an army against the Hittite chiefs."[22]
A few years later, Barlow was indeed to lead an Egyptian army, if a very
small one. Cort, who had also recommended Scott for one of the two posts in
Egypt, lauded Barlow as a "fine experimentalist . . . who has done quite a
little in biometrics."[23] In June 1929, both men were appointed special members
of the International Health Division's field staff in Egypt to see "what, if any,
influence the sanitation campaign had upon the transmission of the two
diseases ankylostomiasis and bilharzia."[24]
Scott and Barlow entered the battle against these diseases with very
different attitudes. Scott was a research scientist for whom the Egyptian
posting was simply a new job, although clearly a fascinating one, to be done
with the best of his considerable ability. Barlow had other motivations.
Originally a missionary physician, he had turned to scientific research. But it

was never disinterested research; the dragon not only had to be found, it also had to be destroyed. He never allowed the disease itself to take priority over the people who suffered from its ravages. "It seems to me to be a real call to service which is too personal in its note and its obligations for me to disregard," he wrote in a letter to the foreign secretary of his mission society, shortly after learning of his appointment. "It is a project which involves thousands of lives and the efficiency of hundreds of thousands of people and therein lies its strong appeal to me. . . . I would like to add this piece of work as one of their contributions to the Cause of Christian Missions."[25] One could never envisage Scott seeing his work in that light.

The two men spent the summer of 1929 at the University of Michigan Biological Station at Douglas Lake, where Cort had set up a summer field program emphasizing work on the parasites of freshwater snails. For many years, many swimmers and waders in Douglas Lake had suffered from an irritating, itching skin rash. In 1927, quite by accident, Cort developed a rash on his wrist after spending a few hours picking and sorting snails from a small collecting bucket. "The next day," he wrote, "the itching continued, becoming almost unbearable whenever the wrist became warm. By the second night, the hand and wrist were swollen and painful and the papules had become definitely pustular." The cause of this irritating but harmless rash, as he soon discovered, was forked-tailed schistosome cercariae released into the water from the snails he had collected. These cercariae are the larval stages of schistosome worms that normally mature in the blood vessels and nasal sinuses of birds. However, these cercariae can accidentally penetrate the skin of some unsuspecting bather, where they are quickly destroyed. In the process, however, a tissue reaction sets in, resulting in what is commonly called "schistosome dermatitis" or, more popularly, "swimmer's itch" (Figure 6.5).[26] These avian schistosomes, with their larval stages carried by freshwater snails, became the means by which many American parasitologists, including Scott, Barlow, and Cort himself, gained firsthand experience with schistosome parasites.

While at Douglas Lake that summer, Scott, Barlow, and Cort devised a research plan for their work in Egypt. The proposed task was of immense scope. Not only were they expected to gain information on the prevalence and the sources of infection of the schistosomes as well as hookworm and *Ascaris*, but also to undertake "broader studies" on the three parasites.[27] Thus prepared, the two men arrived in Cairo in September 1929. Barlow was to remain there for over 20 years.

The campaign

"Just now my work is divided into three branches of activity," Barlow explained in his second Christmas letter to the "Folks of the First Church":

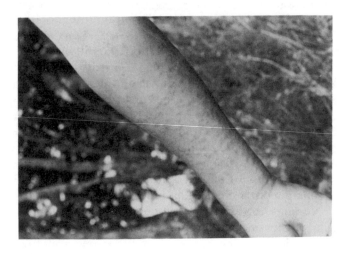

Figure 6.5. Swimmer's itch (my son's arm)

surveying the population for disease, treating infected patients with antimony tartrate ("which does not make them feel too good"), and taking a census of snails. The latter activity, he noted, "I have been doing myself."[28] But already the original program of the International Health Division had been compromised. That original program had seemed simple enough back in New York. One village, Bahtim, was to be sanitized with borehole latrines; a second village, Mostorud, was not. A comparative survey of the two villages for hookworm and bilharzia would then indicate the impact of the latrines on the two diseases.

But there were problems. The original survey of Bahtim, carried out before the latrines were built and before Barlow and Scott arrived, was inadequate, according to Barlow. Furthermore, collecting stools for examination was no easy task. The villagers, who, we must assume, were never consulted, refused to cooperate in the manner expected. They distributed stools from one member of a household into the collecting cans of the rest; they put buffalo stools into cans; they returned cans empty; they put camel urine and even ditch water into other cans. Even worse, the whole plan of operation was compromised by the government promising both villages that they would receive treatment. But the Mostorud villagers then demanded sanitation or they would not accept treatment. Not surprisingly, the program collapsed.[29] Not an auspicious start! But, despite these and other similar problems, a considerable amount of information was collected from 15 villages over the following few years. Four villages received neither latrines nor treatment, two received only treatment, and six received only latrines, whereas three, including Bahtim, received both treatment and latrines. Scott handled the statistical techniques for this program, and devised methods of egg counting from which the prevalence of the diseases was estimated.

By the end of 1931, they were forced to report that "no appreciable effect, due to sanitation, could be deduced," although "Bahtim is a cleaner-smelling, more wholesome village with its latrines than it used to be without them." A year ago, they explained, "one had to tread back-streets in constant danger of soiling one's shoes. Now one can walk anywhere about Bahtim without danger and without taking special precautions about stepping." But, although there had been no change in the prevalence of the parasites, Barlow remained hopeful. "I am convinced," he wrote in this 1931 report, "that our statistics will eventually show a significant improvement in worm diseases."[30]

But Barlow was wrong; no such improvement occurred. Despite repeated warnings from Scott that the sanitary campaign was having little impact on either of the parasites, the officials back in New York remained confident. "Striking success in use of latrines," they noted in 1932; "practical sanitation is being achieved," they reported three years later. Even as late as 1936, they considered the campaign "an outstanding success, that when it is terminated there will be in each of the fourteen provinces and three governments a nucleus of approximately three villages thoroughly sanitated."[31] But what of the parasites and the diseases? On that issue they remained silent.

Clearly, latrine building could no longer be seen as a means of effective control of bilharzia and hookworm; building them had become an end in itself. By 1936, the officials in New York must have been aware of the problems. Scott, in a preliminary report of 1935, had informed them quite bluntly that neither sanitation nor treatment had made any difference to the parasites. In treatment villages, whether sanitized or not, Scott noted, "the rates have all returned to practically their former level within 3 or 4 years of study following treatment."[32] In 1936, Scott returned to the United States, where he remained on the Rockefeller staff for one year working under Cort's direction at Johns Hopkins. There he prepared the final report on the sanitation campaign; the Scientific Directors could no longer avoid the sobering truth.

In villages receiving only treatment, Scott reported, "the entire effect of as much treatment as the people could be persuaded to take had been dissipated within three years." A similar picture emerged for those villages receiving only latrines. Again, Scott noted, "the inescapable conclusion is that sanitation produced no measurable effect on infection with the species of worm parasites under study." It was immediately obvious to Scott why the sanitation program had failed to dislodge the worms. "The crux of the matter," Scott wrote, "is that this sanitation was installed in the houses, while the most important parasites were transmitted in the fields." Perhaps in time, Scott thought, the villagers, having grown used to latrines in the home, might practice field sanitation as well; but "problems which have existed for thousands of years cannot always be expected to yield to solution at the first attempt."[33]

The Rockefeller Foundation has many virtues, but patience is not one of them, and failure was a concept they did not understand. What, then, were they to do when faced with the collapse of their sanitation and treatment campaign? The answer came from Barlow: Kill snails.

From the very start of the sanitation campaign Barlow believed in the efficacy of killing the snail hosts. "While I believe that sanitation is essential and should be carried out to the limit," he noted in his very first report to New York, "I feel that snail study, looking to control, is the one supremely crucial factor in prophylaxis."[34] By the summer of 1930, such a view seemed justified by the news that another Rockefeller employee, Lewis Hackett, had banished malaria from two villages in northern Italy by the application of Paris green, a larvicide that destroyed the larvae of the malaria-transmitting anopheline mosquito.[35] That same summer Barlow learned also that Paris green had been used in Cyprus to kill bulinid snails and that plans were underway to use it there in an antibilharzia campaign.[36] Barlow also knew of copper sulfate and its miraculous success in killing snails from the Dakhla Oasis. He actually visited the site during the summer and became convinced by what he found there: After treatment with copper sulfate (Figure 6.6),

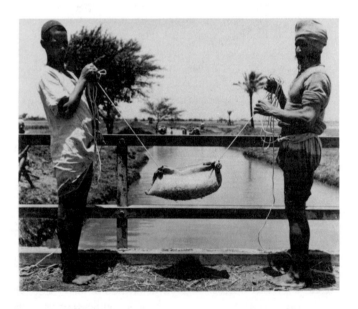

Figure 6.6. Spreading copper sulfate in a gunny sac that was dragged in the canal (Courtesy of the Rockefeller Archive Center)

snails were no longer present in sufficient numbers to be of epidemiological importance.[37] Another set of observations made at this time further convinced Barlow that killing snails gave the best hope of success against the disease. He satisfied himself that the Nile did not transport snails into the canals at every inundation; they lived their entire lives in the canals. To kill these snails would therefore have a dramatic impact on the disease; new snail populations would not be imported every year by the Nile to begin again the cycle of infection.

But how were the snails to be killed? By 1932, he had lost his earlier faith in copper sulfate. Not only was its cost prohibitive, but also Barlow had been shocked to discover that Khalil's experiment with copper sulfate in the Dakhla Oasis was fraudulent. Barlow discovered that the village stream, in which the absence of snails had been attributed to copper sulfate, had in reality been diverted and the old stream-bed filled in, "so that the experiment could hardly be reported as a sulphating experiment at all."[38] But if not copper sulfate, what might work?

Death by drying, perhaps? But here again he had discovered, contrary to what was commonly believed, that snails can survive when left exposed to the air by the drying of canals. Of 262 planorbid snails collected from the mud of a canal left dry for a few weeks during the winter clearance, 216 recovered when immersed in warm water. Thus, from this and other similar experiments, Barlow concluded that "when the closure is over there is a seed stock amply sufficient to repopulate the area fully." Furthermore, he argued, bulinid snails in the Sudan can survive drying for up to seven months. "It does not seem practical then," he wrote, "to attempt to use either the winter closure or the summer rotations as a means for the extermination of the molluscs involved in the spread of schistosomiasis in Egypt."[39]

At this stage, even Barlow became a decided believer in the cult of sanitation, as he informed Heiser in the spring of 1931.[40] But not for long; a new and promising line of attack had opened up. In the previous year, Barlow had accidentally killed his snails in the snail ponds (isolated man-made holes in which snails were kept and bred) by removing the vegetation. He immediately saw the practical implications of this mistake and in 1931 attached to his annual report an article entitled "The effect upon snails of clearing canals of vegetation and snails."

The idea was deceptively simple. At regular intervals, the *fellaheen*, using tools with which they were familiar and without control or supervision, would clear the canals of weeds and snails. From a few rather crude experiments, "that need to be repeated under carefully controlled conditions," Barlow suggested: "It seems to offer a practical solution for keeping schistosomiasis in Egypt below the critical level by using a procedure which is easily comprehended by the fellaheen and which is so simple that they can carry it out without supervision."[41]

The first of these experiments began in April 1934, when, at two-month intervals, a number of canals were cleared of vegetation and snails. By September, the bulinid snails had all but disappeared from the test area and remained low throughout the following year. "The experiment was undertaken knowing one year's clearance would be totally inadequate," Barlow wrote, "yet the results obtained were decisively positive and point encouragingly to the use of clearance as the most important measure in a scheme for the control of schistosomiasis in Egypt."[42]

With their eyes still firmly fixed upon their beloved latrines, the Scientific Directors of the International Health Division paid scant attention to this work, merely noting, in November 1935, that "canal clearance offers hope" and "clearance must be put to the test soon."[43] But the test did not begin for another two years, a reflection of Barlow's unfocused style of research and the Rockefeller Foundation's abiding interest in sanitation. To support Barlow's approach was tantamount to admitting failure.

But the scent of failure was present. Despite much optimistic rhetoric, by 1934 the Scientific Directors were becoming dissatisfied with the events in Egypt; everything seemed to be coming apart. The high hopes generated by the sanitation program were clearly unfounded, and now friction was developing between Scott and Barlow. As a result, in 1934, Cort was persuaded to visit them in Egypt. Both men were in the doldrums. Their work had met difficulties and they were beginning to get on each other's nerves. One can hardly be surprised, for, as Barlow said, "Continued heat and sunshine are not good for Anglo-Saxons. They are inclined to get a bit nervy."[44] Scott wanted to go home, and both men, particularly Barlow, were experiencing considerable problems handling the statistical data. In addition, as mentioned above, Barlow was even losing faith in his belief that in snail destruction lay the best hope for disease eradication.

Cort's visit did much to improve the situation. He not only gave fresh impetus to Barlow and Scott, but finally convinced the Directors to broaden their line of attack. Interviewed on his return to the United States by Frederick Russell, the Director of the International Health Division, Cort reminded him that neither hookworm nor bilharzia was being affected by the borehole latrines. But what *had* been shown, Cort stressed, was the spotty and very localized distribution of infected snails. Locate these sites of infected snails, and "most, if not all of [the disease] could be eliminated." Furthermore, he told Russell, "Scott's work is going along very well and will be the best helminthological survey of Egypt that has ever been made." Although he was less complimentary toward Barlow, who, Cort noted, tended to scatter his efforts and spend too much time on worthless projects, he nevertheless urged the Directors to continue supporting Barlow's work. "I think now he will stick to the main issues," Cort explained, one of them being the snail clearance experiments.[45]

Reluctantly, therefore, the Directors in New York turned their attention from latrines to snails. In 1936, George Strode, the new Director of the East, advised that a large-scale experimental project "to break the cycle of disease transmission by eliminating as far as possible the snail" would begin in 1937.[46]

In 1938, Barlow presented the results of this two-year clearance experiment (Figure 6.7a–c). Every two months, running from May 1937 to December 1938, a team of *fellaheen* cleared weeds and snails from a set of canals in the Bahtim area. The process was cheap and required little skilled labor, although Barlow was honest enough to admit the drawbacks of such a plan. "When I pay a man 3½ piastres (17½ cents) for a full day's work in these sticky, muddy, schistosome-infested canals, under a blazing, pitiless sun, it makes me feel like a snake but it is the wage of the country and may not be tampered with."[47] Then, during the nonclearance months these same canals were surveyed for bulinid and planorbid snails.

The withdrawal

The report of these experiments (see Table 6.1) must have come as a delightful surprise to the Directors – the best news out of Egypt for some time. But

Table 6.1. *Results of Barlow's snail clearance experiments; number of* Bulinus *and* Biomphalaria *snails collected at each site*

	Bulinus snails		*Biomphalaria* snails	
	Clearance area	Control	Clearance area	Control
1937				
Feb	233		1002	
April	623		1479	
June	2015	2085	2939	5549
Aug	409	424	980	1491
Oct	136	131	517	681
Dec	1110	716	2785	2024
1938				
Feb	386		678	
April	576		2167	
June	388	1526	323	2176
Aug	45	366	16	1013
Oct	18	151	3	950
Dec	30	1051	15	1885

Source: Barlow, *Annual Report to the Rockefeller Foundation*, 1938.

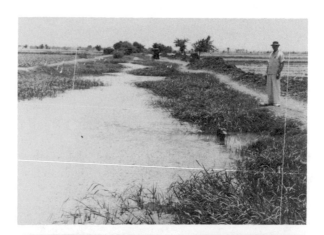

a

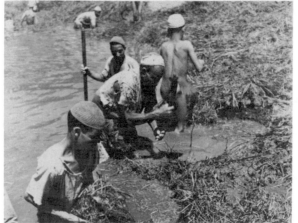

b

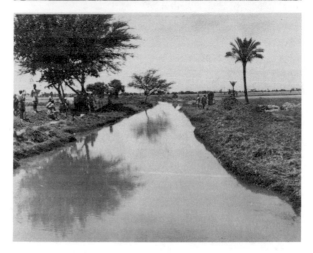

c

their reaction to it was quite extraordinary. Lumping all the December figures together from both snail species, they reported that whereas the number of snails increased in the control area from 2,740 (716 + 2,024) in December 1937 to approximately 2,900 (1,051 + 1,885) in December 1938, the number in the cleared area declined from 3,895 (1,110 + 2,785) to 45 (30 + 15) during the same period. The Directors, at their meeting in November 1939, then made an extraordinary prediction:

On the basis of these experiments, it is estimated that schistosomiasis could be entirely eliminated from Egypt by canal clearance over a period of twenty-five years.

To bring this about, it would be necessary only to "create an organization within the government to continue the work after the withdrawal of the Division's aid."[48] In 1940, the Rockefeller Foundation withdrew from Egypt and the Egyptian Government formed the Bilharzia Snail Eradication Section with Barlow as its Director.

Whether they withdrew for the reasons stated or whether they used Barlow's experiments to justify pulling out of a bad situation is hard to say. Certainly the Egyptian campaign had its critics. Wilbur Sawyer, one of the directors, expressed the most serious reservations:

I have never been happy about our work in Egypt. Unless it can be put on a totally different basis I think we should try and complete our schistosomiasis work and perhaps all our work in Egypt by the time Dr. Barlow leaves the service. The fundamental weakness in Egypt is that our procedure has been different from that in almost any other country. . . . It has not been planned in such a way as to lead step by step to satisfactory local health organizations. . . . I was shocked while in Egypt to see how inadequately the most important problems were studied or tackled.[49]

Sawyer's comments were a little hypocritical. Far from working in step with the Egyptian public health officials, Barlow and Scott had been told to ignore the work of Khalil and the Endemic Disease Section, created in 1928 to direct the work of the antihelminth treatment annexes. From six such annexes in 1924, their numbers grew to 57 by 1930 and 85 by 1940, treating nearly 400,000 patients that year. This lack of cooperation was to bear fruit later on as the Snail Eradication Section also attempted to carry on its campaign independent of the Endemic Disease Section.

Clearly the most valuable contribution made by the Rockefeller campaign came from the data collected by Scott. His 1937 paper, entitled "The incidence and distribution of the human schistosomes in Egypt," has provided the baseline data with which all succeeding surveys have been compared. From an

Figure 6.7. Barlow's canal clearing operations, 1937–8. (a) Barlow examining an uncleared canal; (b) the clearing operation; (c) a cleared canal. (Courtesy of the Rockefeller Archive Center)

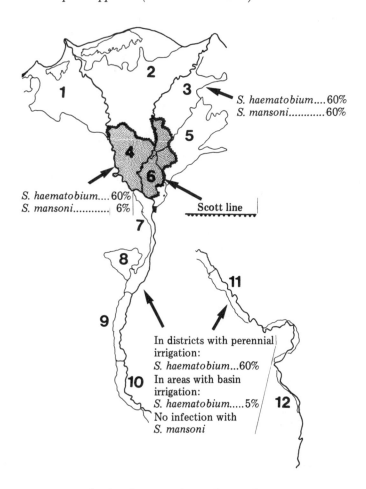

S. haematobium....60%
S. mansoni............60%

S. haematobium....60%
S. mansoni............6%

Scott line

In districts with perennial
irrigation:
S. haematobium...60%
In areas with basin
irrigation:
S. haematobium.....5%
No infection with
S. mansoni

Figure 6.8. The distribution and prevalence of the two human schistosome species in Egypt, according to J. Allen Scott (1937): 1, Beheira Province; 2, Gharbiya; 3, Daqahliya; 4, Minufia; 5, Sharkiya; 6, Qaliubiya; 7, Giza; 8, Fayum; 9, Minya; 10, Assiut; 11, Girga; 12, Aswan.

impressive data base – 40,000 villagers from 125 villages together with figures from 700,000 patients in the various treatment annexes – Scott estimated that about seven million Egyptians out of a total population of 15 million were infected with either or both schistosome species. Among the rural population, the figure was even higher: over 6.5 million infected out of 11.7 million population, or 55 percent.

Scott also showed that the distribution of the disease fell into four sharply divided areas (Figure 6.8). In the Nile Valley south of Assiut, where districts were still under basin irrigation, only about 5 percent of the population were infected with *S. haematobium,* whereas in the area of perennial irrigation between Assiut and Cairo and in the Nile Delta, 60 percent of the population carried that worm. *Schistosoma mansoni* was virtually absent from the Nile Valley south of Cairo, occurring only in the Delta. There, however, its distribution fell into two areas. North of what I shall call the "Scott line," the population was infected as much with *S. mansoni* as with *S. haematobium,* but south and west of this line, only about 6 percent of the population were infected with *S. mansoni.*[50] If nothing else, these figures revealed the full extent of the bilharzia problem in Egypt, and the naive optimism of the previous decade.

Nevertheless by 1940, outside of Egypt bilharzia was not considered to be a serious or widespread disease. At a 1938 meeting of the Health Committee of the League of Nations, Hilmy Bey, the Egyptian delegate, suggested that a bilharzia commission be set up. A meeting of experts set up to examine the Egyptian suggestion believed that no commission was necessary and noted that there were "few tropical diseases in which the etiology is so clear, treatment so satisfactory, or preventive measures so obvious."[51]

7

Into the 1930s: Economics of disease

Before the First World War, tropical medicine was focused mainly on the health of British colonial officials and American army personnel. But after the war, economic factors began to play an increasingly important role. Profits generated by fruit plantations in the tropics of Central America and by mines in the South African Witwatersrand and Southern Rhodesia seemed threatened by workers rendered inefficient by disease. Such concerns were not new, of course. Hookworm had long been associated with worker inefficiency, and General Gorgas's medical work during the building of the Panama Canal had shown the absolute necessity of maintaining a healthly workforce. But in the 1920s, many private companies doing business in the tropics, or recruiting laborers from there, came to realize that profits could be enhanced by recruiting medical staff, by building hospitals, and by sanitizing work camps for their employees. Thus, diverting profits to medical care could represent good and even necessary long-term business investment. So widespread became this belief that the words "Behind every banana and every ounce of gold stands a healthy man" could be used as an epitaph of the 1920s.[1] But, on the other hand, in some economic situations where an inexhaustible supply of cheap labor was available, it was more profitable to limit medical expenses.

In both cases, however, good business practice required that these firms paint their medical endeavors with glowing colors, convincing both themselves and the public that they were founts of medical benevolence. The American public, for example, were asked to believe that their corporations were ambassadors of humanity, adding their share to the considerable blessings of American civilization – another weapon in God's work of tutelage. The medical work of our tropical companies, noted an article in *The World's Work*, "may well be called the most dramatic and spectacular item in the whole tale of 'The Heart of the Dollar.' It has been an important part in the campaign of the white man against the peculiarly malignant diseases of the tropics – a campaign marked by self-sacrifice and unsurpassable courage which makes it as magnificent an adventure as the religious crusades of the

Middle Ages." Every American, urged the author, must feel proud, "as he comes upon case after case in which American corporations abroad are setting foreign capitalists vivid examples of the value of this sort of sympathy and humanity toward labor."[2] Likewise, the medical care offered to African laborers in the South African gold mines was said to be an example of what all communities should strive to reach.[3]

LATIN AMERICA

The United Fruit Company, the largest American fruit company in Latin America, seems to have spent the most money on protecting the health of its workers. By the late 1920s, the Company, founded in 1899 out of a merger between Andrew Preston's Boston Fruit Company and Miner Keith's banana plantation and railway company of Costa Rica, had planted two million acres of land with bananas, sugar cane, cacao, coconuts, and other fruits. It owned 1,571 miles of railway, 187 locomotives, and 5,461 railcars; operated 86 steamships of "The Great White Fleet" (whose motto was said to read: "Every banana a guest, every passenger a pest"); employed 67,000 workers, and had yearly net earnings of nearly $20 million. From these earnings the Company spent $1 million per year for medical expenses, and $500,000 for sanitation and street-cleaning operations.[4]

Modern hospitals lay at the center of these medical operations. The first opened in Panama in 1900, and others quickly followed: Costa Rica in 1904, two in Cuba by 1908, Guatemala a year later, Colombia and Honduras in 1914, Jamaica in 1919, and a second hospital in Honduras in 1921. By World War II, five more hospitals had been opened in Panama, Honduras, Guatemala, and Costa Rica. On entering Golfito Hospital in Costa Rica, opened in 1941, Charles Wilson, Special Assistant to the President of the Company, noted that "the visitor might think he was in the Grand Central Palace, New York, at any exhibition of the very latest in hospital furnishing. . . . It is a public monument to be envied by any city in the world."[5] Similar remarks were made by another enthusiast. "The humanitarian spirit of Uncle Sam's big business," he wrote, "has never been more largely or more happily interpreted than by the medical service of the United Fruit Company."[6] "It is evident to anyone not stone blind," he further noted in 1927, "that the huge investments of American capital in foreign countries are there for purposes of development, not exploitation."[7] Another devotee, after describing swamp clearances, oiled waters (for mosquito larvae), and clean water provision, became exuberant: "This is War, and this is Magnificent! It has all the dash, the brilliancy, the courage, the organization, the discipline, the generalship and the strategy of war, and it has its heroes, dead and living."[8]

This "magnificent war" was also being fought in Puerto Rico. After the occupation by the United States, the government encouraged U.S. investment in the island. There is, the first governor noted as early as 1901, "a surplus of labor accustomed to the tropics," as a result of which "the return of capital is exceedingly profitable."[9] By the 1920s, a tariff-protected sugar empire had been born on the island, representing, by the end of the decade, 65 percent of all exports. Forty-four percent of cultivated land was planted with sugar cane, all in the hands of a small number of American companies: the South Puerto Rico Sugar Company, the Fajardo Sugar Company, the Central Aguirre Sugar Company, and the United Puerto Rico Sugar Company, with combined assets of over $85 million.[10] The Caribbean had become the "American Mediterranean," according to historian Gordon Lewis, and the American citizen was told that "American rule or influence has brought enormous benefits to the Caribbean peoples by way of stamping out diseases, [and] improving sanitation." These sugar companies in Puerto Rico, like the United Fruit Company, invested in the health of their employees by building hospitals and providing medical services for them. As John McClintock, Assistant Vice-President to the United Fruit Company, noted in 1954: "In the underdeveloped areas where American companies have gone, where they have brought great enterprises into fruition, where they are continuing, one of the primary factors was to establish conditions of health where people could not only exist but also could work."[11]

SOUTH AFRICA

Economic interests lay behind the entry of South Africans into the war against tropical diseases, including bilharzia. The discovery of diamonds near the confluence of the Orange and Vaal rivers in 1867, and the uncovering of the Witwatersrand gold reef 20 years later transformed life in southern Africa and had an equally profound impact on disease and medicine. It set up the demand for cheap African labor, and, as in Latin America, it led to claims that the companies hiring this labor were sources of medical benevolence.

"The health of the Bantu mineworker became almost an obsession with the mining companies," wrote A. P. Cartwright in his eulogistic volume, written in 1971 to commemorate the 50th anniversary of the Mine Medical Officers Association of South Africa.[12] Like the American fruit companies, these mining companies built modern hospitals and hired full-time medical staff. By doing so, according to Cartwright, they did much to reduce the extraordinary disease mortality among miners recruited by the Chamber of Mines.

After the Boer War, during which the mines were closed, the Chamber of Mines faced a critical labor shortage. To overcome this shortage the mines began recruiting Africans from areas north and east of the Transvaal. The results were only too obvious. A health report of 1903 showed an annual mortality rate of 57.7 per thousand, 41.7 percent of them from respiratory diseases. Worse again, the report of 1905 showed an almost unbelievable mortality rate of 130 per thousand from Africans recruited from outside South Africa and hand-picked for their physique and good health. That is approximately one-eighth of a workforce consisting entirely of young males died each year!

These "tropical natives" were recruited from Portuguese East Africa by the Witwatersrand Native Labour Association. The recruits, after marching from "rest camp to rest camp" to reach their ports of embarkation, were shipped to Lourenco Marques. Trains then took them inland to the border station of Ressano Garcia, where they were medically examined. Those pronounced fit, after being held in compounds, were then transported to Johannesburg in batches of 1,200, where they were compounded again for three more weeks. A second examination followed. Some were rejected, some were retained for further examination, whereas those passing the tests were led to the all-male mine compounds to begin work. Between 1910, when the Union of South Africa was formed, and 1912, approximately 45,000 Africans were recruited in this manner; 10,000 of these were rejected, and of the 35,000 put to work, 1,449 died (41 per thousand) during that period, 49 percent from respiratory problems.[13]

But despite receiving advice that these figures would be substantially reduced by improving the miners' diets, by providing better housing and bedding, and by building hospitals, nothing was done until 1913. The situation in South Africa differed from that in Latin America. In Africa, there was an inexhaustible supply of cheap labor which rotated through the system every six months; to spend money on health in these circumstances would have unnecessarily cut back on profits. But in 1913, pneumonia killed 31 percent of the African workforce. As a result, the British Colonial Office threatened to prevent further recruiting from their colonies to the north.

Faced with these threats, the Chamber of Mines invited General Gorgas to look over the situation, aware that, years before, pneumonia had wreaked similar havoc among the West Indians hired to work on the Panama Canal.[14] After much wining and dining, Gorgas recommended the most basic improvements – greater hospital facilities, more spacious accommodations in the camps, the provision of one bed per miner, and the provision of water, sewerage, and better food – but he also argued that the conditions in which the recruits had been shipped to the high velt, and not the conditions in the mines, was the major cause of pneumonia. They were sick, according to Gorgas, before they reached the Rand. Thus, in the eyes of the Chamber of Mines, improving the living conditions in the mine compounds was not the most economical way to reduce disease mortality; a better way would be to stop recruiting the most unhealthy miners who, statistics had shown, came from Portuguese East Africa and other tropical areas outside South Africa. In 1913, recruitment north of the Limpopo River was thus banned, and the ability of the mines to recruit more Africans, even when their major source of supply had been temporarily dislocated, was made possible by the famous Native Land Act of the same year. This act not only prohibited Africans from acquiring land outside the 7 percent reserved for them, but also prevented them from working as managers and tenant farmers on estates owned by absentee white landowners. In other words, it drove the reluctant Africans back to the mines, where the major recommendations of Gorgas remained unimplemented. However, one company, the Central Mining Rand Company, took action by appointing Dr. A. J. Orenstein, of Gorgas's Panama staff, to be its "Superintendent of Sanitation," beginning, according to Cartwright, major reforms.

But how major were these reforms? The most detailed information we have of the real conditions in these mines comes from the study of the Southern Rhodesian mines by Charles van Onselen, the son of a mineowner who was given access to the medical records of the companies. By 1890, the British South Africa Company had established itself north of the Limpopo River, anxious to expand into a second Witwatersrand. But it was not to be; there was no gold reef but only a series of small quartz reefs with unpredictable ore levels. The dream ended in 1903 with the collapse of the Rhodesian mining stock. By 1910, however, by maximizing productivity and minimizing labor costs, the mines had recovered their fortunes. African wages and work hours were controlled by the Rhodesian Native Labour Bureau, who kept up a flood of the cheapest labor from the poorest areas of the country and held down their wages. "Fundamentally," van Onselen wrote, "it was the reduction in costs achieved at the expense of African workers' wages that made the most important contribution to the continued viability of the industry."[15]

Costs were reduced also by limiting expenditure on food, housing, and hospitals. Thus although "miner's diseases" such as syphilis were common, the major diseases in the Southern Rhodesian mines came from their wretched living accommodations and their inadequate diet. Tuberculosis was rampant, pneumonia the greatest killer, but hard on its heals came scurvy! Scurvy, a disease of vitamine C deficiency, accounted for 13.5 percent of all deaths in 1908 and was still a problem 30 years later! Annual mortality rates from diseases, given by van Onselen, show a decrease from a high of 65.91 per thousand in 1906 to 21.94 in 1915, with a leveling off after that. According to van Onselen, this decline reflected improved conditions brought about by competition for workers between Northern Rhodesia, Nyasaland, and Southern Rhodesia. But with the end of this competition, there was little demand for further reform, and the death rates were stabilized at "tolerable limits." Reforms took place, therefore, only if profits were not thereby jeopardized.

But, as in Latin America, the same propaganda battle was waged. "The food and accommodation provided [by us] is vastly better than the natives have been accustomed to at their own kraals," the Southern Rhodesian Chamber of Mines fantasized.[16] Similarly, an edition of *The Mining Survey*, published by the Transvaal Chamber of Mines, argued that a migrant laborer was protected from any moral or physical degeneration because "as soon as his economic needs have been satisfied he returns to the tribe. His venture into the world of the European is, therefore, not a complete break with his mode of life, his traditions and custom. It is rather an interlude."[17] Photographs contrasting the primitive tribal settings with that offered to the miner in the compounds, fill the article. The article claimed also that the migrant labor system was set up to benefit the health of the African; returning regularly to the open-air life of the Kraal greatly reduced the danger of tuberculosis and silicosis. And what is one to make of Cartwright's extraordinary claim? "The mine medical officer," he writes,

is more than simply a physician or a surgeon in his job. In a sense he is a medical missionary, too, for in treating his patients he teaches them some of the first lessons of civilization. More than this, every year he sends back to the tribal territories 40,000 men who have had some training in first aid. For that alone the people of Africa have reason to be grateful to him.[18]

Those words were written in 1971.

THE ECONOMICS OF BILHARZIA

However generous the various corporations may or may not have been in providing medical care to their employees, many of the diseases were fostered by the conditions in which the laborers worked. Silicosis, pneumonia, scurvy, and other diseases were generated out of the working conditions in African mines. So, too, with bilharzia; the prevalence of the disease increased, not from working in mines, but whenever men were forced to labor in irrigated plantations. As David Bradley so crisply remarked, "Schistosomes are *the* hazard of irrigation. This is partly because freshwater snails and irrigation engineers have similar ideas of what is ideal."[19] Such was the case, for example, in the irrigated sugar plantations of Puerto Rico, and among the cotton plants of the irrigated Gezira Plain in the Anglo-Egyptian Sudan.

In 1934, under the policies of the New Deal, Puerto Rico was transferred from the War Department to the Department of the Interior, and a complex federal relief program was initiated under the direction of the Puerto Rico Reconstruction Administration, whereby $57 million was poured into the island in a futile attempt to break the sugar monopoly, one of the major causes of the island's ills. Immediately before this period of attempted reform, Ernest Faust, now a professor at Tulane, began a study of *Schistosoma mansoni* on the island, with support from the National Research Council and from the Bailey Ashford Scholarship Fund.

Faust may have been prompted into doing this work from reports that the disease was no longer as benign as formerly reported. Bilharzia, I remind the reader, was not a serious problem when the initial hookworm campaigns of Ashford were taking place. Even in 1916, when it was found to be endemic around the coast of the island and in the sugar valleys to the southeast (Figure 7.1), it was still regarded as benign.[20] In 1927, William Hoffman of the newly opened School of Tropical Medicine in San Juan, discovered the snail host of the parasite, then called *Planorbis guadelopoupensis*, and again hinted that the disease was more widespread than previously believed.[21]

What Faust found, however, changed the picture considerably. Not only was the disease endemic over large parts of the island, but it had become a severe problem in a new endemic area: the irrigated sugar plantations of the southeast region in the vicinity of Guyama, Arroyo, and Patillas.[22] In one *hacienda*, for example, 56 percent of the field workers had feces positive for the eggs of *S. mansoni*. Bilharzia, Faust warned, "is spreading and its incidence [prevalence] increasing."[23] Thanks to the sugar industry, bilharzia had become a serious health problem on the island.[24]

Bilharzia was also in danger of becoming a major problem in the foreign-office-controlled Sudan, where the demands of the Lancashire cotton industry had led to the construction of the Sennar Dam on the Blue Nile in 1925, and the opening of the vast Gezira Plain for irrigated cotton growing. The British had known for many years that the Gezira Plain was ideal for irrigation; the clay soils were impervious to water and the land gently sloped away from the Blue Nile in a northwesterly direction. Also, for many years, the British had been investing in Egyptian cotton, extending the areas of irrigation to meet the needs of the powerful Lancashire cotton industry. But, because of mounting competition from the United States and Germany, Lancashire, at the turn of the century, had been forced to produce more expensive and finer cloths. This required the long-stapled variety of cotton grown in Egypt. But Egyptian productivity had leveled off, and the British Cotton Growing Association, founded in 1902 to promote cotton growing in the British Empire, began pressuring the British Government to finance a new cotton scheme in Gezira. Aware of the great strategic importance of the Sudan, and convinced that the scheme would make one of the Empire's most poverty-stricken countries self-sufficient, the British Treasury reluctantly agreed on a £3 million loan in 1913, and the scheme got underway immediately after the end of World War I.[25]

Whether one accepts Gaitskell's enthusiastic endorsement of the Gezira, which, according to him, was "built for the people of the Sudan by the paternalistic pride of their British administrators and the adventurous enterprise of the British commercial partners," or whether one accepts Barnett's more negative assessment that a basic and unnecessary instability was introduced into the Sudan economy by basing the country's wealth on the export of a single cash crop, whose price was determined by a small number of external buyers, there can be no argument that the scheme created a new health problem – bilharzia.

PUERTO RICO

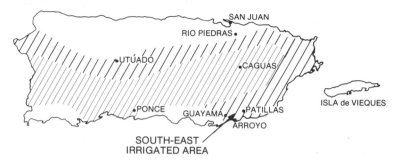

Figure 7.1. Puerto Rico. Hatched areas indicate high ground.

When completed in 1925, the Sennar Dam created an enormous irrigated area much like the Nile Delta, with interlocking waterways and canals. These, as medical authorities recognized at the time, provided perfect conditions for the snail hosts of bilharzia. Not only was bilharzia endemic along both the Blue and White Niles in the Sudan, but also the cotton scheme itself demanded a large migrant labor force, many of whom were carriers of the parasite and many of whom were Egyptians.

Optimism flourished during the early years, based on the optimistic prognostication that the disease could easily be eradicated by killing snails with copper sulfate and treating the victims with tartar emetic. Also, to reduce the likelihood of migrant workers carrying the worms into the project area, quarantine stations and treatment dispensaries, mirrored after those in Egypt, were also established. Within the Gezira itself, the usual combination of treatment, education, and snail killing went on. Naturally, hopes faded as the disease gradually established itself. By 1927, snail hosts of both *S. mansoni* and *S. haematobium* were abundant in the canals, but before the Second World War the authorities insisted that, although bilharzia was present in the irrigated area, it was under control. Nevertheless, although optimism pervaded official reports, even these began to shift their language from "elimination" to the much less optimistic "control" of the disease.[26]

The disease did not establish itself in the Gezira until the disruptions of World War II. It was kept out by the activities of the Sudan Medical Service which seems to have been one of the most efficient in British Africa. Much of this stemmed from the presence of the Wellcome Tropical Research Laboratories which had been set up by H. S. Wellcome in 1903 and formally amalgamated into the Sudan medical department in 1935.[27] But when the exigencies of the war drastically undercut the efficiency of the antibilharzia program, the inevitable happened. Thus the history of bilharzia in the Sudan paralleled the story in Egypt: The same initial optimism led gradually to a profound pessimism as the inextricable link between bilharzia and irrigation schemes established itself.

MEDICAL RESEARCH

It is always a temptation to the scientifically minded medical man to interest himself in investigating one more of the new things for which Africa has been famous from the times of the Romans, but we have to remember that "knowledge puffeth up" unless applied in charitable acts.[28]

Governments, businesses, research institutes, and universities always find it easier to initiate research on problems than to attempt to change the conditions that bring them about. Thus many tropical-based companies played an important role in supporting research in tropical medicine. The mining companies of South Africa, for example, were more amenable to funding research on tropical diseases than on seriously addresssing the health problems of their employees, most of which would have been rectified, or at least drastically improved, by decent housing, good food, and humane policies.

In South Africa, the government and the Witwatersrand Native Labour Association founded the South African Institute for Medical Research. Opened in 1914, it was required to carry out routine bacteriological examinations and to investigate diseases of workers in the diamond, gold, and coal mines.[29] Naturally, lung diseases such as tuberculosis, silicosis, and pneumonia were their prime concerns. But only silicosis, because it afflicted both black and white miners alike, was considered to be an industrial disease, "a trammel and menace to the gold-producing industry of South Africa." Diseases from which only the African miners suffered were believed to have been imported into the mines. Thus, the South African Institute for Medical Research accepted the views of General Gorgas: The African miner was sick before he entered the mines. According to this view, tuberculosis and pneumonia had been introduced into the mines by "diseased natives"; they were not the product of deplorable working and living conditions in the mines and mining compounds.[30] Strictly speaking, therefore, these diseases were neither the concern nor the responsibility of the mineowners. Nevertheless, as I shall explain later, the assumed presence of these "diseased natives" was a major factor in generating medical activity in South Africa and Southern Rhodesia.

In Britain and the United States, companies involved in tropical trade supported schools of tropical medicine which became centers of research activity. As explained in a previous chapter, the Liverpool School of Tropical Medicine was founded with support from the trading companies of Liverpool. Similarly, in North America, the United Fruit Company played a major role in the founding of the Department of Tropical Medicine in Tulane University and, to a lesser degree, in funding research activity at Harvard.

"We are endeavoring to become the commercial power in tropical America," wrote Isaac Brewer in an article in support of founding a school of tropical medicine in New Orleans, and such a school, he added, would appeal "to the business man who has interests in the torrid zone . . . because it will enable him to obtain the greatest amount of labor from his employees and will reduce the number who have to be invalided home."[31] On July 2, 1911, William Gorgas "made much impression in business and shipping circles," of New Orleans when he spoke to them on the need to establish a school of tropical medicine in the city.[32] So impressed were they that the United Fruit Company immediately gave $5,000 per year for five years to establish a chair in tropical medicine in the Medical Department of Tulane. "New Orleans must then, for its own protection and in order that it may do business with the countries to the south of us, need just such a school," commented *The Times-Democrat* on the day the grant was announced.[33] Three weeks later, Creighton Wellman accepted the Chair of Tropical Medicine, Hygiene, and Preventive Medicine at Tulane University.

Tropical medicine began as a department within the Medical Department of Tulane, but, in 1913, it enhanced its status by becoming the School of Hygiene and Tropical Medicine within the newly named College of Medicine, with Wellman as its Dean. The new School not only included on its staff Dr. Robert Swigart, General Superintendent of the United Fruit Company's Medical Department, but was equipped with the aid of a $25,000 grant from the Company.[34]

Problems at Tulane; Creighton Wellman

The important role that Tulane was to play in tropical medicine was hardly preordained by what happened next. During the Christmas break of 1913, Wellman suddenly resigned, "owing to a protracted illness," according to the University press release. The New Orlean's press smelled a scandal, particularly as Wellman, but not his wife, seemed to be missing from their Charles Street home. But their best sleuths were unable to come up with any better explanation than that he had left town after neglecting to settle certain debts.[35] The truth was far more horrifying: He had eloped with 20-year-old Elsie Dunn, daughter of Seely Dunn, a well-known local railroad magnate engaged at the time in building some lines for the United Fruit Company, whom Wellman had met during a tour of their hospitals. As a result of this rapid departure, the School soon descended into a "chaotic state, with lack of organization every day more and more apparent." Other faculty members were "begged" to give Wellman's hygiene lectures, and, in the end, these classes were placed in the hands of a committee.[36] The whole thing became a wonderful scandal that must have enlivened many a faculty cocktail party.

Tropical medicine is a field filled with larger-than-life figures; none more than Creighton Wellman, the Casanova of tropical medicine (Figure 7.2). Born and raised in Missouri, a graduate of Chicago University and Kansas City Medical College, he first comes to our attention as a physician to an American mission in Bihe, Portuguese West Africa (Angola), where he horrified the missionaries by "going native" on numerous occasions. Realizing that "I didn't know what I was doing," he spent the first winter in the London School of Tropical Medicine, where he gained his Diploma in Tropical Medicine. That experience turned his mind toward research, and in the nine years at Bihe, he published many articles in tropical medicine journals and corresponded regularly with the American Society of Tropical Medicine. "All the important things I know today," he wrote in his autobiography, "I learned in Central Africa. It was there I chose to spend my first youth. And it was there I lived fully." He was to live fully many more times in his career!

Wellman and his wife, Lydia, then moved to London where he studied entomology, met many important establishment figures, and clearly gained

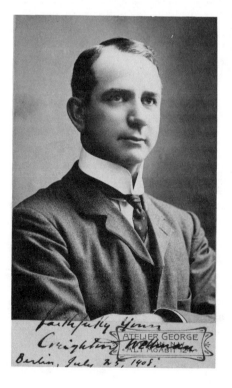

Figure 7.2. Creighton Wellman (Courtesy of the University of Illinois Archives)

prominence in what was still a very small field. After returning to the United States, divorcing his wife, remarrying a golden-haired beauty, and teaching at Oakland Medical College, he was appointed to the Chair at Tulane. He found in Newcomb College (the women's college associated with Tulane) "the largest collection of beautiful girls I ever saw in one place in America." Whether Elsie Dunn was one of them, he does not say, but one night he wrote out his letter of resignation, caught the train to New York at dawn the next morning, changed their names to Cyril and Evelyn Kay-Scott, embarked on the boat to Southampton, and then backtracked to Brazil and Rio.

With money running out and Elsie pregnant, he found work as a book-keeper for a small Singer Sewing Machine Company store in Rio. Discovering that the manager of the store had been embezzling funds, he reported the incident to head office and was immediately promoted to accountant and then auditor for the Brazilian branch of the company! Eventually he was promoted again and settled in Natal as superintendent for the Para District. But that career was not to last. The call of the wilderness, and the interference of Elsie's parents, to whom she had written telling them of her whereabouts, led Wellman (Scott) to move up-country and take up sheep ranching. But fate stepped in again; the sheep flock was wiped out by murrain, and the couple made penniless. Living off his wits for a while, he managed to bluff his way into employment at a manganese mine owned by the International Ore Company of Toronto and before very long found himself manager of the mine.

Growing tired of this life, he returned to New York, where he took up freelance writing without much success. But success began to flow toward Elsie, who found Greenwich Village to her taste. "Bohemianism is like measles," Wellman complained, "it is something you should get over." So he walked out of this long marriage and, after a period in Cape Cod as a real estate manager, moved to Paris where, with much more success, he took up life as a painter. In Paris, he had a passionate love affair with a brilliant and beautiful Frenchwoman, Mademoiselle Elise, who, in addition to being a linguist and a musician, held a doctorate in philology. This period in Paris, was, he wrote, "the emotional highlight of my life." But the affair was not to last; Elise died suddenly, and Wellman found himself back in the United States.

He now opened the Cyril Kay-Scott School of Painting in Sante Fe, New Mexico, which not only flourished but was taken over by Denver University as a summer school, Wellman being appointed Dean of the College of Fine Arts. In Sante Fe he married again, but this, too, was not to last. Toward the end of this extraordinary life, Creighton Wellman, alias Cyril Kay-Scott, wrote his autobiography. Dedicated to his family of 11 children and grand-children, it was called *Life Is Too Short*![37]

The School of Tropical Medicine at Tulane somehow survived the scandal until 1919, when it was absorbed into the Department of Medicine. But tropical medicine did not begin to recover until 1925. Then Aldo Castellani, the Florence-trained physician who had clashed with David Bruce during the infamous sleeping sickness commissions to Uganda in 1902 and 1903, was appointed to head the Department of Tropical Medicine.[38] Three years later, Ernest Faust arrived from Peking as Professor of Parasitology.

Problems at Harvard; the United Fruit Company

With the virtual collapse of the Tulane School of Tropical Medicine, the United Fruit Company turned its eyes north to Boston, their second home and still the site of the Company's head offices. There, in January 1913, following the initiative of Dr. Frederick Shattuck, Professor of Clinical Medicine, Dr. Richard Strong was appointed to the Chair of the Department of Tropical Medicine in the Harvard Medical School.[39]

In many ways the Department was formed in response to the assumed threat that tropical diseases might be carried into the Boston area. With the opening of the Panama Canal, noted a publicity and fund-raising letter, increased trade with Asia and the Americas could be expected. Traders and travelers from these areas, "afflicted with grave pestilential diseases," could very easily introduce them into the United States, it warned, unless the medical personnel in port cities were trained to detect and treat tropical diseases. Recognizing this fact, the letter concluded, Harvard formed its Department of Tropical Medicine. Thus the Harvard Department aimed to instruct its students on "tropical diseases which are likely to be encountered in our cities, especially in the South and East."[40] A few years previously, Dr. Edward Tobey, a graduate of the Liverpool School, who had actually given a course on tropical medicine at Harvard in 1909, used the same arguments in his plea for a Department of Tropical Medicine at Harvard. Our new possessions, he wrote, indicate that "there must be a constant influx of tropical diseases into our so-called temperate zone," brought in by military and diplomatic personnel, travelers, missionaries, and traders.[41] Both Strong and Tobey were fond of stories illustrating diagnostic errors of physicians not trained to recognize tropical diseases. Strong, in particular, was apt to tell the story of a member of Boston's Beacon Hill set, who returned from abroad with malaria, only to be diagnosed as syphilitic by more than one Boston physician!

During the summer of 1914, however, with Tulane in chaos, and anxious to cooperate with Harvard in the study of tropical diseases, the United Fruit Company appointed Strong as Director of its medical laboratories. "We shall," Strong remarked in his acceptance letter, "have the medical and sanitary interests of your company at heart."[42] Strong also planned to establish a small tropical disease hospital in Boston, to cater to returning travelers, missionaries, and those "engaged like the employees, for instance, of the United Fruit Company, in foreign trade."[43] But the Company promised only

$3,000 for such an undertaking, illustrating a general lack of enthusiasm for such a scheme.

More ominously, the United Fruit Company quickly became less than enamored with the Harvard Department. The Company simply could not understand the necessity of trying to carry out research on tropical diseases in a New England city. The Company offered cooperation, but only "if they would do their work in the tropics instead of attempting to make 'water run uphill' and do their work here [Boston]," noted F. R. Hart in an internal memo to the Company Vice-President.[44] The Harvard faculty felt much the same way, and refused to accept any financial responsibility for the Department. To do so, the Dean of Medicine informed Harvard's President, "would endanger the development of other more important departments of the School."[45] By the summer of 1916, the Department was facing financial difficulties. Its endowments had fallen away considerably, and its bank balance had dropped from $24,578 in June 1914, to only $4,159 two years later.[46]

In 1915, somewhat in desperation, Strong applied for an annual $50,000 grant from the Rockefeller Foundation, whose International Health Board was about to move into the field of tropical medicine. The problem of making the tropics productive "through the energy and science of the white man," Harvard noted in its application to the Rockefeller Foundation, "is mainly a problem of medicine." Schools of tropical medicine have been active in Europe, they pointed out, but Tulane has failed, "for reasons doubtless familiar to you." Harvard, they claimed with some justification, has built up "the only real and living school of Tropical Medicine in the Americas."[47] It may seem strange, they agreed, to locate a school of tropical medicine in New England, but, as Strong had noted earlier, research is best done in temperate regions and by sending individuals on research expeditions to the tropics. "It is a well-known fact," he wrote, "that the mental activity of those who live continually in a tropical country tends to be reduced, at least temporarily."[48] But the Harvard brief went one step beyond that modest and understandable claim. "The climate of Boston," they pointed out in obvious reference to New York and Baltimore, "is such that serious work is more easily done during the summer there than in the Eastern Seaboard cities further south." But nothing came of the application; the timing was wrong. The General Education Board was then preoccupied with debates over a new institute of hygiene. The Department at Harvard was saved, in the end, by a $100,000 gift from Mrs. Frederick Shattuck.

But even with that gift, financial and prestige problems continued to haunt tropical medicine at Harvard. In 1922, for example, tropical medicine was demoted from a school to a department within the School of Public Health, which was opened that year with an endowment from the Rockefeller Foundation, and many of its classes were transferred to other departments.[49] In addition, with little support forthcoming from the University, the Department was still forced to seek aid from the United Fruit Company. But the relationship was never a happy one; only a handful of people believed that Boston was a suitable location for such a department. Thus, when Strong died in 1938, the inevitable happened, and the Department of Tropical Medicine was amalgamated with the Department of Tropical Pathology under Tyzzer.[50]

Economic interests also played a key role in tropical medicine on the West Coast of the United States. In 1914, at the University of California, the Hooper Foundation for Medical Research began offering lectures and research classes in tropical medicine. Fourteen years later, Alfred Reed was appointed to the Chair of Tropical Medicine, and in 1929, the Pacific Institute of Tropical Medicine was founded. Funded by a "Shipowners' Fund" to which ten businesses contributed, and modeled on the Hamburg Institute for Tropical Medicine, it was set up "for special service to shipping, import and export business, tourist traffic, missionary activities, and international relations," and "to rendering a type of service to commerce and shipping which is not now available elsewhere on the West Coast." With eyes fixed on the Orient, one of its founding documents reads:

American sanitary and medical science must pave the way for commerce. Students from these countries educated at this Institution and returning to their own countries, mean easier and quicker introduction of American commerce and better international relations.[51]

In the words of Reed, institutes of tropical medicine were the "advance agents of commerce."[52]

NATIVE RESERVOIRS OF DISEASE

During the 1920s, diseases endemic to the African and South American populations were considered important if they interfered with the working efficiency of the laborers. But these endemic diseases could also generate concern if they were assumed to be a health threat to the white population. Such occurred in Southern Africa. There, particularly after the claims by the mining companies that their migrant labor force was diseased even before they were hired to work, white South Africans and Southern Rhodesians had become greatly disturbed by the threat posed to their health by the diseased Africans who surrounded them. Annie Porter warned of the danger in her first report to the South African Institute of Medical Research. The African, she noted, "becomes a potentially dangerous nuisance to non-immune hosts, and a disseminating centre for a number of gastro-intestinal troubles as a result of his promiscuous habits." White children, she warned, were particularly liable to infection by parasites passed to them by their African nurses. Indeed, she concluded, "it seems very probable that infected natives serve as reservoirs of disease."[53] Similar concerns were expressed in Southern Rhodesia. "The native is the reservoir," noted the 1931 report of the Southern Rhodesian Public Health Department, "from which the white man, who is obliged to live in close proximity with him, becomes infected."[54] In that same year, C. T. Loram, Chairman of a South African committee set up to investigate the possibilities of training Africans in medicine, took up the cry. "There are hordes of natives in many centres," the report noted, "who have little chance of medical treatment and the untreated sick become a menace to the rest of the community."[55] The threat came not so much from specific diseases, but from the "disease-ridden natives" who carried these afflictions. The whites began to see themselves as a threatened enclave, surrounded by a sea of ignorant, filthy, diseased, rural black Africans. Clearly, therefore, the health of the rural African population was of concern; action had to be taken.

In South Africa the African population received little or no medical care. Whereas, in the 1920s, 1,500 physicians looked after 1.5 million whites, only 900 served the needs of 4.7 million Africans. To prevent further deterioration in the health of their labor supply, and to guard against the spread of disease from this rural population into the white population, 1,000 extra physicians were needed, according to the Loram Committee. Obviously, the report concluded, that number of physicians could never be met by the two existing medical schools at Johannesburg and Capetown.[56]

The answer, according to C. T. Loram, was to set up a Government Native Medical Service to staff a series of centrally located hospitals surrounded by village nursing stations. African nurses, midwives, and health assistants would obviously be needed, but the central hospitals would also require African physicians to cater exclusively to the needs of the African population. But in that society, as well as among the white settlers of Southern Rhodesia, this issue was clouded by a racial nightmare: the possibility of whites, and particularly their womenfolk, one day being examined, touched, and treated by African physicians. Indeed, the unthinkable had actually happened. In 1927, Dr. Silas Molema, an African physician with a Glasgow medical degree, had actually attended white patients in the Mafeking Hospital. The hospital nurses, with the support of the physicians, went out on strike. Episodes like that could be avoided in the future, Loram hoped, if African physicians were employed only within an African health service.[57]

In South African terms, Loram was a liberal, who believed in equal rights for all "civilized" persons. But Africans, having not yet reached such a lofty pinnacle, "remained a subject race in need of betterment. Therefore, whites had to decide what was best for Africans." He believed that the so-called separate-but-equal black school system in the American South provided a suitable model for South Africa. In 1914, he had spent time at Columbia University Teachers College, visited Tuskegee and other black schools, and had eventually gained his doctoral degree from Columbia for a dissertation on

"The education of the South African Native."[58] In keeping with this philosophy, Loram rejected any notion that the African physician be trained at a lower level than his white counterpart. But a purely African medical school on black American lines required more capital than the South African Government would be willing to invest; thus the Committee recommended that African medical students be trained at a non-European branch of Witwatersrand Medical School in Johannesburg. In the context of South Africa, that involved separate lecture rooms, separate clinical facilities, and, of course, separate patients in separate wards.

The Loram Report allowed the authorities at Witwatersrand University to extricate themselves from a dilemma that had long plagued them. Although viewing themselves as an "Open University," willing to admit nonwhites "on a footing of equality with whites," they nevertheless did their very best to exclude blacks, particularly from their medical school where the problem of ward teaching was a particularly touchy issue.[59] The doctrine of "parallelism" seemed one way to reconcile their "liberal" image with reality. Thus, they submitted a brief to the Loram Committee agreeing to undertake the training of African students, but "in view of the strong prejudices of the community, non-European students cannot be admitted to the existing medical classes for European students; but they must be taught in separate classes."

Edward Thornton, one of the most influential members of the South African medical profession, was totally opposed to the Loram scheme. In 1927, he had represented South Africa in a League of Nations Health Organization study tour of French West Africa, and had been much impressed by what he saw. Native practitioners would be a menace, he argued to the Loram Committee and to a subsequent meeting of the Medical Association of South Africa. They would "combine the wisdom of medical practitioners with the art of witch-doctoring," and would represent an added threat should they attend white patients. Surely, he argued, the medical needs of the natives could best be met by African health assistants, not by "opening the profession to a specifically subsidized invasion by natives."[60]

The Loram Report and Thornton's well-known opposition to it generated a heated debate in South African medical circles. Not unexpectedly, the profession was opposed to any inferior second-grade medical training; "near doctors" were anathema to the medical profession in South Africa as well as everywhere else. Subordinate assistants were one thing, but medically trained Africans implied an inferior grade of physician who would automatically lower the "prestige of the medical service."[61] The Medical Association of South Africa, at their annual general meeting of 1930, played the liberal game. They expressed support for an African medical service and agreed "that no distinction on ground of colour be made in the qualifications of medical men, nurses or health visitors." But equally, they were not in favor of Africans actually receiving this uniformly high standard of medical training at that particular time. A motion to establish a "medical school for the natives" was withdrawn, and instead they requested their Federal Council to formulate proposals for a rural health service.[62]

A year later, after receiving comments from the various branches of the Medical Association, the Federal Council forwarded a final memorandum on the issue to the Union Government. All physicians must receive the same standard of basic medical training, they argued, but with so few Africans prepared for such training no warranty existed for spending money to have them trained in South Africa. There were other problems, too. It would be unfair for the Government, they argued, to provide financial assistance for Africans to train abroad, thus offering them advantages not shared by Europeans. In addition, they noted, white patients and white medical students would face grave difficulties if Africans and coloreds were admitted to teaching hospitals. "It has been suggested," the report noted, "that their hospital training should be undertaken solely in Native wards. It must be remembered, however, that the Native wards of the hospitals furnish very important material for the training of European students." Instead, the Medical Association concluded, all that would be needed to upgrade the quality of African services would be a three-year course in a school for nursing aides.[63]

Meanwhile, the Rockefeller Foundation had reacted in a surprisingly favorable manner to the Loram Report. For nearly ten years they had been pressured by various officials in South Africa to provide financial support for a new African medical school, and so, in 1924, Dr. W. S. Carter, Associate Director of Medical Education for the Rockefeller Foundation, prepared a lengthy report on the issue after spending a month in South Africa. He agreed basically with the views of the Medical Association of South Africa: To train Africans for medicine "seems premature at present"; second-grade African physicians were unacceptable, and Africans should be trained as public health nurses.

It seems to the disinterested observer that a few scholarships, which would enable qualified natives to take the course in medicine in the University of Edinburgh, would be a safe and less costly educational experiment than the establishment of a medical school for them. . . . Nursing education for the natives is more urgently needed at the present time than medical education.[64]

Thus, in 1926, two years before the Loram Report appeared, the Foundation concluded "there is nothing for us to do in South Africa at this time."[65]

With the receipt of the Loram Report, however, Carter now agreed that an African school at Witwatersrand was "worthy of aid from the foundation." Following negotiations with Loram, the Foundation received a request for a £65,000 capital grant. In 1929, a rather suspicious Rockefeller Foundation agreed to the request, forwarding a cablegram to Loram: "Rockefeller Foundation willing to assist seventy thousand pounds for building if proper plan is worked out by government."[66]

But a proper plan was never worked out by the Government; profound changes had taken place in South African politics that made any such scheme unthinkable. In 1920, with a fall in gold prices reducing the profits of the mine companies, the Chamber of Mines threatened to cut costs by hiring even more cheap African labor to replace the better paid semiskilled whites. As a result, the miners struck, to fight for a "White South Africa." Although suppressed by the ruling South African National Party, generally considered to be the party of mineowners and industrialists, the miners had their revenge two years later. In 1924, the Afrikaner's Nationalist Party, led by General Hertzog, supported by the Labour Party of the white industrial workers, won a famous electoral victory on a platform of white privilege and segregation of the races. The Nationalists, with backing from white labor, began to establish a segregated state, and Loram was forced to resign. The Minister of Native Affairs, after reference to what he called the "Carnegie Trust," announced to the House of Assembly in Capetown that "at the present time we are not prepared to go in for that branch at the Witwatersrand University to train native doctors."[67] Loram, however, now Superintendent of Education in Natal, continued to correspond with the Rockefeller Foundation, arguing for patience and displaying an extraordinary degree of optimism. Once the franchise had been removed from the "Cape Natives" (a major concern of the Nationalists), he confidently predicted, the Government "will then salve their consciences by giving the Natives certain material benefits, among which will be more Higher Education, including I honestly believe, training in Medicine and Public Health."[68] Two years later, however, he could only offer hope that a new government would come into power. Meanwhile, he noted, the South African medical profession sees any African physicians as competitors, "and is not above making use of the government's anti-Native feeling to prevent this being done."[69]

In 1934, however, after years of parliamentary stalemate between the Nationalists under Hertzog and the South African Party under Smuts, the two formed a United Party which took over the government, winning the prewar 1938 election in a landslide. With the appointment of Jan Hofmeyr to the Ministry of Education and Health, Dr. Edward Thornton was asked to prepare another report on the contentious issue. As a result, a scheme to train "medical aides" at Fort Hare was initiated. "It would now be possible," Hofmeyr announced, "to proceed with one of the biggest forward steps in native welfare which had been taken for a very considerable time."[70] Thus, in 1936, with a £75,000 gift from the Chamber of Mines, a five-year course for medical aides was established at the South African Native College at Fort Hare. "We are standing at the beginning of a new period, a new era in the development of the Bantu races of the Union" announced Senator F. S. Malan at the foundation stone ceremony, but, he was quick to add: "My message to you is to use what has been given you, to build on what you have got, and not to be tempted to become agitators or mere propagandists, but to be practical in your activities . . . place yourself in the position of the other man, and show restraint, discretion, and judgement."[71]

Over the Limpopo River, the Rhodesians were apprehensive also about their diseased rural Africans, reflecting perhaps the move away from a mining-based economy to an agricultural one. Also, in 1923, following a referendum in which 59.4 percent of the voters, the vast majority of whom were white, voted for self-government, and 40.6 percent for union with South Africa, the country had been formally annexed to the British crown and granted the peculiar status of a "self-governing colony." The British retained responsibility for foreign affairs and for any legislation pertaining to the African populations. In theory, although not in practice, the British remained as "trustees" to the African in Rhodesia.

In 1928, the annual public health reports began to insert a section entitled "Health of the Native." The health of African miners was obviously the major rationale for this section, but the health of those living in the rural African reserves was quickly to become a concern also. "The native is the reservoir," noted the 1931 report "from which the white man, who is obliged to live in close contact with him, becomes infected. As instances may be cited, diseases of the type of malaria, dysentery and various intestinal worms, such as *Schistosoma*." This realization that the Africans represented a serious health hazard, together with the realization that "broadly speaking, the problem of the health of the native is as yet untouched," galvanized the whites into action. There must be, they argued, "a systematic medical control of the natives." The country should be divided into medical units, the medical authorities argued, each with a central hospital run by Europeans, ringed by dispensaries manned by low-salaried African orderlies. And, in the true spirit of the times, the reports noted that "it is considered desirable that the native should bear the cost of his medical care."[72]

By the mid-1930s, the white settlers of Rhodesia had opened 25 African base hospitals. "Apart from all humanitarian reasons and to place it at its lowest level," William Blackie, Director of the Public Health Laboratory in Salisbury, wrote, "it is reasonable to regard this enterprise as an insurance for the protection of the health of the European and an investment by the nation for the better maintenance of its labour supplies in quality and quantity."

I am no sentimental negrophilist. . . . But no matter how much we may dislike it, the native will not permit us either to ignore or forget him unless under penalty of extreme peril to ourselves, since, for a great number of the diseases which worry us, the native provides the infected reservoir. . . . If I can succeed in awakening the public conscience to this regard, I shall feel that I have performed a greater service to the European community than to the native people."[73]

One of the African diseases that seemed to threaten the health of the white community in South Africa and Southern Rhodesia was bilharzia.

BILHARZIA: A THREAT TO THE WHITE POPULATION

The public health authorities in Rhodesia had long expressed concern about bilharzia. "This is a serious disease, which is more or less endemic to Rhodesia," the 1921 public health report noted, although treatment of white school children by tartar emetic, they noted, "have robbed it of much of its danger." But, with "independence," the overriding concern with the well being of the white population became very explicit. Bilharzia, the 1923 report noted, "seems well under control among Europeans, though of course the natives are commonly infected." But these diseased Africans were a menace, the report noted, as they prevented the whites from enjoying their right to swim in safety! Attacking the disease, the same report noted, "might help to free the country of infection and enable us to bathe safely." Two years later, an inspection of white school children revealed that bilharzia was not spreading among them, only 24 cases being noted. But in 1927, a 7.5 percent prevalence of the disease among the boys of Prince Edward School, Salisbury, was said to be "disquieting."[74]

In 1927, William Blackie, a helminthologist from the London School of Tropical Medicine and future Director of the Rhodesian Public Health Laboratory, arrived in Rhodesia with a Rhodesian Research Fellowship to investigate helminth infections in the colony. A preliminary survey of white children revealed that bilharzia was the most serious helminth disease in the country, and, given the threat posed by African "reservoirs of disease," a massive helminth survey of the population in the African reserves was clearly called for. His 1930 survey of the African population revealed both *Schistosoma mansoni* and *S. haematobium* to be present, with the prevalence of the latter reaching over 20 percent in some areas.[75]

With an African population of over one million, and a white population which then stood at 48,400, the contact between these "diseased natives" and the white population had increased, according to Blackie. "Since the Native is slow to adopt the sanitary measures of the white man," he wrote, "there must necessarily be increased opportunities for acquiring his diseases." But the presence of widely spaced infected Africans, and the danger of infection from *Schistosoma matthei*, another species of schistosome endemic in cattle, sheep, baboons, and monkeys, rendered control difficult. But "a considerable amount of schistosomiasis could be prevented, particularly amongst European children," he concluded, by treatment of these children and "by the destruction of snails within a mile or two radius of the towns and townships."[76]

Bilharzia was also well known in South Africa. Dr. G. A. Turner, medical officer to the Witwatersrand Native Labour Association, first discovered the high prevalence of bilharzia among mine recruits. "There is probably no disease," he wrote in 1910, "which causes the inhabitants of the Province of Mozambique so much distress and anxiety as bilharziosis. Every evil under the sun, amongst others impotency in men and sterility in women, is attributed to it." Over 20 percent of those recruited from Mozambique, Lake Nyasa region, and Zululand, contained eggs in their urine, Turner reported, while liver autopsies revealed rates approaching 50 percent.[77]

With the formation of the South African Institute for Medical Research, the parasitologist Annie Porter took responsibility for surveying African laborers for protozoan and helminth parasites. In 1919, she began a 12-year study of bilharzia. Although forced into many mistakes by her inability to identify the snail intermediate hosts, and to distinguish the human schistosome larvae from those of other schistosomes, she was basically correct in describing the distribution of the disease in the Union. Bilharzia was endemic in the Transvaal, she noted, roughly north of the Mafeking–Pretoria line; in Natal; and in the Cape Province, east of the Drakensburg escarpment and north of the Sundays River and Port Elizabeth (Figure 7.3).[78] In 1931, she married and left South Africa to become a research assistant at MacDonald College, affiliated with McGill University in Montreal, where her husband, Dr Fantham, had gained an appointment. With her departure, research on bilharzia came to a halt, and for the next 18 years the Department of Parasitology of the Institute limited itself to routine examinations of mine workers' urine and feces.[79] But no attempts were made to treat the mine workers. According to a government pamphlet on the disease published in 1926, any treatment campaigns would have been uneconomic and impracticable, given the rapid turnover of miners drawn from an inexhaustible supply.[80]

But, in the story of bilharzia, South Africa is unique. Surveys during the 1920s revealed that the disease was a problem among the children of poor Boer farmers in the Transvaal, representing the only Europeans in Africa to be seriously threatened by the disease. In South Africa, bilharzia is a disease of both black and white. But whereas the South African Government and mineowners took no action in regard to Africans infected with the disease, the response was immediate when white children were found to be infected.

To the recently elected government dominated by the Nationalist Party intent on establishing a "white aristocracy" of workers, the presence of disease-ridden poor whites, their own kith and kin, whose children carried bilharzia, was a matter of urgent concern.[81] In 1927, Afrikaner schoolchildren were collected together in "summer camps" at various sites throughout the

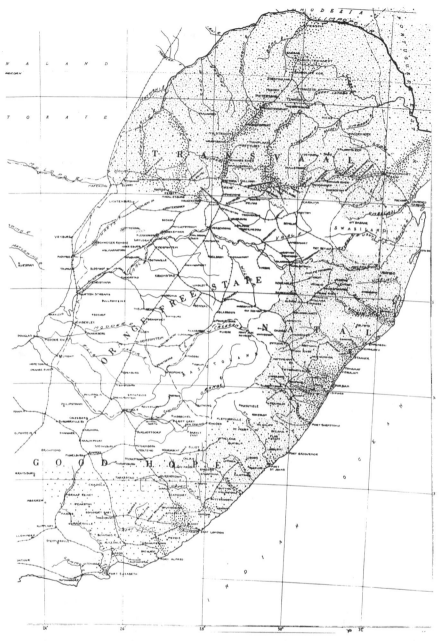

Figure 7.3. Distribution of bilharzia in South Africa. From Anne Porter, *The Larval Trematoda Found in Certain South African Mollusca* (Courtesy of the South African Institute of Medical Research)

Transvaal, and given the standard intravenous injections of tartar emetic. By 1929, a Transvaal Bilharzia Committee had been formed to oversee the "summer camps," to set up educational and publicity programs, and to post English and Afrikaans signs at swimming holes warning children of the danger in the water. By 1932, with enthusiasm for the treatment camps in decline, the Committee decided to press for bilharzia-free swimming pools in the schools of white farm children in which the water could also be used for irrigation. Although in the Transvaal a brief and unsuccessful attempt was made to open a similar camp for African children, in Natal, where white farmers were more wealthy than their Transvaal counterparts and bilharzia was limited to the African population, no attempt was made to copy the Transvaal example. Bilharzia would be attacked only if it infected the white population.[82]

If the South Africans were unwilling to spend money to treat Africans infected with bilharzia, they were certainly not prepared to attack the economic factors that increased the seriousness of bilharzia and other diseases. But, again, a different set of rules operated for the white community. In 1927, the year in which summer treatment camps opened in the Transvaal, the Nationalist–Labour government and the Dutch Reform Church requested the assistance of the Carnegie Foundation in an investigation of "poor whitism." The Carnegie Commission, reporting in 1932, painted a picture of landless rural "bywoners," – poor settlers with small land holdings, unskilled laborers, and pioneer-type nomads. Usually of Dutch-German extraction, poorly educated if not illiterate, speaking only Afrikaans, and weakened by disease, they remained isolated from the mainstream of European progress, psychologically unable to adjust to modern conditions.[83]

Bilharzia, or "human redwater disease" as it was known locally, was reported to be one of the major health problems among the children of poor whites. "We have no hesitation whatever in stating," the report noted, "that, as a school disease, 'red water' ranks but slightly inferior, as far as its debilitating power is concerned, to hookworm disease and malaria."[84] But the recommended solution to these health problems, including bilharzia, was not to be insecticides, molluscicides, or tarter emetic. "Poverty and unsatisfactory diet," the report concluded, "generally had a more detrimental effect than malaria or other diseases." The economic system, not disease, was the root cause of all other problems. The system created poverty and ignorance among the poor whites, which in turn led to malnutrition, and the weakening of resistance to disease.[85] Even though the children of these poor whites were treated with tarter emetic, the South African Government was made aware that the root problems were economic. For the first and only time, a European-styled government set out to eliminate a bilharzia health problem by economic and social means. They introduced a series of measures aimed at increasing the prosperity of the "poor white" Afrikaner community and eliminating the economic threat posed by the equally unskilled African. These included farm credit programs, improvements in farm marketing, inducements for farm resettlements, and recognition of Afrikaans as an official language, thereby opening up new opportunities for unilingual Afrikaners.[86]

By the 1920s, concern over the health of various indigenous populations within the British and American empires had grown. But most of this concern was self-serving; it was driven by the belief that unhealthy workers were inefficient and that "diseased natives" could threaten the health of the white population. Also, the notion that, however self-serving the motives, this foreign investment in the tropics had nevertheless brought nothing but improved medical benefits to the employees of the companies involved, needs to be tempered. Profits determined the degree of such benefits, and the conditions in which some of these workers lived and worked were often such as to encourage the spread of disease. But these companies did encourage training and research in tropical medicine. By the 1920s, four centers of tropical medicine in Britain and the United States were supported by business interests: Liverpool, by various Liverpool trading concerns; Tulane and, to a lesser extent, Harvard, by the United Fruit Company; and the Department of Medical Zoology at the Johns Hopkins School of Hygiene and Public Health, more indirectly, by the Rockefeller Foundation. Also, in South Africa, the mining companies had helped form the Institute of Medical Research.

Bilharzia grew in importance during the 1920s. New irrigation schemes in Puerto Rico and the Sudan created conditions for the spread of the host snails, and, in Southern Africa it became one of the endemic diseases that threatened the health of the white community. Tartar emetic and copper sulfate were the usual answers, but when the "poor whites" of the Transvaal were found infected with the disease, the problem was attacked economically. Only then were they prepared to admit that diseases were not simply induced by pathogens. But for the first and only time, those suffering from bilharzia were white, not black.

8

The 1930s: Empires in transition

By the beginning of the 1930s, tropical medicine had entered the doldrum years. With the exception of programs supported by the International Health Division, neither the British nor the American Government showed much willingness to invest in the discipline and continue the fight against disease; there were enough problems at home. But, by the beginning of World War II, imperial policies of both the British and American governments began to change, and, as a result, the war against tropical diseases recovered its momentum.

THE BRITISH EMPIRE

Financial restraints of the penny-pinching British Empire naturally curtailed any excessive expenditures on medical matters. Between 1918 and 1929, the British Government invested only £15.84 million in the colonies, representing 0.028 percent of the gross national product (Table 8.1). Although the number of African hospitals gradually increased during this period, most of them were supported by the missionary societies. From the records collected by these hospitals, however, colonial officials began to learn of the diseases endemic to the Africans themselves, rather than simply those that had long been known to be a threat to Europeans. Bilharzia can be numbered among them.

In Nigeria, for example, where the first case of bilharzia was noted in 1908, the disease was thought to be more widespread than the records indicated, but still not a serious problem. These records were assumed to be unreliable because, as noted in 1910, the Nigerian "does not feel prompted to seek medical aid." Similarly, when, in 1922, the medical authorities of Uganda first noted bilharzia, they reported "very little suffering," and on those grounds assumed the disease to be more widespread than the health returns indicated. The Nigerian report of 1922 was the first to note any physical deterioration and pain associated with the disease; a Uganda survey of the same year noted also that suffering and disability did occur, and concluded that "economically,

Table 8.1. *British expenditure on the colonies, 1918–39*

Year	GNP[a]	Colonial expenditure[a]	%GNP
1918	5467	0.16	0.003
1919	5583	0.28	0.005
1920	5894	0.77	0.013
1921	4779	3.06	0.064
1922	4206	1.98	0.047
1923	3975	4.73	0.119
1924	4005	0.72	0.018
1925	4266	0.77	0.018
1926	4156	0.83	0.020
1927	4399	0.70	0.016
1928	4426	0.89	0.020
1929	4512	0.95	0.021
Total 1918–29	55,668	15.84	0.028
1930	4368	1.97	0.045
1931	4046	2.23	0.055
1932	3901	1.68	0.043
1933	3931	1.97	0.050
1934	4167	1.46	0.035
1935	4394	1.85	0.042
1936	4593	1.93	0.042
1937	4822	1.06	0.022
1938	5085	1.93	0.038
1939	5414	3.03	0.056
Total 1930–9	44,721	19.11	0.042

[a]Figures in £millions.
Source: Modified from S. Constantine, *The Making of British Colonial Development Policy*, 1914–40, p. 275.

it [bilharzia] must be viewed with concern."[1] But, beyond these few remarks, nothing was done about the disease in either of these two countries.

But records from Nyasaland indicated a more serious problem. Prior to the 1920s, only a handful of cases were reported each year. Indeed, in many hospitals bilharzia was simply subsumed under the category of a "fluke" disease. In 1922, however, 131 African outpatients were diagnosed with the parasite, a number that steadily increased during the decade to reach 230 by 1924, and 736 two years later. By 1931, with over 4,000 cases reported, bilharzia was, for the first time, listed as one of the major African diseases, with a prevalence of 8.27 percent.[2] But this increase in numbers may not have represented any actual increase in the prevalence of the disease during the decade. It was more likely the result of a series of surveys carried out by two individual medical officers in the protectorate. The first survey occurred in 1922 when Captain W. Dye of the Royal Army Medical Corps found 75 percent of the population in the North Nyasa District, near the shore of Lake Nyasa, to be infected with *Schistosoma haematobium*.[3] Then, at the end of the decade, a Dr. W. Gopsill found *S. haematobium* in the Lower Shire District and, in a very crude publication, claimed that *Melanoides tuberculata* must be the snail host of both schistosome species because it was one of the common snails in the region and was found to harbor forked-tailed cercariae.[4]

These amateurish surveys of African health, carried out by British medical officers with the necessary drive and enthusiasm, seem typical of British activity in Africa at that time. Any serious research was left to the pundits back in London and medical researchers in the white communities of Southern Rhodesia and South Africa. In addition, any costly campaigns to rid Africans of disease were out of the question, given the financial constraints of the Empire. Neither was "trusteeship" alone a sufficient reason to break these financial shackles, as an earlier helminth survey of Nyasaland had already indicated.

This 1912 survey of the North Nyasa District was carried out in response to what was seen as the inefficiency of laborers from the Ankonde Tribe. As expected, the survey revealed a very high incidence of hookworm disease, which had long been blamed for this inefficiency. But because, as the author noted, very few of the tribesmen seemed "much the worse for it," he concluded that "the inferiority of the Ankonde as workers cannot possibly be ascribed to ankylostoma infection." The Ankonde were racially immune to hookworm, the report claimed, and thus their inefficiency could not be attributed to hookworm. Clearly, therefore, the report went on to say, there was little reason to embark upon a costly and extensive campaign against hookworm because, in this case, any money spent on a campaign would not be repaid by an increase in worker efficiency. Concern for the well-being of the African population was not a sufficient reason to initiate a health campaign. Instead, the report concluded, there should be no policy change; the British should continue gradually to improve African sanitation and treatment of the more serious cases in African hospitals.[5]

In the 1930s, however, British expenditure on the colonies increased to £19.11 million (Table 8.1). In terms of the GNP, this represented a 50 percent increase over the expenditure of the previous decade. This increase reflected the impact of the first Colonial Development Act which received Royal Assent in 1929. But this act was not directed at colonial development per se, but was linked to British problems at home. Concern over mounting unemployment in Britain during the 1920s led some of those who did not subscribe to the prevalent view of British colonial policy as outlined by Lord Lugard to argue that a policy of colonial development, involving the spending of British money, would create demands for British goods and thereby help reduce this unemployment. This idea was consistently opposed by the Colonial Office whose duty, according to one official, "is primarily to watch over the interests of individual colonies, and not directly to foster British trade at their expense." It was opposed also by those in support of British trusteeship, to whom the Empire was not, in the words of the *Manchester Guardian*, "an estate to be exploited for the benefit of the British taxpayer."[6]

But the most significant resistance came from the British Treasury. As unemployment increased in the early 1920s, and as demand for British exports declined, the Treasury put in place a policy of financial restraint. According to this traditional policy, when times are tough, as they were during the 1920s, it becomes necessary to consume less and spend less. It would be, therefore, financially irresponsible to spend money on colonial development.

With the return of Baldwin's Tory government in 1924, however, L. S. Amery, a supporter of imperial development, became Colonial Secretary. He set up the Empire Marketing Board to encourage consumption of imperial products, and advocated imperial economic development as a long-term answer to Britain's economic problems. Once again the Treasury opposed the idea, but in the 1929 election campaign, in which both the Liberal and Labour parties viewed unemployment as the major issue, the Treasury acquiesced to a new policy. Colonial development became the Tory's answer to the opposition's criticisms of continuing high unemployment. Immediately before the election, the Prime Minister pledged support for a colonial development fund. But to no avail; the Government was defeated, and the second Labour Party Government came into power.

The new Government immediately rushed through the first Colonial Development Act "for the purpose of aiding and developing agriculture and industry in the colony or territory, and thereby promoting commerce with or industry in the United Kingdom." But there was no comprehensive plan of colonial development; the Colonial Development Advisory Committee, set up to advise the government on the schemes to be supported, merely reacted in an ad hoc fashion to projects submitted to them by the individual colonies. Most historians now agree that colonial development per se was not the goal of the act, but a means of reducing the high unemployment levels in Britain. By granting money for colonial development with the stipulation that all orders be placed in Britain and all goods be British made, the government believed that British exports would be stimulated and employment generated for British workers. As the Colonial Secretary Lord Passfield, the former Sidney Webb, noted during the reading of the bill in the House of Lords, "The principal motive for the introduction of this measure is connected with the lamentable condition of unemployment in this country, and this is an attempt to stimulate the British export trade."[7] This interpretation is supported also by the way the money was spent. In the 11 years the act operated, 1929–40, fully

30 percent of the money was spent on internal transportation and communications and 10 percent on water supply and water power – two areas that would require importing much British material. Agriculture and fisheries, on the other hand, were granted only 6 percent and 2 percent of the total budget, respectively.[8] The makeup of the Advisory Committee also supports this interpretation. Chaired by B. Blackett, a Director of de Beers and the Bank of England, it consisted mainly of businessmen as well as Ernest Bevan, then General Secretary of the Transport and Allied Workers Union.

On the other hand, however, the second highest amount, 16 percent, was spent on public health, an area that could hardly be expected to enhance British exports to a great degree. But even here British interests were involved. At the first meeting of the Advisory Committee, Lord Passfield warned them that schemes must be "economically advantageous," and then added: "I do not mind what form the advance takes, but even if it never came to a money advantage, if it did yield an advantage to the Colony's public welfare it may be worth doing even if it pays no pecuniary dividend at all." Thus, as he said later in the meeting, with obvious reference to public health, "If we can increase the productivity of the African natives, they will buy more things from us."[9] Blackett, too, saw public health in the same light, and may have been responsible for its relatively high profile.

In the 11 years the act operated, approximately £9 million in grants and loans was recommended. A little over £6.6 million of this was spent, however, representing only £600,000 per year. Most colonies seemed to have received a small slice of the pie for hospital and sanitation schemes, although the amounts were always small. Nyasaland, for example, used the money to build new hospitals, child welfare clinics, and rural dispensaries, and to improve village water supplies.[10]

This was an empire on the cheap, and, in such an empire, any involvement in tropical medicine was necessarily limited, unless, of course, finances could be provided by the Rockefeller Foundation.[11] And behind any scheme that was approved lurked the British unemployed. As late as 1939, for example, a sleeping-sickness survey in Bechuanaland was granted special permission to use locally obtained non-British transport, with a warning for the future that "as far as possible, only vehicles of British manufacture should be obtained."[12] As Constantine has so correctly concluded, "Whatever the undoubted value of aid to the colonies themselves, the primary function of the Colonial Development Act was to ease the economic difficulties of the United Kingdom."[13]

THE AMERICAN "EMPIRE"

Tropical medicine in the United States also passed through a lean period in the 1920s and early 1930s. This decline in interest is illustrated by the activities of the American Society of Tropical Medicine. By World War I, the American

Society of Tropical Medicine had clearly established itself as a successful, albeit very small, professional body that included among its members almost all the eminent figures in the discipline. But after the war, the Society seemed to stagnate. In 1921, for example, it had an active membership of 107, the same as it had been in 1909. With the launching of the *American Journal of Tropical Medicine* in 1921, however, its membership began a slow climb to reach 181 in 1925, 252 in 1930, and 412 in 1935.[14] Even so, with the flush of empire diminished, the First World War at an end, and finally the depression, there seemed little interest in the subject, and financial support was almost nonexistent. In an attempt to counter this disturbing trend, the leaders in the field called together a conference, sponsored by the Leonard Wood Memorial (a fund directed at leprosy in the Philippines), to formulate plans for a revival of the Society's fortunes and a general attack on tropical diseases.

The membership agreed to found the American Academy of Tropical Medicine whose role was not only to educate the public, further knowledge, and be a general source of expertise, but more significantly to receive research funds and administer research grants. Membership of this elite 50-member Academy, founded in February 1934 with Theobald Smith as President, was restricted to any U.S. citizen "who has conducted and published meritorious original investigations," and "whose scientific interest is, to a definite degree, devoted to one or more problems in this field."[15]

To meet their financial goals, the Academy turned initially, without success, to the Leonard Wood Memorial. But although the Directors of the Wood Memorial refused financial help, they did offer some timely advice by suggesting that the Academy set up a special fund-raising branch: the American Foundation of Tropical Medicine. It should be made very clear, Perry Burgess, President of the Wood Memorial warned, that the American Foundation of Tropical Medicine would only solicit funds, whereas the Academy – the experts – would administer them. No medical men, he argued, should be members of the board of the Foundation. In addition, he warned, because philanthropy was no longer as popular as it had once been, specific financial details had to accompany all requests for financial help.[16] Armed with this advice, Earl McKinley, Secretary of the Academy, forwarded a dossier to all institutions with a potential interest in tropical medicine, asking for their views on the matter.[17]

In 1935, after the joint meeting of the American Society and American Academy of Tropical Medicine in St. Louis, described by one enthusiast "as one of the great moments in the development of tropical medicine in the United States," the Foundation was created. Presided over by Perry Burgess, it included the presidents of Johns Hopkins, Columbia, and the University of California, together with numerous American business executives such as Harvey Firestone and Francis Hart of the United Fruit Company.

At its first meeting, Mr. Pierce of Pierce and Hedrich presented what he called "a carefully worked out case for tropical medicine." Tropical medicine represented an appealing case, he wrote, "one of the great unfinished tasks in the field of medical science." But to obtain funds, he warned, it was necessary to be very specific in terms of goals and needs.[18] Unfortunately, the members seemed unable to follow this advice. "The research projects submitted by the members of the Academy are, for the most part, entirely too vague," the progress report of the Foundation noted one year later, "they do not appear to be specific enough to warrant their use for the purpose of raising funds for their support." In addition, the report continued in its forthright manner, there were so few research projects submitted "that perhaps there is not the *real need for support of research* in tropical medicine among American workers that we have been led to believe there was." What we need now, the report urged, was a "*really concerted effort.*" It was not sufficient to request "\$5,000 for research on malaria," it warned; fund raising needed "*detailed reasons*" for "*the needs.*"[19] Clearly, from the tone of the report, tropical medicine in the United States and its empire was enjoying no better support than in the British Empire. These were not vintage years.

During the 1930s, however, both the British and American governments faced mounting criticisms over the nature of their respective empires. By the end of the decade, partly as a result of these criticisms, both governments began to change their policies toward the tropical territories which they controlled, and, in the process, the problems of tropical diseases again became important to them. Thus, whether in Africa or Latin America, the fortunes of tropical medicine again appeared to be on the upswing.

BRITISH CRITICS OF EMPIRE

During the 1930s, those who realized that the British Empire of wardship had no future, grew more persistent in their criticisms. The comments of the ex-colonial French administrator Hubert Deschamps were as applicable to the British Empire as they were to the French. "Like parents who refuse to see their children grow up," he wrote, "one administered from day to day without thinking about the evolution that one ought to be conducting."[20] Consisting of renegade colonial officials, missionaries, and a small knot of Labour Party parliamentarians, these critics were united in a belief that British influences had been destructive, and that the dual mandate needed to be supplanted by a single mandate: the preparation of the colonies for self-government.[21] The 1930s were, in the words of Constantine,

a watershed during which the morality of colonialism and the record of Britain's achievements were subjected to fierce criticisms at home and abroad. The stability of the empire was also threatened, initially from within by social disturbances and burgeoning nationalist movements. . . . Protective trusteeship and the civilising mission in the colonies had sown economic stagnation, social unrest and political dissent.[22]

A group of British academicians from Oxford University, where colonial history had a rich tradition, were particularly vocal in their criticisms. In 1920, Reginald Coupland was appointed Beit Professor of Colonial History at Oxford. He became a leading proponent of a multiracial commonwealth, in which the African nations would become full members of a British-centered club, not tools of imperialist economics.[23] Coupland and others began pressing for an inquiry into the conditions in British Africa, and eventually, with financial backing from the Carnegie Foundation, Malcolm Hailey (Figure 8.1), then Governor of the United Provinces after a long career in the Indian Civil Service, was asked to direct such a survey. To gather the data, Hailey brought together a team of British researchers, among whom Dr. E. B. Worthington (Figure 8.2), a Cambridge University zoologist with African experience, reported on science and medicine.[24] Worthington's report, published separately as *Science in Africa*, provided the basic scientific and medical information for Hailey's more famous *African Survey*. Both authors, as will be discussed in later chapters, called for reforms in all areas of British administration of Africa, and an end to the idea of colonial self-sufficiency.

The year 1938 became pivotal in the history of the British Empire. In that year, not only were Hailey's *African Survey*, and Worthington's *Science in Africa* published, but also William MacMillan's fiercely critical *Africa Emergent* appeared. The British public had been made painfully aware of the validity of

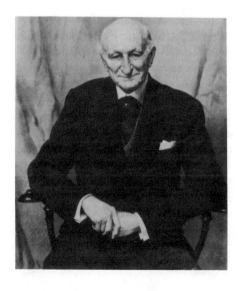

Figure 8.1. Lord Hailey. Reprinted with permission from E. Worthington, *The Ecological Century* (Courtesy of E. Barton Worthington)

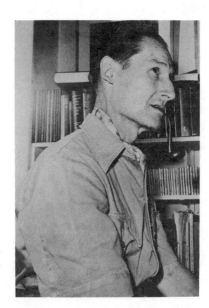

Figure 8.2. E. Barton Worthington. Re-printed with permission from E. Worthing-ton, *The Ecological Century* (Courtesy of E. Barton Worthington)

these criticisms by the West Indian riots of the previous year. These riots, leaving 39 dead and nearly 200 injured, had not only shattered the compla-cency of the British toward their Empire, but had seemed to provide a cogent vindication of MacMillan's earlier book, *Warning from the West Indies*. Pub-lished in 1936, and immediately republished in Penguin paperback after the riots, MacMillan warned that unless the British Government took responsibil-ity for a complete reconstruction of West Indian society, the poverty, igno-rance, and disease on the islands would lead to massive economic and social destruction. In 1938, he repeated the same message for Africa. The Imperial Government, MacMillan warned, must immediately take financial and politi-cal responsibility for the economic, social, and educational development of Africans. The "untouched problem of health," MacMillan claimed, was one of the major "roots of backwardness," and almost all Africans were infested with some type of intestinal worm. In particular, he warned of the dangers of bilharzia in South Africa. "As far south as Pretoria," he reminded his readers, "and anywhere north or east of Johannesburg, bathing . . . carries the risk of bilharzia," and everywhere poor nutrition prevents them [from] withstanding the onset of disease.[25]

Also in the year 1938, Malcolm MacDonald, son of Ramsey MacDonald, was appointed Colonial Secretary in Neville Chamberlain's Tory Govern-ment. He, perhaps more than any other person, was responsible for the birth of the new Empire and a new Colonial Office. The old Empire of indirect rule, trusteeship, and colonial self-sufficiency collapsed as the Colonial Office redefined its role. It became an agent of social and political development; colonies were no longer to be left to manage their own affairs within the crippling limitations of their own budgets, but were to be "developed" with financial aid from the British Treasury. Clearly, with disease viewed as a major impediment to African development, tropical medicine could not but profit from this new approach to empire.

The Colonial Development and Welfare Act (1940)

In February 1940, only a few weeks after the debacle of Dunkirk, the Colonial Office presented a draft statement to the Cabinet. "All was not well with the Colonial Empire," it read, "we need an active policy of colonial development."[26] A day later, it forwarded a telegram to all the colonial governments. "The Government proposes," it read, "to proceed with their policy of development as far and as fast as the exigencies of the time permit. His Majesty's Government are trustees for the well-being of the peoples of the Colonial Empire. . . . The primary aim of Colonial policy is to protect and advance the interests of the inhabitants of the Colonies." The old principle of colonial self-sufficiency is to be revised, it warned, and in its place the colonies will be eligible for a yearly grant of £5 million from the British Treasury with an additional £500,000 available for research.[27]

On May 21, 1940, Malcolm MacDonald rose before Parliament to present the Colonial Development and Welfare Bill, "to make provision for the development of the resources of Colonies, Protectorates, Protected States and Mandated Territories, and the welfare of their peoples." Progress in the past has been hampered by financial restraints, he informed the House, but this bill "breaks new ground. It establishes the duty of taxpayers in this country to contribute directly and for its own sake towards the development of the colonial peoples." Economic development including health and education would be given priority, he stressed, and to this end an Advisory Committee on Colonial Development and Welfare and a separate Advisory Committee on Colonial Research would be established. "It is our destiny," he concluded, "to complete the great work for our Colonial peoples to which we set our hands long ago."[28]

The bill met overwhelming approval in what can only be described as a rather guilt-ridden House of Commons and House of Lords. Creech-Jones, speaking for the Labour Party, spoke of the end of "platitudinous talk about trusteeship," and the importance of research, which, up to then, had been paid for by Rockefeller money. "If we are Empire builders," he informed the House, "we should appreciate the importance of research and be prepared to pay for the fact." This bill "is our chance," he noted. Sir Francis Freemantle of St. Albans waved the flag of Tory paternalism with his remark that "we are the parents of these young and backward nations," and urged the government to develop an educational system that "will not spoil them, but will develop their minds." A few were less complimentary. Colonel Wedgewood reminded the House that a war was going on; this is a "prewar bill," he complained, "and every other speaker also seems to have partaken in this playacting." Mr. Stephen of Glasgow Camlachie saw other factors at work. This money, he was sure, would be used "to try to improve the holdings of British Imperialism in these Colonies, and very little of it will go to minister to the needs of native peoples." The colonies, he argued, were really plantations for the British, and the money would be used as a subsidy to find markets for the British ruling class. But Mr. Stephen was a member of the radical left; the vast majority supported the bill which gained Royal Assent on July 17, 1940.[29]

The bill was received with rapture and enthusiasm by some of the colonies. The Gold Coast Youth Conference felt "a deep sense of appreciation to his Majesty's Government," while the *Sierra Leone News* wrote of "an outburst of gratitude everywhere among Colonial subjects," that "will rivet still more tightly than ever the bond of loyalty between the Empire and all who will be helped by these provisions." But the *Bahamas Tribune* was almost guilty of bad taste: "One feels like bellowing 'Britannia Rule' so the whole world might hear."[30] As Earl de la Warr said in the House of Lords a few years later, "We in this country should be feeling that we have given to the world a new conception of the word 'Empire,' and a new meaning to the word 'Imperialism.'"[31]

AMERICAN CRITICS OF EMPIRE

The British were not the only people to hear that their empire needed to be changed. Also during the 1930s, although to a lesser degree, the American "empire" came in for much criticism. Dollar diplomacy and "tutelage," Secretary Ickes remarked, had often created "more widespread misery and destitution and far more unemployment . . . than at any previous time."[32] Critics pointed out also that any medical benefits enjoyed by the employees of American companies in the tropics had been only an accidental by-product of their business activities.

In Puerto Rico, for example, the self-serving propaganda of the 1920s had been replaced by a more realistic picture. Small landholders, the American public now learned, had been forced to sell out to the large American companies with their centralized sugar factories; subsistence crops had been replaced by cash crops; and, with inflated prices of imported food, the peasant had been driven to near starvation. Puerto Rico, Luis Muñoz Marin agonized, "is a land of beggars and millionaires, of flattering statistics and distressing realities. More and more it becomes a factory worked by peons, fought over by lawyers, bossed by absent industrialists, and clerked by politicians."[33]

Even the medical system of these companies, praised so lavishly during the 1920s, appeared now to be seriously flawed. A Brookings Institute report of

1930 included an interview with the Puerto Rican sociologist, J. C. Rosario. The company hospitals, he told the interviewers, are

established for the purpose of giving medical attendance to workers. The attendance is free to all laborers. If their families need medical attendance they get it, but for this they have to pay a fee. If they do not have money, the factory pays and then makes a small weekly discount from the laborers wages until the account is settled.[34]

In addition, the cane worker was forced to pay 50 cents per week for any medicines prescribed for him. But the average cane worker received less than $1 per day in the 1920s. It was now becoming apparent that American humanitarian medicine was delivered at a price that represented a considerable fraction of the laborer's wage. And for those living beyond the tentacles of the sugar, coffee, and tobacco companies, the situation was even worse. "No physicians ever come here," said one *jibaro*; "What are we going to do, Señor?" said another, "the poor have to resign themselves to their fate."[35]

But one can also argue that these companies not only did very little to better the health conditions of the Latin American poor, but actually made their conditions worse. They did so by creating social conditions in which diseases flourished. Only the company town with its clubs for "Yankees," its golf courses, and bowling alleys were sanitized. Alongside them lay the civil towns, with open sewers, bars, and whorehouses. Puerto Rico itself had become, according to Luis Marin, "Uncle Sam's second largest sweatshop," and sweatshops harbor ill health, however many hospitals are attached to them.[36] As "an eminent authority on tropical diseases" (I assume it was Bailey Ashford) told the interviewers of the Brookings Institute:

The problem here is fundamentally economic and not sanitary. No doubt improvements in water supplies, sewage disposal . . . will have an appreciable effect, as will also the systematic work in rural sanitation being carried out in connection with the hookworm campaign. But I fear we shall not see any great fall in the death rate as long as 1. there is an excess of labor with a big proportion of the people unemployed a great part of the year; and so long as 2. food costs are more here than in the United States, while the wage of the common laborer averages less than a dollar a day. Under such conditions insufficient food, an unbalanced diet, and crowded housing will remain, and T.B., malnutrition, intestinal and other infections will take their toll.[37]

By the late 1930s, the Americans, like the British, were poised to renew their war against tropical diseases. But this change did not come about in response to these criticisms but rather as a result of new policies toward Latin America, initiated by the Roosevelt administration. In this new policy, to quote historian Bryce Wood, "tutelary democracy began to be regarded as inconsistent with the principle of self-determination championed by Wilson at Versailles, and the use of marines for the protection of business enterprise came to be opposed by influential leaders in both the major political parties."[38] The American empire, like the British, was about to change.

Gradually the United States began to look for other ways than force to protect American lives, property, and business investments. In 1933, and again in 1936, the United States signed articles renouncing any intervention, "directly or indirectly, and for whatever reason, in the internal or external affairs of any other of the parties."[39] In its place the United States began to implement a so-called Good Neighbor Policy, in return for which the U.S. Government expected reciprocal action from Latin American countries. In other words, the United States would carry out policies favored by the Latin-American countries, in the belief that by doing so these countries would reciprocate by actions beneficial to the United States.

Few felt the immediate impact of these policies more than those Americans who were members of the American Society of Tropical Medicine. In 1939, the year in which membership in the Society passed the 500 mark for the first time, the Secretary of the American Foundation of Tropical Medicine noted that "the time is peculiarly appropriate for a major effort in the field of tropical medicine in the Western Hemisphere." To take advantage of the situation that had arisen as a result of the Good Neighbor Policy, the Secretary recommended that the Foundation devote its energies toward medical teaching and research in the Latin-American republics. Grants should be given to American medical schools to set up postgraduate courses in tropical medicine, he argued, and graduate fellowships should be established for Latin Americans to study in the United States. Furthermore, he urged, financial support for the *American Journal of Tropical Medicine* and the *Journal of Parasitology* would enable both to be distributed to South and Central America.[40] Not surprisingly, the Council of the American Academy of Tropical Medicine unanimously approved the Secretary's recommendations, and the American Society of Tropical Medicine expressed "its sympathetic interest in the activity of the American Academy of Tropical Medicine in increasing inter-American cooperation on the fields of tropical medicine and parasitology."[41]

By 1940, eight $1,000 fellowships in tropical medicine had been granted for a six-month postgraduate course at Tulane, but two years later, some donors withdrew their support, and the Foundation ran out of money to finance more Latin-American fellowships.[42] Although these scholarships were guaranteed finally by Nelson Rockefeller, the Coordinator of the Office of Inter-American Affairs, a new situation had by then arisen: The Americans had entered World War II.

The outbreak of World War II only a few years after the Good Neighbor Policy was first enunciated changed the nature of this policy and in doing so health and medicine came to play an even greater role. With the German threat, reciprocity from the Latin-American countries could no longer be simply anticipated; vital interests were at stake. To prevent German infiltration into South and Central America, the passive policy of good neighborliness had to be replaced by a more active process of "continental solidarity." To counter the Axis threat, the United States decided to buy war material from Latin America so as to provide these countries with foreign exchange and to help them achieve full employment. The United States also decided to support cultural programs which, together with the economic projects, "would tend to prevent discontent and disorder and thus eliminate a fertile field for Nazi propaganda."[43]

A Division of Cultural Relations was established in 1940 to coordinate these activities. It financed projects whose priority was set by their potential impact on continental solidarity. Medical projects were given the second highest priority; although having only "secondary defense significance," they nevertheless had "direct propaganda effect." The importance of these medical projects to the program became apparent two years later, when a special Institute of Inter-American Affairs, under the direction of Dr. George Dunham of the U.S. Army Medical Corps, was founded to coordinate these medical and sanitary programs. His mandate included the improvement of health conditions in strategic areas as well as more general health and sanitation campaigns throughout Latin America. These health campaigns were carried out, not only to increase the potential productivity of Latin American countries, but also to demonstrate the "tangible benefits of democracy."

By war's end, the United States had spent over $20 million on 800 health projects in Latin America, which ran the gamut from campaigns against specific diseases, through hospital construction, to training Latin Americans in U.S. medical schools. The "overall objective," Dunham told members of the American Foundation of Tropical Medicine in 1945, after the German threat was over, "is to promote economic development and progress," needed to ensure future stability in order to develop U.S. markets.[44]

The United Fruit Company also continued its well-publicized battles against tropical diseases by arguing that healthy workers not only produced more fruit but would be less likely to fall prey to Nazi propaganda. In 1942, Charles Wilson, between 1930 and 1935 a Special Assistant to the President of the Company, published *Ambassadors in White*, which, while purporting to be a history of American tropical medicine, was in fact a glowing account of the United Fruit Company's work in tropical medicine. The United States, he reminded his reader, belongs to the American Hemisphere, but "not the hemisphere of any imperialist dream, but the America of mankind, still the new-found land, still the community of freemen determined to stand or fall by their humanity and their freedom."[45] But, he went on to stress, this "hemisphere solidarity cannot be built on a sick man's society."

Since the Monroe Doctrine we have considered that it is our job to help protect the Southern nations from political aggressors. Today, and even more urgently, it is our job to help Latin American nations protect themselves against the fifth column of disease.[46]

This "insidious and ubiquitous column of disease," he wrote, is "more dangerous to us of the north than anything out of *Mein Kampf*."[47]

Their concern over German totalitarianism was not engendered only by fear of profit loss. In 1930, the United Fruit Company had been taken over by Sam Zmuri, or Zemurray as he came to call himself (Figure 8.3), a Bessarabian Jew who became involved with the agonies of the "final solution" and the founding of Israel. He bought and financed *The Exodus*, for example, and stole, from under the noses of the German guards, a couple of boats that were being built for the Company in Bremenhaven and which the Germans were planning to confiscate. He had immigrated to the United States in 1892, when 15 years old, and had lived for a few years in Selma, Alabama. He first realized the profits that could be gained from bananas, by buying up cheap, overripe ones at the quay side in Mobile and selling them "immediately" at a profit. With this money, "Sam, the Banana Man," as he was called, formed the Cuyamel Company with a 15,000-acre banana plantation in Honduras. In the 1920s, after a series of episodes that read like some adventure story that one would find in the famous British *Boy's Own Paper* (including a successful coup in Honduras involving Sam Zmuri, Manual Bonilla, General Lee Christmas, and Guy "Machine-Gun" Molony), the Cuyamel Company became the

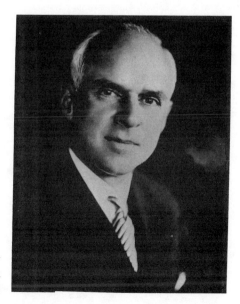

Figure 8.3. Sam Zmuri or Zemurray (Courtesy of the Middle American Research Institute, Tulane University)

United Fruit's most serious competitor for the U.S. banana market. In 1929, however, Sam sold his interest in the Cuyamel Company for United Fruit stock worth $31.5 million and thus became the Company's largest shareholder. But the depression reduced the value of the Company's holdings, and so, after obtaining enough proxies from disillusioned shareholders, he took over the Company. Not surprisingly, a company headed by Zmuri saw itself in the vanguard of the struggle against the Nazis in Latin America, and viewed its medical work as an important component of this struggle.[48]

Changing imperial policies in London and Washington held promise for tropical medicine. The British seemed set to substantially increase their investments in the well-being of their colonial subjects, while, at the same time, the American Government and its corporations were beginning once again to address health problems in South and Latin America. By the end of the decade, the practitioners of tropical medicine in Britain and America could look forward to a brighter future.

But there was a more immediate war to be won as, once again, American troops and troops of the British Empire were posted to tropical zones and again faced the menace of tropical diseases.

9

Bilharzia: World War II

The Second World War served tropical medicine well. The subject became important again as the allied armed forces found themselves once more battling tropical diseases. Its practitioners matured overnight into experts, whose opinions on medical matters were of vital importance. In addition, by the end of the war, bilharzia began to be listed as a serious tropical disease world-wide; it could no longer be ignored.

"The war has placed our Society in a position of real importance," announced Dr. Thomas Mackie, President of the American Society of Tropical Medicine, in his presidential address of April 1941, eight months before Pearl Harbor and the German declaration of war. Members of the Society served on committees of the National Research Council, and the Public Health Department, and most significantly advised the Surgeon-General's Office on control and treatment of tropical diseases to which U.S. personnel could be exposed, were they to become involved in the war.[1] The war, when it came, also acted as a powerful fillip to the Society, which, up until then, was still very much a rump group of the Southern Medical Association.[2] Membership jumped from 546 in 1941, to 674 in 1942, 901 in 1943 and 1,213 in 1944, and money became available for research. In 1944, for example, the American Foundation of Tropical Medicine obtained $75,000 for use in teaching and research, $15,000 of which went to Tulane. In addition, the Firestone Rubber Company donated $25,000 for research on trypanosomiasis in Liberia.[3]

In a report of 1944, Andrew Warren of the American Society of Tropical Medicine listed seven tropical diseases as being of particular importance in the future: malaria, amoebiasis, filariasis, hookworm, leishmaniasis, schistosomiasis, and echinococcosis. This list was of major significance in the bilharzia story; for the first time the disease had been counted as one of the major health problems of the world. Until that time, bilharzia had hardly been noticed by the Society. Papers on the disease had been presented in 1906, 1915, and 1916; and, in 1913, a discussion entitled "Is the importance of intestinal parasites in tropical pathology exaggerated?" led Charles Craig to conclude that hookworm was the only parasitic worm of any importance. "*Schistosomum*," he wrote, "is important; but its locale is limited and the number of cases is small."[4] But, in 1944, this disease, which had been ignored by the Society and had also failed to gain any mention in Harold Scott's two-volume *History of Tropical Medicine*, published out of the London School of Hygiene and Tropical Medicine in 1939, had suddenly been elevated to one of the seven most serious tropical diseases. Since then, it has never fallen from this high plateau.

This increase in status could not have occurred simply because of bilharzia's general impact on the allied armies in the war. Only 42 cases were reported by the British and Commonwealth armies in Egypt and the Middle East, and the British medical history of World War II dismissed the disease with a shrug: "By the application of simple precautionary measures based on knowledge gained during the war of 1914–18," the history noted, "there was no repetition of the outbreak which then occurred in Egypt."[5] Similarly, the Australian history reported that "infection by the *S. haematobium* or *S. mansoni* did not prove an appreciable risk in the Middle East."[6]

The medical authorities of the Indian Army, on the other hand, expressed more concern. By one of the quirks of natural history, none of the schistosome-bearing snails is endemic to India, and although cattle schistosomes are common, the human population is spared the ravages of the human parasites. The Indian authorities naturally wanted to keep things that way. But in August 1944, 23,152 men of the 82nd West African Division, with British officers and some NCOs, arrived in India directly from Nigeria. But before embarking, some of the British came down with the disease after bathing in a lagoon in Epe, near Lagos. In May and June, the British who had been exposed to the contaminated water were admitted to hospital and treated, whereas the African troops were given only a cursory examination and treated in the lines. But so many of these African troops were found with schistosome eggs in their feces, that, after arriving in India, all of them were thoroughly surveyed and, if infected, given a course of treatment. Of 21,338 African troops examined, 3,640 – or 17 percent – were pronounced positive, with a high of 26.7 percent in one of the Nigerian brigades.[7]

The American Army reported over 2,500 cases of bilharzia, but such a number is miniscule compared with those of malaria and venereal diseases, to say nothing of the battle casualties suffered during the bloody war with Japan.[8] Nevertheless, because of one campaign the disease seems to have impinged on American consciousness and thereby brought to the front line of tropical diseases. That one campaign took place in the Philippine island of Leyte, very near the end of the war.

THE LEYTE CAMPAIGN

The potential dangers of bilharzia to American troops had been minimized in a series of technical bulletins put out by the U.S. War Department in the latter stages of the war. Only in Northeast China was bilharzia listed as a "disease of special military importance." Elsewhere, including Southeast China, Japan, and Egypt, the disease was downgraded to one of "potential military importance," whereas in Formosa and the Celebes it was considered merely as "a serious disease of nonmilitary importance but likely to affect small numbers of troops." In July 1944, three months before the Leyte landings, publication of *TB MED* 68 revealed that the disease in the Philippines was confined to Mindoro, East Leyte, and North Mindanao, and that it, too, was "a serious disease of nonmilitary importance but likely to affect a small number of troops."[9]

A series of publications in Philippine journals during the 1920s and 1930s had indicated the seriousness of the disease. Autopsies by Mendoza-Guazon led him to suspect that schistosomiasis japonica "is a menace to this country and is probably endemic"; in 1932, M. Tubangui found *Oncomelania quadrasi* to be the intermediate host. In 1941, following a survey of the islands, Tubangui and his associate revealed the extent of the problem. Bilharzia, they discovered, was endemic on the east side of Minoro, the whole of Samar, the northern tip of Mindanao, and in the Leyte Valley (the coastal plain lying to the east of the central mountain chain of the island); 25,000 to 33,000 Filipinos – or 20 percent of the rural population – were estimated to be infected.[10]

By the summer of 1944, with General MacArthur's forces in New Guinea, and those of admirals King and Nimitz in the Marianas, two possibilities presented themselves for future action in the war. Japan could be reached either by a two-pronged pincer attack through the Bonin Islands on the right and Formosa and China on the left or, as MacArthur favored, by a more direct approach from New Guinea, through the Philippines, and north into Japan.[11] After much to-do, agreement was reached at the 1944 Quebec Conference to take the Philippine route by first invading South Mindanao in November 1944, and then Leyte a month later.

In August, however, a group of fast-carrier forces under Admiral Halsey managed to bomb and shell Japanese air bases in Mindanao without opposition. As a result, a decision was reached to forego the invasion of South Mindanao and jump directly north into Leyte – to switch, therefore, from a site without bilharzia to one in which the disease was endemic.

At daybreak, on October 20, 1944, the main American forces entered the Leyte Gulf (see Figure 9.1). Landing near Tacloben, on the northern front of attack, the Xth Corps consolidated the beachhead before moving west, across the northern end of the Leyte Valley, to capture Carigara on the north coast of the island. Three days later, on November 4, they reached "Breakneck Ridge," approximately 20 miles north of the Japanese headquarters at Ormoc, and scene of the most vicious fighting of the campaign. Meanwhile, the XXIVth Corps, after landing on the southern edge of the landing beach near Dulag, moved across the Leyte Valley and over the central range of hills to

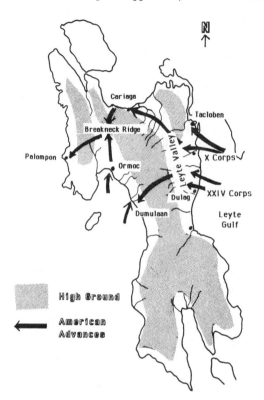

Figure 9.1. The Battle of Leyte

capture Dumulaan on the west coast of the island. On Christmas Day 1944, with the capture of Palompon, the last port to be held by the Japanese, an official communiqué finally announced: "The Leyte–Samar campaign can now be regarded as closed except for minor mopping up operations."[12] Out of 257,766 men who took part in the operation, the U.S. Army sustained 15,584 casualties with 3,508 killed. In the same period, 84 men had been admitted to the 118th Field Hospital with suspected bilharzia, and by May 1945, the total number of cases had increased to about 1,000.[13]

According to Ferguson's account, U.S. medical personnel were not told of the change of plans that resulted in the early invasion of Leyte. But even if they had, there is little evidence to suggest that they would have done very much about the situation. "Before December 1944," Ferguson wrote, "interest in schistosomiasis had been to a certain extent academic. It was felt by some Medical Department personnel that the disease would not be of military importance in Leyte."[14] Indeed, of course, that was exactly the message of *TB MED* 68, and that was exactly what happened: 1,000 cases out of a force of 257,766 men represented only 0.388 percent of the total American troop strength in Leyte. Nevertheless, the Americans overreacted to an extraordinary degree.

According to Ferguson's account, the medical staff in Leyte learned of Tubangui's survey only a week after landing on the island, despite the fact that *TB MED* 68 referred specifically to that work. But, whether that statement is true or not, members of a malaria unit began immediately to survey the civilian population for schistosome eggs, to search for the snail intermediate host, and to initiate education programs warning troops of the potential hazards of the disease.[15]

On November 18, the 118th General Hospital, manned by the medical staff of the Johns Hopkins Medical School commissioned in the officer reserve corps, landed in Leyte, set up their hospital in Kaboynan, and began admitting patients two weeks later. Anticipating some cases of bilharzia, a disease with which they were not familiar, they planned to gain experience by treating some Filipino patients with antimony drugs. But in December, the disease suddenly appeared among American troops admitted to the hospital: 80 cases in December and 155 in January. By the end of January, the hospital's adjutant could report, "The situation regarding manpower is becoming critical. [A] number of cases of schistosomiasis have been diagnosed. In spite of early warning about swimming or bathing in freshwater a great number admit to swimming in nearby river."[16]

Fearing a major epidemic, a major military operation against bilharzia geared into action. An extensive educational program got under way with posters (see Figure 9.2), cartoons, radio broadcasts, and mobile demonstration laboratories. Their messages were clear: "Stay out of freshwater streams, ponds and rice paddies," "Don't wade or bathe in unsafe waters," "Don't drink unpurified water," and "Don't wash vehicles in unsafe water."[17] In February, the 5th Malarial Survey Unit and a Medical Research Unit arrived and were attached to the Johns Hopkins General Hospital. Their officers (F. Bang, N. Hairston, O. Graham, and M. Ferguson) were detailed to study the epidemiology of the disease, the control of the snail host, chemotherapy, and prevention of infection in the military. Then, in April, a Subcommission on Schistosomiasis, appointed by the Army Epidemiological Board in Washington, arrived to study the problem with objectives similar to those of the 5th Malarial Survey Unit: to study the distribution and epidemiology of the disease, to develop methods of protecting the troops from infection, to control the snail host, and to improve diagnostic techniques. Directed by Ernest Faust, the Subcommission consisted of W. H. Wright of the National Institutes of Health, D. B. McMullen of the University of Oklahoma, Major G. W. Hunter, III, and sergeants P. Bauman and J. W. Ingalls. Then, a month later, incredible as it may seem, three officers from the Naval Medical Research Unit No. 2 arrived in Leyte to carry out a much smaller investigation into the

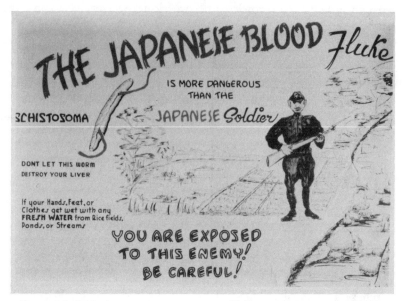

Figure 9.2. U.S. Army poster, warning of bilharzia in Leyte (Courtesy of Edward Michelson)

epidemiology of the disease. The American military, it seemed, never did things by halves!

Of these men, only Bang was a physician (M.D. degree from Johns Hopkins). The rest had a broad set of qualifications and interests that distinguished tropical medicine in the United States from the purely physician-centered discipline in Britain. Graham, for example, was an entomologist with the U.S. Department of Agriculture, whereas Wright, with a Diploma in Veterinary Medicine and a Doctorate from George Washington University, was employed by the U.S. Public Health Service. Ferguson and Hunter both held a Doctorate from Illinois, the latter a student of H. B. Ward, and McMullen had received his Doctorate under W. W. Cort at Hopkins. These were the men who were to put bilharzia on the academic map of the United States by publishing their wartime findings in the *American Journal of Hygiene* and the *American Journal of Tropical Medicine*.

It quickly became apparent that combat-engineering companies involved with road construction and bridge building had been hit hardest by the disease. A road paralleled the landing beaches of the XXIVth Corps, on the west side of which lay a continuous marsh with numerous streams and sloughs. Although infantrymen became infected by wading and swimming across these watery barriers, engineers, standing for long periods in water while bridging these marshes and streams, proved to be the major target for infection. By early February 1945, of 164 cases diagnosed in the XXIVth Corps, half came from one engineer batallion alone. The 5th Malarial Survey Detachment concentrated its survey activities on this batallion. The figures were stark: 62 percent of those infected in the batallion were members of bridge and road construction units, although such personnel made up only 21 percent of batallion strength; as many as 89 percent of strictly bridge-building units came down with the disease. A minor survey in the area revealed the familiar story: 76 percent of villagers in two barrios with schistosome eggs in their stools, and a spotty distribution and low numbers of infected snails.[18]

The spotty distribution of infected snails attracted the attention of the Naval Research Unit. Not surprisingly, they reported that "infestation of snails takes place only near the immediate locality where human feces drain into the water inhabited by *Schistosomorpha quadrasi.*" In one swamp, joined to a nearby village by a drainage ditch, they found 21 percent of those snails crawling among fecal material to be infected, whereas 30 feet away, only 3.1 percent carried the larval stages, and only 1.3 percent were infected at the edge of the swamp. Schistosomiasis was not a disease of rice workers, they noted, but of children. By 15 years of age, they estimated, virtually all of the children carried a worm load.[19]

Members of the Schistosomiasis Commission also focused their attention on the snail host; they collected 16,447 snails from four stations in Leyte in order to determine their life cycles and pattern of infection. The snail species *Oncomelania quadrasi* breeds throughout the year, they reported, takes about four to five months to mature, and is susceptible to infection immediately on hatching.[20]

Naturally, the overriding concerns of all three teams of investigators in Leyte were military. How could future outbreaks be prevented? Could chemical impregnation of uniforms prevent penetration of the cercariae? How could infected troops best be cured? Not surprisingly, members of the Commission believed that control could best be achieved by eliminating the snail hosts. To test the efficacy of various chemicals, they constructed three types of outdoor test plots in a 12-acre field rich with snails: 85-sq.-inch "small natural" plots, bordered on the sides by U.S. Army-issue dehydrated food cans, were used to screen out chemicals that were of no value; 25-sq.-foot "natural" plots, and 25-sq.-foot "pond" plots, consisting of diked pits dug down below water level, into which two to three thousand snails were added, were used to test potentially useful chemicals. Nineteen chemicals were tested, including the old standbys, copper sulfate and Paris green, and the new wonder chemical DDT. The latter was found to be useless, whereas dinitro-cyclo-hexyl-phenol and Paris green, each used alone, proved to be more effective snail killers than copper sulfate, copper carbonate, copper guanylu-rea, calcium arsenate, and calcium cyanamide. But in terms of cost, the fertilizer calcium cyanamide came out on top: 54 cents per 100 square feet compared to 72 cents for copper sulfate, and a little over $1.50 for Paris green and the phenol compound. By treating with any of these successful chemicals, they concluded, the snail population would be reduced to a degree where "the possibility of an infection reached a vanishing point." Thereafter it would be necessary only to dust or spray small foci of snails that remained after the initial campaign.[21]

The possibility of protecting troops from infection by impregnation of uniforms with effective chemicals generated a series of rather imaginative, but repetitive, experiments by both the Malarial Unit and the Commission. By smearing chemicals on the shaved exposed skin of experimental rats before applying a cercarial suspension (Figure 9.3c), they found that many miticidals and insect repellents such as dimethyl phthalate, dibutyl phthalate, and benzyl benzoate appeared to prevent cercariae from penetrating the skin. Also, both untreated Byrd cloth, used as a wind and cold protector by the U.S. Army, and olive drab woolens, acted as efficient barriers to cercarial movement. Cercariae, for example, put into an inverted bag C (Figure 9.3a) of the material in question, failed to move into the outer vessel. Also, more suitable

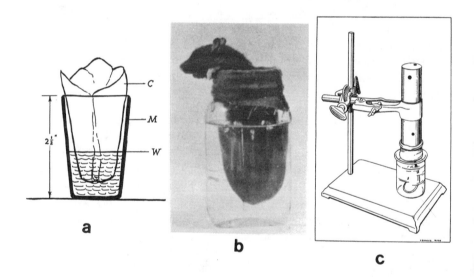

Figure 9.3. Laboratory work in Leyte, I: (a) method of testing for cercarial penetration of fabrics; (b) method of exposing anesthetized rats to cercariae; (c) method of testing liquid and ointment repellents to cercariae by coating rat tails. a,b, From M. S. Ferguson et al., "Studies on schistosomiasis, V," *American Journal of Hygiene* 44 (1946); c, from W. H. Wright et al., *American Journal of Hygiene* 47 (1948), with permission of the *American Journal of Epidemiology*

tropical clothing, when soaked in various chemicals and passed through numerous washes, prevented the movement of cercariae from one vessel to the other. They also placed anesthetized rats inside the cloth bags to be tested (Figure 9.3b). "This arrangement," they noted, "was comparable to a man with trousers closed at the bottom standing in infested water." The combination of new cotton khaki and dibutyl phthalate proved to be the most effective barrier, capable, for example, of preventing movement across the barrier after ten washings. Protection, members of the Malarial Unit concluded, would best be achieved by impregnating uniforms with dibutyl phthalate, benzyl benzoate, or a mixture thereof, and by smearing these chemicals on exposed skin.[22] Members of the Commission came to similar conclusions after a set of very similar experiments.[23]

Meanwhile, work at the 118th Hospital showed how little bilharzia therapy had changed in 25 years: Tartar emetic appeared still to be the drug of choice. "Patients treated with tartar emetic," their physicians reported, "had fewer recurrences than a comparable group treated with Fuadin."[24] Surprisingly, perhaps, the mode of action of these antimony drugs was still unclear. Thus, in an important series of tests, members of the Commission analyzed the effect of antimony on the schistosome worms in experimental guinea pigs (Figure 9.4). After four weeks of treatment, they noted, the adult worms migrated to the liver, became smaller, lost their gut hematin (the gut of feeding schistosome worms becomes blackened with breakdown blood products), and their ovaries and yolk glands degenerated so that few, if any, eggs were present in the uterus. But, these worms were not dead, they discovered; even after four weeks of continuous treatment, half the shrunken worms in the liver of the guinea pigs were still alive. "Relapse following treatment," they noted, "is nothing more than a recovery of vitality on the part of the worm when the concentration of antimony is no longer damaging to the worm." Relapse cases in the 118th Hospital, they noted, indicated that the worms took about 18 days to recover their egg-laying powers after treatment stopped, and 28 days passed before mature eggs appeared once again in the feces.[25] Clearly, the old view that the disease could be completely cured by injections of antimony was no longer warranted.

From the medical viewpoint, the acute nature of the disease among American troops in Leyte made this outbreak particularly significant. For the first time, the disease was seen in its very early stages, not in its chronic form. Indeed, in many cases the disease was recognized even before the worm eggs had reached the feces, and disease symptoms were noticed that had rarely been reported before, and never in such quantity.

Bilharzia, Faust and his colleagues revealed, passed through three consecutive stages in its development. The first, the incubation period, coincided with the penetration of the cercariae into the skin, their passage via lymphatic or venous vessels into the heart and lungs and eventually into the liver where

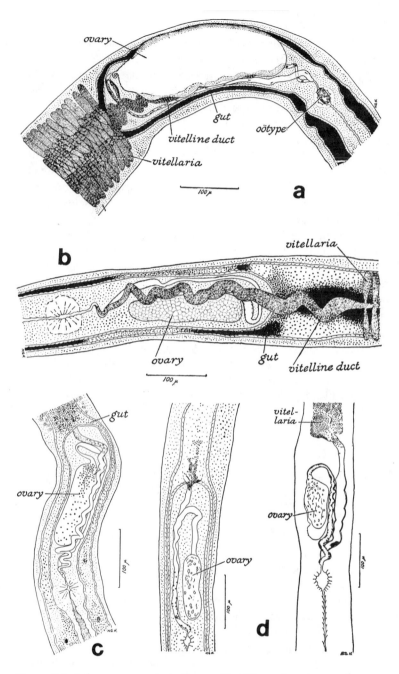

Figure 9.4. Laboratory work in Leyte, II. Effect of antimony drugs on female schistosome worms. (a) The normal reproductive system of the worm; (b) after one week of treatment; (c) after two weeks of treatment; (d) after four weeks of treatment. From F. B. Bang and N. G. Hairston, "Studies on schistosomiasis japonica IV," *American Journal of Hygiene* 44 (1946), with permission of the *American Journal of Epidemiology*

mating occurs. Symptoms of the disease were so varied at this stage, Faust reported, that "many skilled medical officers, who had been indoctrinated with information concerning the endemicity of the disease on Leyte but without previous actual experience, failed to recognize the signs and symptoms of the disease."[26] On initial exposure, Faust reported, there might be sharp needling pains at the sites of cercarial penetration, followed a few days later by a bronchial cough. Then, after two weeks or more of no apparent sickness, severe urticaria could develop, and for the first time, the patient might feel unwell. There could be, for example, a lose of appetite, lethargy, night fevers, and tenderness in the upper abdomen, all of which could suggest many diseases other than bilharzia. But a rise in the number of eosinophils (a type of white blood cell) by the end of the incubation period would immediately indicate a parasitic infection.

The problem of diagnosing the disease at this early stage, when therapy would be most effective, presented one of the most important and baffling riddles to the teams on the island. One hope, given the unreliability and variability of physical symptoms, lay with serological work. But extracts of *S. mansoni* injected subcutaneously failed to produce the characteristic antigen wheal in troops known to be infected with the parasite, although better results were obtained on chronic civilian cases. The flocculation test, however, where the parasite antigen was added to a patient's serum on a microscope slide and then examined for clumping, seemed a little more encouraging: Ninety of 104 individuals known to be carrying the worm proved positive in the test.[27]

Locating eggs in the feces of lightly infected acute cases proved to be a major headache as well, and much effort was spent on finding more effective means of locating the schistosome eggs. Direct smear methods, whereby fecal material was simply mixed with saline and the sample examined under the microscope, obviously gave poor results; it was all too easy to miss the eggs. Methods were needed to concentrate the eggs. Flotation methods, in which eggs floated to the surface of fecal samples mixed with zinc sulfate, proved unreliable. Sedimentation techniques proved the most effective, although often cumbersome and time-consuming. In its simplest form, fecal samples were mixed repeatedly with water, allowed to settle, with the clear fluid poured off each time. Eventually, the eggs concentrated enough in the sediment so that microscopic examination could give reliable results. The most effective of the various sedimentation methods tried came from the acid–ether technique, whereby egg concentration went hand in hand with the removal of fecal debris, fat, and mucus. Basically, in this method, the fecal sample was mixed with hydrochloric acid, strained through gauze, decanted, and a mixture of acid and ether added. This mixture was then centrifuged, and the sediment examined.[28] Hunter introduced another variable in this technique: The feces were first emulsified with a mixture of sodium sulfate and hydrochloric acid, strained through gauze, centrifuged repeatedly with fresh batches of acid and sulfate, and decanted each time before the final acid–sulfate mix, ether, and a detergent were added.[29]

All these findings were reported back to the military authorities in Washington during the war, and many accounts of schistosomiasis japonica, particularly those pertaining to the very practical problems of diagnosis, appeared in the *Bulletin of the U.S. Army Medical Department* as soon as the war ended.[30] In 1945, the War Department published *TB MED* 167, entitled "Schistosomiasis japonica," which provided an excellent summary of what was known of the disease at that time, much of it derived from work at Leyte. Whatever one thinks of the American reaction to this disease in 1944, it is clear that those who worked on the problem added immeasurably to our knowledge of bilharzia.

Americans were not the only troops to be infected in Leyte. Some members of a 560-strong Australian airfield construction squadron, after using a river adjacent to their camp for swimming and washing, came down with the disease, and a subsequent check revealed that nearly half of the squadron had eosinophilia.[31] But, as the Australian history explained, "The handling of the affected men aroused considerable discussion. On the one hand, the Royal Australian Air Force felt that the unit was isolated and was carrying out very good work with a high morale, that most of the men did not feel ill, and that their mild infections could be treated while they continued to work. On the other hand, the U.S. troops affected were mostly sent to the 118th General Hospital on Leyte."[32] Once in the hospital, these men were either detained for a lengthy examination or evacuated to the United States. As a result, some American troops deliberately exposed themselves to contaminated water, and a black market in infected stools got underway. Obviously, none of this sat well with the Australians, although in July 1945, the entire Australian squadron and all Americans with bilharzia were evacuated home. Neither is there a record of what the Australians thought of the "famous fifty" from the Johns Hopkins Hospital.

Although, according to information obtained by the hospital, only 30 of the bilharzia cases admitted could be considered severe, so many troops suffered from an unexpected degree of invalidism that a psychiatric evaluation was requested on 50 patients who had been hospitalized for an average of 105 days following treatment.[33] Most had been cleared for light duty, and only 13 showed physical symptoms characteristic of the disease. But "subjective" symptoms such as fatigue, shakiness, headaches, abdominal cramps, and blurred vision were rampant.

Nothing was known, wrote the psychiatrist in his report, about the effects of the disease on patients after brief exposure. "One did not know," he wrote, "how to be sure a patient was cured, or what part of the symptoms of a given patient at a given time were due to the parasite, what part to the treatment, and what part to the emotional reactions." As a result, he concluded, an atmosphere abounded "in which rumors flourished and disability-producing attitudes throve."[34]

All the patients were confused about the disease and resentful of the treatment they had received, the psychiatrist explained. Many felt that they were "guinea-pigs" in an experimental drug program, and few had any confidence in the medical officers. "I guess they're writing a book about it," one man told the psychiatrist; "I know I'm being used as a guinea pig. I felt kinda peeved at first, but I can't do much about it," reported another. They faced, also, a stream of totally confusing information. Outside the hospital, in an attempt to dissuade men from swimming in freshwater, highly alarmist radio broadcasts talked of the "disastrous effects of schisto." But, as another patient said, "They tell you in the hospital schisto isn't serious. On the radio they say it kills. That breaks down the morale of the fellows who got it. Either the radio or the doctors are screwed up about something."

Special attention must be devoted to the emotional reactions to the disease, the psychiatrist concluded. Physicians must not only attack the worm, but maintain "the proper therapeutic atmosphere" of faith in the physician and an expectancy of recovery. The patient, the report stressed, should rely on the physician for information on the disease, and the physician, in turn, should emphasize "those aspects of the disease which lend themselves to an optimistic interpretation." Only one-third of the patients fully understood, he noted as an example, that flukes cannot multiply in the body. But optimism, he warned, must be "consistent with accuracy"; patients gain no confidence in a physician who tells them that schistosomiasis is no worse than a common cold. Other advice permeated the 24-page report: Physicians must be consistent with one another and with other authorities; vacillation about prognosis, which keeps the patient "in a demoralizing turmoil of hopes and fears," should be avoided; and, above all, "the obvious first requisite is to regard each patient as an individual." But, in the middle of a ferocious war, it is hard not to feel sympathy with medical officers who were being asked to give special attention "to combatting emotional reactions which impede recovery, such as anxiety, resentment, and confusion." I must say that it is hard to imagine any sergeant-major that I have known putting up with the antics of the "famous fifty," much less allowing a report to be written about them!

In reality, whatever occurred in Leyte, bilharzia turned out to be "a largely preventable disease,"[35] and the words of the technical bulletins proved true: Bilharzia in the Philippines, as well as in Egypt, turned out to be "a serious disease of nonmilitary importance but likely to affect small numbers of troops."

But, immediately before and after their return to civilian life, members of the Malarial Unit and the Commission published their Philippine findings in academic journals, and thereby did much to raise the visibility of the disease. The Leyte campaign not only put bilharzia on the map, but did so at a time when members of the American Society of Tropical Medicine were expressing concern about the future status of their profession. Bilharzia was "discovered" at a very opportune time.

PART II

A brief interlude: Social medicine

10

New ideas

There were always those who could not accept the underlying belief that diseases were the most basic problems of the tropical world, "the supreme ill of human life," as Gates had written. To such people good health could not be defined simply as the absence of diseases, and could not be achieved merely by eliminating them or their pathogens. To this group the social conditions in which people lived and worked were a major cause of disease.

These views were widely held throughout the nineteenth century. Before the acceptance of the modern germ theory, the general interrelationship between disease and social conditions was generally assumed. But some physicians, such as Rudolf Virchow and others, expanded these views into a doctrine that medicine was basically a social science. Society, according to these writers, must ensure the conditions necessary for its citizens to enjoy a healthy existence. But, since poor health was due as much to social and economic conditions as to contagia, miasma, decaying matter, and such, then society must ensure that its people were free from misery, poverty, hunger, and ignorance, both at home and in the workplace. Epidemics of disease, Virchow warned, indicated the existence of social and economic problems within the diseased community, and thus measures to promote health must include social and economic reforms. The scope of medicine must be enlarged, he argued; it must intervene in the social, economic, and political life of the community.[1] But such social views had been undermined by the rise of bacteriology and parasitology and by the notion that the sick were merely bearers of disease-causing pathogens. The victims and their environment had been replaced by the pathogen and the disease as the major focus of concern.

Proponents of these social views gained little support until the 1930s, although a major confrontation between the social and the scientific approach to disease had surfaced during the 1920s. Members of the Malaria Commission of the League of Nations had attacked the idea that malaria could best be eradicated by the elimination of mosquitoes, a view adhered to by Lewis Hackett of the International Health Board who had been sent to examine the problem in 1924. The discovery of the mosquito cycle, noted members of the

Commission in that year, "has not in fact provided sanitarians with a unique, practical and definite solution of the problem." There were other factors involved. Housing and feeding, they noted, affected both resistance to infection and mortality. "Malaria," they concluded, "is a social disease and, equally with tuberculosis, is liable to be influenced and even partly eliminated . . . by proved measures of social hygiene."[2] The terror of malaria, Professor Swellengrebel noted in the same report, can be reduced by combining quinine therapy with methods that foster economic improvement. Italy, the country on which he reported, had moved in that direction by a process of "bonification," or swamp drainage and land resettlement. Such a process, he pointed out, was not a campaign to eliminate the breeding sites of mosquitoes, but "measures of social hygiene meant to improve the hygienic condition of the population, to increase their general well-being and ultimately their resistance to malaria, results in the form not so much of lessened prevalence of the disease as in a lessened severity, evidenced by a reduced death rate."[3] The second report of the Commission, published two years later, was even firmer on the issue. Attempts to eradicate the disease by killing mosquito larvae were rarely justified, they concluded; the best approach was to reduce the prevalence and severity of the disease by "improving the economic and social conditions of the people and their general well-being and standard of life."

Hardly anything has retarded the effective control of malaria so much as has the belief that, because mosquitoes carry malaria, their elimination should be the object of chief concern and expenditure. . . . Since the advent of the new knowledge of the transmission of malaria by mosquitoes, there has been a tendency to forget that there are many methods of dealing with the disease, and that some of them are effective even without any attempt being made to reduce mosquitoes.[4]

Such social views had retreated from the malarial battleground by the late 1930s, but had gained ground elsewhere. In Britain, for example, lobby groups such as the Children's Minimal Council, the Committee against Malnutrition, the National Unemployed Workers Movement, and numerous social scientists began to argue that despite the obvious triumphs of modern medicine, the health of many members of society was less than adequate. The Women's Health Inquiry of 1939 found, for example, that 31.2 percent of working-class wives had a "very grave" health status. A new approach was needed, they argued, and the promotion of health had to be separated from the cure and prevention of disease; the latter did not necessarily lead to the former.[5]

In 1935, two physicians, George Williamson and Innes Pearse, opened the Peckham Health Centre in London as an "experimental human research laboratory designed to test their idea that the social situation of the family was the main source of either healthy growth and development, or disease and social disintegration."[6] The health of local families, who had paid a fee to join, became the main emphasis of the Centre. Members were required to submit to regular health checks designed to measure their capacity for family and social life. The Peckham Centre was a health center, featuring such things as recreational facilities, and, according to its founders' ideas, was separate from medically oriented "therapeutic centers."

Ideas, such as these, reappeared in greater force after the Second World War, following what Jane Lewis has called a social awakening by many British academicians and politicians. At Oxford University in 1942, for example, John Ryle became Britain's first Professor of (so-called) Social Medicine.

To those trained in laboratory-centered medicine, social medicine was and remained an exasperatingly vague and broad concept. What constituted social medicine was expressed most succinctly by Ryle in a radio broadcast over the South African Broadcasting Company. "We know," he said, "that the greatest savings of life and many of the great improvements in popular health, especially in infancy, childhood and young adulthood, come not from medicines and surgical operations and hospitals, but from improvements in sanitary, domestic, nutritional and working conditions."[7] The nation's health, therefore, could best be improved by social change, although some others, the "racial hygienists," favored selective breeding as an answer to these same medical concerns.

Modern medicine, John Ryle wrote, shortly after taking office, has become so technical and objective, so filled with consultants and narrow specialists, that sight of the patient as an individual has been lost. Medicine is now scientific, he concluded, "to the exclusion of the most important science of all – the science of man – and the most important technique of all – the technique of understanding." As a result, he argued, the modern physician is only vaguely aware that illnesses "have discoverable origins in social, domestic, or industrial maladjustments, in fatigue, economic insecurity or dietary insufficiency." More social security, better food and houses, better facilities for open-air recreation, better education, and more cultural opportunities, Ryle argued, would bring more benefits to the people and to the state than any further advances in curative medicine.[8] Similarly, in the United States at the same time, Henry Sigerist of Johns Hopkins University was arguing that disease was related to a host of social factors such as housing, nutrition, sanitation, and working conditions.[9]

In the broadest sense, social medicine called for reform in all areas of human existence inimical to good health, whether economic, social, or even genetic. And to some, at least, the medical profession had to assume leadership in this reform; only they possessed the expert knowledge and information upon which such reform could be based.

Ideas from social medicine infiltrated into the medical world of the British Empire. "Whether at home, in India, or in the colonies," Ryle concluded, social medicine "may shortly become our most urgent common interest." There was certainly some justification for Ryle's statement, for by the 1930s the British Colonial Office was beginning to realize that disease was not the most fundamental problem in the tropical world, the cause of all other evils. Poverty and malnutrition were beginning to impinge on its conscience.

BRITISH IMPERIAL HEALTH PROBLEMS

Lord Hailey recognized the problems of malnutrition in the Empire. In the past, he argued in his *African Survey* of 1938, medical attention had concentrated on the grave diseases of the tropics, but at present, another approach was gaining ground. Quoting then from an Indian report of 1935, he wrote:

No preventive campaign against malaria, against tuberculosis, or against leprosy, no maternity relief or child welfare activities, are likely to achieve any great success unless those responsible recognize the vital importance of this factor of defective nutrition and from the very start give it their most serious consideration. . . . Abundant supplies of quinine, and the multiplication of tuberculosis hospitals, sanitoria, leprosy colonies, and maternity and child welfare centres are no doubt desirable, if not essential, but none of these go to the root of the matter. The first essentials for the prevention of disease are a higher standard of health, a better physique, and a greater power of resistance to infection.[10]

Thus, he concluded, "medical science must be in Africa increasingly concerned with the relations between nutrition and health, and with advising on the medical aspect of social policies bearing on the question of subsistence." To do this, he went on, the health services in Africa should not restrict themselves to the application of modern science to the cause and relief of disease, but should help to organize social and medical campaigns with the limited resources available, by encouraging, for example, "the education of Africans to take part in health activities, and the co-operation with other social services." Administrators in Africa should ask, he wrote, "whether the attack on poor nutrition may not be the most important factor in reducing disease."[11]

These statements were not entirely surprising. Colonial officials had already established a link between malnutrition and disease.[12] In 1925, heavy stock losses in South Africa had been blamed on poor nutrition, and, in a subsequent survey, the diets of two African tribes were also examined, and a tentative link was made between diet and health. A more thorough survey followed, and in 1931, John Boyd Orr, the future first Director of the United Nations Food and Agriculture Organization (FAO), and John Gilks of the Kenyan Medical Department published their findings. The Masai tribe, they pointed out, were on average 5 inches taller and 23 pounds heavier than the Akikuyus; whereas the Masai ate milk and meat, the Akikuyu were limited to cereals and fruit with a low calcium intake. Their disease statistics were equally startling (see Table 10.1). The loss of health and efficiency attributable to a poor diet is of considerable economic importance, they warned, and "a general improve-

Table 10.1. *Prevalence of disease in the Masai and Akikuyu tribes*

Disease	Masai (%)	Akikuyu (%)
Bronchitis	4.0	28.0
Pneumonia	0.0	3.0
Tuberculosis	1.0	6.0
Ulcers	3.0	33.0
Malaria	2.0	18.0
Helminths	2.0	5.0

Source: Boyd Orr and J. Gilks, *Studies in Nutrition.*

ment of agriculture and animal husbandry amongst the Akikuyu will also certainly be accompanied by an improvement in the health and working capacity of the natives themselves."[13]

The Governors of British Colonial Africa, meeting in 1947, were also aware of some of these new ideas being broached about disease. Medicine in the past, they complained, was geared to the medical needs of government officials. There had been a bias toward curative work, and the only common practice they could discern was the wholesale construction of hospitals. "Unfortunately the erection of permanent memorials, in the form of hospitals," they noted, "exercises some subtle fascination not confined only to the medical department," and medical policy had been based "on the satisfaction of the most obvious demands on the medical staff, without full consideration having been given to the problem of the medical needs of the territories as a whole."

Diseases in the colonies were different from those in Britain, they noted; many of the chronic community diseases that constituted their major problem were related to malnutrition. Nevertheless, they complained, the sufferers "are dealt with piecemeal at dispensaries or hospitals." But these methods had not worked. Too much emphasis had been placed on curing specific diseases rather than addressing the various factors that caused diseases. Single-disease campaigns had often failed, they noted. "In the first place, the people were passive agents of the campaign, rarely understanding what it was all about and perhaps a little resentful at the work they were forced to do for their own good. In the second place, it took no account of the fact that whereas one disease might be an important and widespread factor in ill health, other factors also existed which remained untouched." Some campaigns they noted, with obvious reference to the Rockefeller Foundation's campaigns against hookworm, "have today their memorials in the stark ruins of latrines, mostly unused, still studding the countryside," and, "like all regulations impressed from the top, had no permanent effect on the lives of the inhabitants." What was needed, the Governors argued, was the provision and protection of water supplies; adequate provision for conservancy and refuse disposal; measures against disease-carrying insects; improvement of houses and prevention of overcrowding; improved agricultural methods; cultivating the right food crops; provision of adequate infant and child welfare clinics, suitable antenatal clinics; adequate provision for regular home visitors, and so on.[14]

In other words, they urged, "medical effort must be expended in the way which will most benefit the community and not the individual."

The Governors also realized that in most colonies a hard choice would have to be made between "extensive attacks on community-wide disease with reliance on simple accommodation for the treatment of the sick, and the spending of money freely on large well-equipped hospitals and expensive specialist staff." But they were clear on how the choice should be made: "It is better to deal with widespread disease amongst the people than to deal with the herniae and bronchitis and such like complaints of the individual."

In 1933, a conference of Indian- and African-based physicians came up with the same startling conclusion: "In an undernourished population," they wrote, "the mere treatment of disease . . . will achieve but negligible results. The first need is a continuous supply of sufficient and well-balanced food for the native to resist infection and the next is the improvement of housing. Both aspects depend on the economic status of the community."[15] Virchow could not have agreed more.

The colonial medical policies of His Majesty's Government were clearly being shaken at their foundations.

THE ROCKEFELLER FOUNDATION

In the aftermath of World War II, many organizations undertook an examination of their future goals and priorities. The Rockefeller Foundation was no exception. In 1942, even before the war had ended, Alan Gregg of the International Health Division had been asked to prepare a memorandum on the subject of social medicine as part of a general policy review. Gregg, in his report, did what Ryle had cautioned not to do: He confused social medicine with "socialized medicine," or the economic accessibility of medical care.

According to Gregg, the provision of good medical care to a large number of people had become the basic problem for the future.[16] Medical care had become so effective, Gregg warned, that the public, many of whom could not afford the services of a physician, were beginning to believe that medical care was "like life, liberty, and the pursuit of happiness – a civic right, a public necessity." Social medicine, he concluded – quite wrongly of course – was concerned with what he called geographic and economic accessibility of this care.

Throughout 1944, the Scientific Directors of the International Health Division believed what they called "health insurance or social medicine," to be one of the future new fields to be explored.[17] But although agreeing that such "socialist" concerns could not be ignored, they believed them to be controversial and "revolutionary in character," and had little sympathy with them. There was, according to E. L. Bishop, "too much emotion, too little sense," while Harry Mustard noted that "it was unfortunate that so many proponents of this idea are such unpleasant people." W. Halverson even remarked, from what data it is not clear, that 35 percent of Californians did not want health insurance! By the end of 1944, however, Gregg had finally realized that social medicine was not equivalent to socialized medicine.[18] Thus, in a somewhat confused state, the Scientific Directors agreed that "social medicine" (whatever that meant) should be examined, and to that end asked Dr. John B. Grant (Figure 10.1) to study the issue.

John Grant, the self-styled "Rockefeller Bolshevik," was born in China, the son of a Canadian medical missionary. After undergraduate studies at Acadia University, a small liberal-minded Baptist college in Nova Scotia, he graduated in medicine in 1917 from the University of Michigan, and joined the staff of the International Health Board who posted him to their hookworm campaign in North Carolina.[19] In 1919, after a short period in China, he was

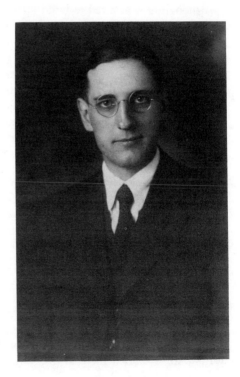

Figure 10.1. John Black Grant (Courtesy of the Rockefeller Archive Center)

sent to Puerto Rico to oversee a hookworm and malaria survey. "Oh! I'll tell you," he told his interviewer years later,

I've been to a lot of places in the world where they had hookworm, some hookworm, but in Puerto Rico, once you got off the plains area, the majority of people you met would have that peculiar color that heavy infestation gives in hookworm, that no other disease does. . . . Their legs would be swollen, their abdomens swollen, and yet they were trying to carry on their daily work, and you wondered, how? They had haemoglobins of 20 or 30. You just didn't understand how they carried on . . . Oh, that was . . . ! And the poverty!

In 1921, Grant returned to China as a faculty member of the Peking Union Medical College. But, like most medical employees of the Foundation, he was first required to spend time at the Johns Hopkins School of Hygiene and Public Health. While there, he began to be stimulated by the ideas of the British Fabians and Sir John Newsholme, who saw disease not simply in terms of pathogens but also as indicators of social and economic disorder. Thus his return to the diseases, poverty, and problems of "the sick man of Asia" came at a crucial time in Grant's life, and he quickly came to realize that the Peking College, a Rockefeller showpiece of Western medicine, was totally irrelevant to the real needs of China.

Although he was hired to build up a college health service for the faculty, students, and staff, he slowly expanded his work beyond this very narrow mandate, and moved the College toward an interest in Chinese public health work. By 1923, he was offering undergraduate classes in public health, and two years later he was appointed Head of the Department of Preventive Medicine and opened the Peking Health Center. In 1932, to cut a long story short, the College moved into the area of rural health. They drew up an agreement with James Yen's Mass Education Movement at Tinghsien, in which they agreed to provide experts in public health, to act as the Tinghsien base hospital, to train public health nurses, and, most significantly, to become a teaching center for rural health.

To Grant, and to Selskar Gunn who was sent out by the International Health Division to report on China, the Johns Hopkins-type of medicine practiced at the Peking College was totally inappropriate for China. "It is doubtful," Gunn wrote in his report, "if the stereotyped medical education now being given at Peking Union Medical College is really meeting the medical and public health needs of China." Both Grant and Gunn knew that health could not be separated from broader social issues; that the state must maintain a decent standard of living before an adequate level of community health could be attained; and that in the final analysis the question of health was a question of economics. Thus, in Grant and Gunn's opinions, any future Rockefeller involvement in China "should be limited to those projects which are part of a unified medical program which in turn should constitute one aspect of a larger plan of social reconstruction," integrated "with other branches of human endeavor, looking towards a general raising of the economic and social level of the masses."[20] The Rockefeller Foundation was learning first-hand some of the major platforms of social medicine, although by 1944 they seemed to have forgotten Grant and Gunn's message.

But, in 1935, they listened and gave lukewarm support to a short-lived China Program. Two years later, with the occupation of Peking by the Japanese, the Program collapsed and Grant moved to India, where he tried out his ideas in the All-India Public Health Institute. He returned to the United States in 1941, where he began again to voice strong opinions in favor of this new social approach to medicine, during the very period when the International Health Division was becoming preoccupied with debates over new policies and new programs.

In September 1945, a few months after agreeing to his new assignment, Grant visited Britain, Canada, and Sweden. Most countries, Grant reported, had developed health insurance programs, but the next stage, he argued, must be "directed toward removing the causes of social ills."[21]

In 1947, with these ideas in mind, Grant set out on a reconnaissance to examine medical care in 12 countries. Curiously, he failed to mention in his report that he actually visited 13 countries, and that in this "missing country," he found what he had been looking for – "one of the most forward looking and comprehensive health plans of any country I'd been to, or have been to since."[22] That country was South Africa.

SOUTH AFRICA: A NATIONAL HEALTH SERVICE

When Grant arrived in South Africa, the United Party, formed by a fusion of Smut's South African Party and Hertzog's Nationalist Party held power, while the more extremist Afrikaner politicians had split away to form the Purified National Party. It was a period of relative liberalism in that troubled country. Under the influence of Jan Hofmeyr, who more or less ran the home affairs of the government, they managed to pass through a small number of social reforms that helped, in a miniscule degree, to ameliorate the conditions of the African population.

In the summer of 1942, the government agreed to set up a National Health Service Commission, "to inquire into, report and advise upon the provision of an organized National Health Service, in conformity with the modern conception of "health," which will ensure adequate medical, dental, nursing and hospital services for *all* sections of the people of the Union of South Africa." The Commission was chaired by Henry Gluckmann, a physician and United Party member, who had been pressing for such a commission for some time. He was especially concerned with the inadequate health care delivered to the African community and with the heavy emphasis on curative medicine in the

South African system. He was also aware that new ideas were abroad in the 1940s, in particular, that medical treatment would "succeed only if simultaneously the social and economic background of the patient is fully appreciated." What was needed, according to Gluckmann, was a new system that promoted good health as much as it cured and prevented disease.[23]

Initially, at least, the possibilities of installing such a medical system in South Africa seemed brighter than in any other country. It went without saying that such a system would apply particularly to the African community which was virtually doctorless. Thus, to set up any "socialistic" medical system would be less likely to threaten the financial well-being of the medical profession. Probably, for that reason, the Medical Association of South Africa threw their support behind the ideas of Gluckmann.

In 1943, after sending a questionnaire to all their members, the Medical Association presented a brief to the Commission. The provision of mere "doctoring," they noted, was no solution to the health problems of South Africa; "freedom from want and poverty will do more to build up a healthy community than any amount of curative medical services." The Government must address the whole problem of social security, they urged, in which health was only one part. If the state was willing to meet its obligations toward nutrition and housing, they announced, the medical profession was prepared to surrender some of its independence to become "socialized" to some extent. The majority of members agreed, the brief continued, that there should be a National Health Service free to all, financed by the state, in which, naturally, private practice should also be maintained.[24] But members of the Medical Association were only partly in tune with ideas of "social medicine" emanating from Britain. Their vision of a health service was far narrower in scope; it was limited to the provision of curative and preventive medical care by general practitioners working in "health centers," who, if "socialized," and placed on a salaried basis, would necessarily expect the same rate of pay as their peers in private practice.

Gluckmann's 3.5-million-word report was presented to Parliament in February 1945. It was an extraordinary document; one can fully understand why Grant was so impressed. Echoing the words of the Medical Association, it warned that health needs could no longer be met by "doctoring" alone. Instead, the report argued, services must be provided by the state not only to cure, prevent, and rehabilitate, but also to promote and safeguard health.[25] Ill health, the document stressed, was "first and foremost" caused by "the economic poverty and the social backwardness of the greater part of the Union's population." Thus

reforms in the public health and medical services will probably bring about very little improvement in the nation's health, unless accompanied by drastic reforms in other spheres as well. . . . It would be unreasonable and unsound to expect the health services forever to make good the deficiences of the socio-economic system.[26]

The medical service itself, the report noted, was marked by the "pitiful inadequacy" of preventive services, which took less than 1 percent of the health budget. The present health service, was, the report concluded, "NOT organized on a national basis," was "NOT in conformity with the modern conception of 'health,' and was NOT available to all sections of the people."[27]

The modern concept of health to which Gluckmann subscribed involved what he termed nonpersonal and personal health services (see Table 10.2).[28] The National Health Service was to take over responsibility for the personal health services and was to be organized around a multitude of health centers. These centers were to be, Gluckmann claimed, laboratories of social medicine, dedicated to the belief that the promotion of health was the best method of preventing disease. They were to be administered by a team of general practitioners in group practice aided by teams of nurses and other health workers, whose services went beyond the provision of curative and preventive medical care to include nutritional, recreational, and cultural training. In addition, the services were to be freely available, funded by a universal health tax.

Table 10.2. *Personal and nonpersonal health services in South Africa, 1945*

Personal health	Nonpersonal health
Promotive services	Housing, and town planning
Adequate wages	Water supplies
Nutrition	Drainage
Education	Sanitation
Physical exercise	Food handling
Industrial hygiene	Abatement of nuisances
	Regulation of offensive trades
Preventive services	
Ante- or postnatal clinics	
Infant welfare clinics	
Nursery schools	
Child guidance clinics	
School health	
Workers' health clinics	
Routine medical examination of all groups at prescribed intervals	
Curative services	
Rehabilitation services	

Source: The Health of The Nation, Part 1, Chapter 3.

The John Gray Community Health Centre attached to the University of Witwatersrand was a model health center. It not only provided curative and preventive medical services to a white Afrikaner working-class community in the city, but also hired dietitians and recreational supervisors (Figure 10.2). The former managed a community restaurant and provided instruction in cooking and nutrition; the latter organized group outings, physical activities, films, discussion groups, and cultural activities for children and adults. Gluckmann envisaged similar health centers springing up throughout South Africa, but most attention was focused on the services to be provided for the African population. According to Gluckmann's report, each of these African health centers would require two African physicians and seven African health assistants – well below the number of physicians planned for the white centers. The necessity of providing physicians for these health centers would therefore require a fourth South African medical school. It was to be located in Durban.

The report was well received by the Medical Association of South Africa. The report, noted the first editorial in the *South African Medical Journal* to address the issue, is a solid work, "completely in accordance with the principles demanded by the medical profession." There is, the editorial noted further, "throughout the report a complete recognition of the supreme role played by poverty and ignorance . . . in the genesis of ill-health." The scheme was, they concluded, one which the medical profession "may safely accept."[29] Similar views were expressed by the Federal Council of the Medical Association, who agreed, at their meeting in 1945, to cooperate fully in the new scheme as long as the state played its part in dealing with the social causes of ill health.[30]

But would the Government play its part? Initially, the Government took a fairly positive, if cautious, approach. The scheme was "ideal," they noted, but to adopt its entire recommendations would demand far-reaching changes, "for which the country is not ready." They were not willing to address the nightmare issues of Union–Provincial jurisdiction, involved in setting up any truly unified national system, but they were ready to establish those parts of the scheme that were "within the framework of the constitution." They were willing, therefore, to open health centers limited to serving the needs of the sick poor, 40 of which were in operation by 1948, and to build the new medical school at Durban.[31]

Gluckmann, at least, felt satisfied; the Government had not killed the report. Gluckmann was appointed to chair a Health Centres Advisory Committee, and in 1945 he became the first Minister of a newly formed Ministry of Health. According to the annual public health report, this ministry was no longer concerned simply with sanitation and infectious diseases, but also with a wide range of health issues including social and economic problems.[32] The Government agreed also to set up an Institute of Family and Community

JOHN GRAY COMMUNITY HEALTH CENTRE (UNIVERSITY OF THE WITWATERSRAND)

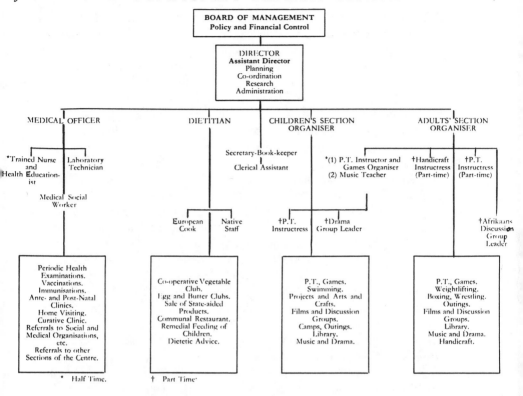

Figure 10.2. Organization of a South African community health center (Reproduced from Third Report, John Gray Community Health Centre, in J. A. Ryle papers, Wellcome Unit for the History of Medicine, Oxford University)

Health, adjacent to the site proposed for the new African medical school, in order to train health auxiliaries for the health centers. The future looked quite bright.

Meanwhile, in December 1947, Grant had returned from his world tour and had presented his final report to the Scientific Directors of the International Health Division. He reminded them that

health of body and mind is a basic human need. A healthful community is a basic social need. *Social medicine*, which has as its aim the meeting of these needs, is committed to a program of curative and preventive measures for the protection of the individual and the community. . . . It is also prepared to advance beyond these measures to the promotion of positive health.[33]

For this to be achieved, Grant explained, minimum standards of nutrition, housing, recreation, education, and social security, as well as freely accessible medical services, had to be established.

Society, Grant argued, had to establish goals of health care rather than medical care, and he pressed forward the idea that there must be social welfare legislation, including family allowances, maternity benefits, and home help; housing policies; and national food policies as well as universal accessibility to medical care. Such a program, he continued, "must focus from health community centers rather than from hospitals," in which general practitioners practice in groups supported by teams of social workers and other health professionals. Medical education also needed to be changed, he warned, so as to include what he called "social-pathological diagnosis." The inescapable conclusion, Grant wrote, was that "the full development and maintenance of man's mental and physical capacity will require the building up of a new scientific discipline . . . in social physiology, pathology and therapy," and that "the social and medical sciences, must extend and refocus their existing interests."

In 1950, following this activity, a Commission of Review was set up to examine the programs of the Rockefeller Foundation. From the start, they promoted the idea that the International Health Division should begin an "interdisciplinary attack" upon what they called "human ecology," rather than, as in the past, limiting themselves to the eradication of specific diseases.[34] In their final report, they explained that after World War II the International Health Division had entered a third stage of development in which "it was agreed that for too long [they] had avoided consideration of the socio-economic factors in public health," and that "an approach to public health problems, without regard for social and economic welfare of a people, was unrealistic." Everything must be integrated, they stressed, and the study of human ecology should involve "the recognition of the interrelatedness of things."[35] As a result of this report and fully conscious that the World Health Association was asserting itself in an area previously occupied by the International Health Division, the Foundation decided to close out the Division and to combine its work with the Division of Medical Sciences to form the Division of Medicine and Public Health.

In the 38 years since the formation of the Rockefeller Foundation, $409.8 million had been spent – $120.8 million on medical sciences and medical education including the Peking Union Medical College. Of the $96.9 million that had been directed toward public health, $91.4 million had been used by the International Health Division and its predecessors.[36]

The Rockefeller Foundation had clearly responded to the social concerns of the postwar era. The program of the new Division, the final report of the Commission noted, "should be directed, wherever possible, toward the elucidation of the ecological factors and recognition of their relative importance in promoting social advancement," and "medical care must be directed not only to the care of the sick, but also to the prevention of disease."

These new ideas were also incorporated into the constitution of the World Health Organization, which began to organize in 1946 and whose assembly first met in June 1948. "Health," according to that constitution, "is a state of complete physical, mental, and social well-being and not merely the absence of disease or infirmity."[37]

"The pump is primed," Grant had concluded optimistically in his final report, and "the universal establishment of this pattern of health care as a 'social science in the service of society' would usher in a new era which would be momentous in human welfare and happiness."[38]

11

Bilharzia: Pessimism in Egypt (1940–1955)

Take up the White Man's Burden –
    The savage wars of peace –
Fill full the mouth of famine
    And bid the sickness cease;
And when your goal is nearest
    The end for others sought,
Watch sloth and heathen Folly
    Bring all your hope to nought.
                                    Kipling

During the late 1940s, the broader definitions of health began to impinge on
the bilharzia problem in Egypt when the Rockefeller Foundation was again
asked to oversee another attempt to destroy the schistosome worms. By then
the optimism of the previous decade had collapsed as both parasite and snail
proved intractable against the two chemicals antimony tartrate and copper
sulfate. The Rockefeller Foundation had been wrong in their earlier prediction; bilharzia was not to be eliminated in 25 years. That the Rockefeller
Foundation had been invited back into the battle was itself an indication of the
failure of the two Egyptian departments set up to eradicate the disease: the
Endemic Disease Section and the Bilharzia Snail Eradication Section.

SNAIL ERADICATION

Although the failure of these government sections was highly probable given
the tools at their disposal, it became an absolute certainty when Claude
Barlow remained in Egypt to become Director of the Snail Eradication
Section. Barlow and Dr. Mohammed Khalil, who became Director General
of the Endemic Disease Section, were mortal enemies. Khalil had graduated at
the top of his class in 1917 by a huge margin and had then gained a Diploma in
Tropical Medicine from the London School, working under Leiper. With
much justification, he regarded himself as a world authority on bilharzia.
Why, then, should he tolerate the presence of yet another foreign expert?

Egypt, he believed, should be run by Egyptians.[1] Thus, rather than working in concert, the two agencies became extensions of two individuals locked in a futile power struggle against each other. The disease was forgotten as each set out to show the superiority of his own section and to castigate the workings of the rival section. Meanwhile, the *fellaheen* continued to pollute the canals with viable schistosome eggs and the miracidia continued to find snails to infect.

The altercation between Khalil and Barlow came to a head in 1939 when the Minister of Health, realizing the imminent withdrawal of the International Health Division, asked Barlow to remain in Egypt as director of a new agency that was to be set up to eliminate bilharzia from Fayoum Province. Barlow agreed to this on the understanding that he would be given a three-year contract with no drop in salary and that the "Bilharzia Destruction Section" would be an independent section of the ministry with its own director, subdirector, staff, and budget.[2] Obviously irked by this decision, Khalil complained to the Prime Minister himself. As a result, both men were ordered to present their views to a special ministerial committee set up to study the question.[3]

Disagreements over the impact of drying on snail mortality, on the role of the Nile in transmitting snails, and on the relative merits of copper sulfate or canal clearance surfaced at the meeting. In addition, Barlow made known his criticism of Khalil's work with copper sulfate in the Dahkla Oasis. Finally, however, after additional ministerial meetings that, in the opinion of Barlow, "had such a political scent that it developed into a positive stench," the government decided to set up a new agency, but also to divide the Fayoum region into three areas. In one part, all methods of killing snails and the parasite would be used; in the second, only copper sulfate would be applied; and in the third, canal clearances would be carried out.[4]

Barlow remained dissatisfied. "I'm still in the fight against schisto," he told his wife in late October, "but they can count me out entirely if I have to fight politicians as well as snails."[5] Nevertheless, despite continued opposition from Khalil, Barlow accepted a three-year contract to direct an independent Bilharzia Snail Eradication Section, after threatening to take up the chair of biology at what I assume to be a fictitious American university. Moderately satisfied, Barlow then took a well-deserved leave in the United States, where he signed his contract in the Egyptian Embassy, returning to Egypt in October, 1940.[6]

While Barlow was away on leave, the Egyptian government changed and Khalil made his move. He was promoted to Director General of the Endemic Disease Section by the new government, which at the same time relegated Barlow's unit to a temporary experimental project under Khalil's jurisdiction. Discovering what had happened, Barlow issued a statement to the Minister of Public Health. "BILHARZIASIS is the most IMPORTANT disease of Egypt," he passionately exclaimed, which "can be eradicted only by killing its snail hosts."

While *experimenting* with methods, which need no further trial, Egypt suffers under the burden of this scourge. . . . Had Prof. Khalil vigourously attacked this disease when he first took up his work with the Egyptian Government he might now be seeing the end instead of the beginning of its eradication. He combats those who try to do the work while doing nothing lasting and effective himself.

"NOTHING SHORT OF A PERMANENT SECTION should be considered," he added; "I am only interested in a Section which will be permanent and which will get right down to the urgent business of killing snails and so rid the country of untold suffering and death." If that were not the wish of the Government, he concluded, they ought to ask for his resignation.[7]

Barlow's outburst naturally reached the desk of Khalil, who forwarded a critique of it to the Prime Minister, Hussein Sirry. "Now that more than 4 months have passed since the appointment of Dr. Barlow on October 1, 1940," Khalil wrote, "he did not do any work at all and refused to begin unless his request to consider the Bilharzia Destruction Section as a permanent section . . . be granted."[8] Sirry's reply to Barlow was brutal and to the point: "The request is refused; Dr. Barlow is to be informed. If he wishes to remain, well and good, if not he has to send in his resignation."[9]

Barlow wrote bitterly to the Undersecretary of State of the Public Health Ministry, complaining of his treatment and pointing out the impossibility of working under a man who "has always held different views to my own on the subject and has always strongly opposed my methods."[10] The reply was evasive: "The question of changing the credit to a permanent one will receive due consideration in the future."[11] Finally, as a last resort, Barlow sent a complete account of the sorry story to the American Ambassador in Cairo, with the request that the matter be taken up with the Prime Minister "so that he could see the full facts of the case rather than the distortions of Prof. Khalil." Barlow's maneuver was successful, and in August he was promised his permanent section. Thus, one can assume that the American Ambassador interfered at a very sensitive time in Egyptian history: The British had taken control again in order to defend the Suez Canal against the Afrika Korps, regarded by many Arabs as potential liberators from British rule. Khalil had been forced to retreat by foreign interests beyond his control.

Khalil continued to make life difficult for Barlow; transport, personnel, and supplies were constantly denied, putting Barlow under considerable strain. Why did Barlow stay in the face of these obstacles? Sometime during the dark days of 1941, he put that question to himself. "There is only one reason," he wrote:

I am not my own master. I am under a dictatorship. Not the dictatorship of the Director of the Section, nor the Government. I am under the dictatorship of the bilharzial snail and so are we all, whether we like it or not, and I do not wish to leave until I have accomplished what I set out to do: BREAK THAT TYRANNY.[12]

Those involved must work together, he noted in another similar memo. "If we fight each other, we can't fight the snails. The effort which we put into personal fighting is just that much effort lost for the fight against bilharzia."[13]

With the permanent section in place by the end of 1941, Khalil lost some of his control, the arguments subsided to some extent, and work began seriously in the Fayoum area. This is a deep depression in the Libyan Desert into which water from the Nile enters by the Bahr Youssef Canal. From this canal, the water first radiates into smaller canals before draining out into the brackish Lake Qaroun. The first annual report of the Bilharzia Snail Destruction Section, as it was now called, was full of optimism. Canal clearance was feasible in canals less than 1.25 meters wide, it reported, whereas in large canals, after as much weeding as possible, copper sulfate was applied by dragging a 10-kilogram sack backwards and forwards across the width of the canal. "The results have been remarkably good," the report concluded.[14]

The work of the Bilharzia Snail Destruction Section continued to expand under the leadership of Dr. Abdel Azim, who took over when Barlow's contract expired at the end of 1943, although he remained as an expert advisor. But what was so striking, given the historical background of the section, was the gradual phaseout of canal clearance as the major weapon against the snails and its replacement by copper sulfate. This was made very plain in the Seventh Annual Report of the Section; clearance had become secondary to copper sulfate treatment.

Clearance of streams from vegetation, which is sometimes indispensable to permit the dragging of the bags of $CuSO_4$, is widely used whenever copper sulphate is not available in quantity, as it reduces the amount of sulphate necessary for killing snails.

Almost 30 years after Chandler's statement: "From the point of view of expense, harmlessness, and convenience in use, copper sulphate is preferable to any other *substance* which has been tried or suggested for destroying snails," his words still hold true. Since the beginning of the snail control work, this section has used copper sulphate for the chemical treatment of infested waters.

Honor was paid to canal clearance in a small passage. "Regular competent clearance of small distributaries would seriously impair their function as snail nurseries," the report notes, "but the task is beyond the material possibilities of the section."[15]

In 1949, two articles reviewing the Egyptian work against bilharzia appeared, one by Khalil and the other by Aly Shousha, the Undersecretary of State of the Ministry of Public Health, Egypt's first delegate to the WHO, and a supporter of the Bilharzia Snail Destruction Section.[16] "It is hopeless to try to eradicate the disease by treatment," Shousha wrote, noting that in 1945 the 94 antihelminth annexes (59 of which were mobile units) had treated 388,485 patients with bilharzia. "Control of the disease by prevention of pollution and by propaganda is equally hopeless," he added. "The only hope of control lies in the destruction of the intermediate snailhosts or vectors of the disease."[17] To that end, Shousha explained, a snail destruction unit had been formed under Barlow that now employed 10,000 men. Using data that measured the percentage of streams containing infected snails, he claimed that the Bilharzia Snail Destruction Section, using all known methods, "is making good progress."[18]

According to the Bilharzia Snail Destruction Section, by 1946 only 2 percent of the streams in Fayoum Province contained infected snails, whereas four years previously one-quarter of them harbored these snails. But such figures were obviously unreliable. Failure to locate infected snails in a stream meant very little, given their very localized distribution. Also, given the obvious desire to boost the section's work, only a very honest investigator would classify a stream as infected that yielded only one or two infected snails from hundreds collected.

Neither was Khalil impressed with the section's work. In 1947, as Khalil explained in his article, Dr. Hilmy visited Fayoum at Khalil's request, to check on the positive claims made to the Egyptian Parliament. But how could it be described as a success, Khalil wondered, when 60 percent of the Fayoum canals still contained bulinid snails – missing the point, deliberately or otherwise, that the Destruction Section claimed only to have reduced the number of canals with *infected* snails. Nevertheless, there was considerable justification in writing:

There is no scientific or moral justification in claiming before Parliament an imminent success while 60% of the main branch canals in the Fayoum are still harbouring snails. This shows that the name of eradication given to the section is a term of ridicule confronting the Egyptian Nation.[19]

Khalil poured scorn on the claim that the number of canals with infected snails had fallen to only 2 percent. The percentage had appeared to fall, Khalil claimed, simply because more and more small canals had been added to the list. "The Eradication Section was deliberately adding every year thousands of small channels free from snails to lower the percentage of infected streams and thus change failure to success on paper."[20] Furthermore, Khalil noted, Hilmy also examined 347 children born after the eradication campaign began, and found 62.8 percent of them with schistosome eggs. "The Snail Eradication Section has been working in Fayoum for 7 years and this is the result," Khalil concluded disdainfully, "Something is fundamentally wrong."[21]

In 1949, the Bilharzia Snail Destruction Section seemed to admit that something was indeed wrong and changed its name to the Bilharzia Snail *Control* Section; eradication of bilharzia had not taken place. Khalil naturally poured scorn on this name change, which, in his view, represented a failure in the *raison d'être* of the section. Name change or not, Khalil remarked, "The fact is that the 'Bilharzia Eradication Section' is attempting control with the methods meant for eradication."[22]

Barlow's copy of Khalil's article is filled with angry, rather trivial marginal comments. In an unpublished memo, Barlow described the article as "a slanderous and scurrilous general attack upon the Bilharzia Snail Control Section."[23] But by this stage, Barlow must have grown tired of his feud with Khalil. Khalil died in 1950, and, in that same year, with his advisor contract expired, Barlow was asked to review the bilharzia problem in South Africa. While there, he wrote about his life in China. "After 20 years of clinical practice," Barlow explained:

I decided that it was futile, since it saved lives and gave relief but it did nothing about the basic control of disease. At the age of 54 with a wife and four daughters I gave it all up, went back to college, got my doctorate in science and have been working ever since on Preventive Medicine. It has been a satisfying life.[24]

Perhaps it had been, but the last few years in Egypt had not been happy ones; the hostility between Khalil and Barlow had ruled out any cooperation between the Endemic Disease Section and the Snail Destruction Section. To the very end, Khalil never forgot his failure to control Barlow's section; his 1949 article ends with these words: "The Endemic Disease Section can profitably carry out the control measures against bilharziasis, malaria, and ancylostomiasis by the same personnel under the supervision of the medical officers of its units."[25] Today, Barlow is a forgotten man in Egypt. In a recently published book on the disease by Mohamed Abdel-Wahab, Scott's picture is included and his work praised; yet Barlow is not mentioned.[26]

The whole rather tragic scenario was perfectly understandable and an example of how personal differences, exacerbated by the political climate in a country growing tired of foreign political manipulation, can become an integral part of medical history. But while men argued, the disease grew steadily worse.

RETURN OF THE ROCKEFELLER FOUNDATION

In 1940, *Anopheles gambiae*, one of the major African vectors of the malarial parasite, began moving down the Nile to Egypt. Despite obvious signs of a forthcoming catastrophe, the Government remained totally unprepared for the major epidemic that ravaged the country in 1944, leaving tens of thousands dead in its wake. After much acrimonious debate, the Government turned to the Rockefeller Foundation for advice. As a result, Dr. Fred Soper, who had earlier directed a successful campaign against the same vector in Brazil and who was in Cairo at the time with the U.S. Typhus Commission, outlined a plan to eradicate the insect from the Nile Valley. By following this advice, a team led by Aly Shousha managed to wipe out the mosquito in six months.[27]

The contrast between this campaign and their own increasingly futile attempts to eradicate bilharzia was strikingly obvious. So they turned again to Soper and the Rockefeller Foundation. But this was 1946, not 1929. The Rockefeller Foundation was feeling the winds of social change in medicine; the step-by-step eradication of each disease was no longer seen as the solution to Egyptian health problems. John Grant had been appointed to investigate the issues of "social medicine," and Dr. George Strode was now Director of the International Health Division. "I think the village offers the real opportunity in Egypt," Strode informed Soper "and I should like to see a broad program developed."[28] Clearly, the Rockefeller approach had changed. They were no longer concerned only with one or two specific diseases, such as hookworm and bilharzia, and neither were they concerned only with building latrines. They were looking at the village as a diseased social unit, whose problems, they believed, could best be addressed by setting up "health demonstration areas" in which a simultaneous attack could be joined against a range of diseases, environmental problems could be tackled, and long-term programs to promote health could be developed. Thus, wishing to gain an up-to-date knowledge of the disease situation, but suspicious of the accuracy of the Egyptian public health reports, Dr. John M. Weir (Figure 11.1) was detailed to visit Egypt and prepare a report.

Missouri-born John Weir had joined the International Health Division in 1939, having graduated with both an M.D. and a Ph.D. in pathology from the University of Chicago. After work in Jamaica and Columbia and two years of service as a malariologist with the U.S. Army, he had passed through the usual training at Johns Hopkins before disembarking at Alexandria on February 23, 1947.

Although quite positive toward the antihelminth treatment annexes, described by Weir as "inexpensive realistic centers that serve their purposes well," he was less kind toward the Bilharzia Section. The parasite had not been eradicated, he pointed out, and the idea that the Section had acted as a control vehicle by decreasing the level of snail infection and breaking the cycle of transmission was based on wishful thinking. "When one asks what level is sufficiently low to prevent transmission through the snail host, one is unable to obtain any concrete answer," he explained, and there was no evidence that the disease had decreased, and no attempt had been made to learn whether, indeed, a reduction in snails leads to any reduction in disease. As in the earlier campaigns against bilharzia, the disease itself had again become the forgotten part of the equation; counting became the operative act, whether it was the number of latrines built, people treated, snails killed, or canals cleared of snails.[29]

The International Health Division, through Weir, proposed a study to develop effective health care and sanitation of Egyptian villages by demonstrating that "a village sanitation and health program based on modern local

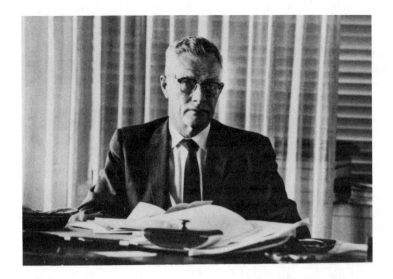

Figure 11.1. John M. Weir (Courtesy of the Rockefeller Archive Center)

health and preventive medical practices can be developed in Egypt which will effectively reduce the high morbidity in the villages at a cost that is within the economic resources of the local community and the government."[30] Five villages of Qaliubiya Province, grouped around the village of Sindbis, were eventually chosen. In them, Weir proposed to construct wells, pumps, showers, latrines, septic tanks, and laundry facilities; to begin a fly-killing operation using the new wonder-chemical DDT; to organize a comprehensive health center; and to initiate preventive campaigns against mosquitoes, lice, fleas, and snails. Weir painted a gloomy and accurate picture of conditions in these villages:

The villages are in reality rural slums for the personnel who farm the surrounding area. They are composed of mud brick materials of the roughest type. The usual house is composed of one main court or room which houses the water buffalo, fowls, and humans plus a storeroom and baking room. The roofs are constructed of a network of poles on which cattle dung and reeds are placed for drying in preparation for the fuel of the baking oven. The floors are of mud, filthy from centuries of accumulated excreta of animals and men. . . . In any village in any part of Egypt the rooms are filled with swarms of flies which cover the people, animals and walls. Water supply is usually taken from adjoining irrigation canals which also serve for defecation, bathing and laundering. In each house or directly in front of the entrance from the street, each family maintains a manure heap composed of dry dirt and the excreta of the animals and the women. These are periodically removed to be spread on the fields for fertilizer and are of great economic importance to the villager. Such structures and habits are universal in rural Egypt.[31]

Nevertheless, Weir estimated that the project would be completed in only three years. Dr. Bruce Wilson, in forwarding the plan to New York, was positively ecstatic. "I am confident," he wrote, "that the IHD [International Health Division] can play a large role in determining the logical solution to the village problems, problems which have baffled the health officials since 2980 B.C. when Dr. Imhotep applied his rudimentary medical knowledge and oriental magic to the problem."[32]

The two-year initial survey of the Sindbis villages, "said to be the most comprehensive and carefully integrated study ever made of the external factors which determine health in rural Egypt," revealed a horrific picture.[33] The average house received a sanitation score of only 21.2, whereas the perfectly sanitized Rockefeller house, somewhat reminiscent of those seen on American television sets, would score 106.5. With the usual diagnostic methods, schistosome eggs were found in 60 percent of the population, but more refined techniques revealed the parasite in 205 of 215 villagers examined, indicating, according to Weir, a true prevalence of 95.3 percent.[34]

Weir's diary tells the tale. One month following the start of the survey, it had become clear, he wrote, "that the original survey made by the Government in 1942 bears no relation to reality as might have been expected since the bulk of the information was gathered while sitting in the Omdah's house drinking tea." One month later, having disclosed that 50 percent of the children born in one village had died by their fifth year, he vented his anger at the same group. "I am completely hopeless about the prospect of ever developing a real public health interest or attitude in the Government employees. They seemed to have a deeply ingrained feeling that the villagers are animals and should be treated as such."[35]

In 1949, they began to take action in the villages. Throughout the period, Weir was continually frustrated not only by changes in government personnel and the usual habit of politicians worldwide "to pass up fundamental sanitation for showy and useless procedures," but also by "swarms" of WHO personnel who were beginning to take an interest in the scheme. There were also problems with his survey team who "seemed totally unable to work independently with any efficiency."[36] Nevertheless, the measures taken began to better the situation. By 1951, the average sanitation score had increased from 21.2 to 37.7, largely owing to the provision of a water supply and latrines (Figure 11.2).[37] But this time, the figures were not used to hide the stark reality. "Such installations," Weir wrote, "do not appear to have a marked effect upon the death rate in infants and therefore presumably little or no effect on the rate of dysenteries in infants."[38] Although fly control by various insecticides proved effective against many crippling eye diseases, the development of insecticide-resistant fly populations made it impossible to maintain the advantage. In addition, as Khalil had noted many years before, some of the social problems of bilharzia treatment came to light. Over 200 individuals who

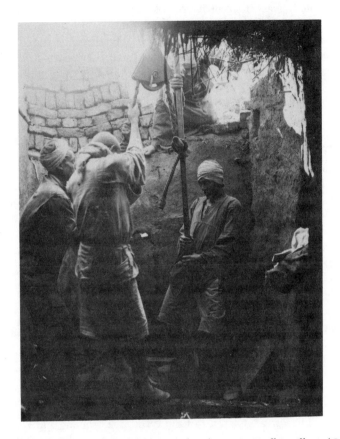

Figure 11.2. Installing latrines inside a house in Sindbis village (Courtesy of the Rockefeller Archive Center)

had failed to complete their treatment with 12 injections of Fouadin were asked why: 24 percent failed to return because of the severity of the drug reaction, but fully 61 percent could not return for economic reasons. As daily paid laborers they could not afford to lose the time during the morning when the treatment clinic was open.[39] The clinics, in other words, were operating at times convenient to a group of city-trained professionals unaware of the financial plight of the rural poor, who were unable to take days off work to secure treatment.

In the spring of 1952, with the project drawing to a close, Dr. Weir gave an "off the record" interview with Alvin Ross of the *New York Times*. Never one to pull punches, even Weir was disturbed to find the interview written up in the paper's May 1 edition. The major discovery of the Rockefeller Foundation, the paper noted, was "that provision of clean water and sewage disposal without fly control has no effect on the death rate." Four days later, under the headline "EGYPTIAN VILLAGE PUT AMONG WORST," the *Times* reported that "the Egyptian village is close to being the most unsanitary place to live of any civilized part of the world" – worse, even, than the villages of India and China.[40]

The 1952 publication of Weir's formal report in the *Egyptian Public Health Association Journal* also generated considerable reaction. "It is unfortunate that the outlook for improvement of health in the villages appears to be so hopeless," commented the Associate Director of the newly named Division of Medicine and Public Health, which had been formed the previous year following the closure of the International Health Division. "One is left with the feeling," he wrote, "that sanitation in Egypt is one of the world's insoluble problems."[41] Many people are saying, a WHO official noted, that "the Rockefeller Foundation has demonstrated that environmental sanitation is of no effect in impoverished and overcrowded countries; so why waste money and build false hopes by doing anything in this futile field?"[42] Marshall Balfour of the Rockefeller Foundation was not impressed. "Without meaning to be cynical," he wrote, "I find no conclusions in the summary that could not have been reached by a competent and experienced observer after one weeks visit to Egyptian villages. Unless there is something more than an evaluation of health, we are fanning the air, at least in a country such as Egypt." Reiterating earlier criticisms of the International Health Division's work in Egypt, Balfour questioned again whether they had contributed much to the welfare of Egypt.[43]

The Egyptian officials were furious at both the report and the *New York Times* article. Dr. Tarraf, Director of the Qaliubiya Training and Demonstration Centre of the WHO, who had taken over the Sindbis project in 1952, argued that the statistics were exaggerated and the report was "not conclusive in its description of the present general state of the Egyptian village." The Minister of Health refused to allow an Arabic translation of the survey without changes and generally protested the unfavorable publicity generated by the report. In 1956, the Israeli Government, via the agency of the U.S. Navy, requested a copy of the report for use in its anti-Arab propaganda.[44]

In 1953, at a time when the sensitivities of the Egyptians were being stretched to the limit, the U.S. Embassy in Cairo put together a film, called "The Wakening," in which Weir unsuspectingly took part. Not only had the Egyptians recently passed through a period of anti-British riots and the final coup by Abdel Nasser, but were, at that time, enduring a protracted discussion with the British that would lead finally to the Anglo-Egyptian Treaty of 1954. The film, as Weir quickly realized, was planned as a piece of crude propaganda, in which the United States received most of the accolades. He therefore wrote to New York, requesting that the State Department be informed that the Rockefeller Foundation was "not an agency of the American Government."[45] But no protest was made, and the film appeared. As the Egyptian paper *Al Misry* headlined: "AN AMERICAN GIVEN CREDIT FOR IMPROVING HEALTH OF VILLAGERS."

Very few seemed capable of understanding the real message of Weir's report, most succinctly described in an 1953 interview when Weir was at Cornell Medical School. "All problems of public health in Egypt," he told the interviewer, "are subsidiary, in the final analysis, to the economic problem."

The sanitation of the community depends on the sanitation of the individual home, and that in turn is related to deep-rooted customs of land tenure, taxation, housing standards, and living conditions. As long as animals live under the same roof and on the same floor with the family, the people will have flies as their constant companions, and as long as they have flies they will have dysentery, typhoid, and other infections which are born of such conditions. As long as whole communities don't have enough to eat, they'll have pellagra. Public sanitation and public health measures can alleviate the conditions to a degree, but in Egypt the economic problem is the basic one.[46]

"The only possibility of improvement," Weir similarly concluded in his published report, "must be that of rebuilding villages along sanitary lines . . . such a process will be costly and must necessarily be a long term program extending over many decades and coordinated with educational, economic, and social improvements."[47]

In 1954, some WHO officials, after expressing concern that the Weir report had generated rumors on the ineffectiveness of sanitation, received a brutal missive from Weir. "There is little advantage," he wrote, "in providing a well and a latrine for a family that sits at the side of their bed and makes mud pies out of cow dung."[48]

The wheel had turned again. Convinced initially that the social problems of the American South were a result of poor education, the Rockefeller philanthropies had moved into the educational arena only to discover that disease and not illiteracy lay at the heart of the problem. Now, the International Health Division and its modern offspring, created to rid the world of disease, were being told that the real problem lay in the socioeconomic conditions of the Third World. But few were ready to listen. Weir's opinion, Dr. Tarraf noted, "is inconsistent with the country's financial potentialities,"[49] although at that very time an international team of experts was conducting feasibility studies on the engineering possibilities of an Aswan High Dam that was far beyond the country's financial capabilities, and would, if built, dramatically increase the burden of bilharzia once again. These were not happy times in Egypt.

The Sindbis project was as close as the International Health Division came to implementing some of John Grant's proposals. But the project died.

As Grant noted in 1949, the literature is "almost redundant" with plans to extend beyond medical care into health care, yet "nowhere up to the present time, has the concept been experimented with, much less demonstrated."[50] And then, at the bottom of the page, in red type, he wrote these lines:

In the evolution of the welfare of communities, are the democratic or the totalitarian countries going to be the first to provide adequate health care.

Five months later, the People's Republic of China was proclaimed in a country where the seriousness of bilharzia was equal to that in Egypt.

12

Bilharzia: Victory in China?

What the Gods failed to cure is not insurmountable to the Communist Party.   *Chinese Medical Journal*

Malnutrition; appalling child mortality rates; high prevalence of malaria, kala-azar, and venereal diseases; a total absence of rural health care; and few physicians typified China on October 1, 1949, when the People's Republic of China was proclaimed from the new capital in Peking. Over ten million people were estimated to be infected with "big belly" (Figure 12.1), the peasant name for bilharzia, endemic to 11 provinces along the Yangtze River valley and some of the south coastal areas. Oxen, horses, donkeys, mules, pigs, goats, sheep, dogs, cats, and mice also carried the dreaded worm. The havoc wreaked by the disease had become part of Chinese folklore: a village near Shanghai with only 461 inhabitants remaining from an original 1,000, 449 of whom had bilharzia; "The Village of Widows," in Kiangsi Province, where acres of potentially productive land had gone to weed. "Scourged by famine, the people survived on seaweeds in spring, wild herbs in summer, husks in autumn, and handouts in winter. Many ended the nightmare of their existence by suicide."[1] After the Chinese People's Liberation Army occupied Shanghai during the Civil War, the troops were required to learn to swim in order to prepare for future battles in the southern provinces. As a result, several thousand acute cases of bilharzia appeared, military training was suspended, and the barracks were transformed into hospital wards. Thus, according to an article in *Harper's Magazine*, the blood fluke had saved Formosa, and *Schistosoma japonicum* "turned out to be a precious ally of America and Nationalist China." In the six months that passed before the Chinese army returned to full fighting strength, the U.S. Seventh Fleet had appeared on the scene, and the opportunity to destroy the Nationalists had vanished.[2]

Health care in these early years was firmly in the hands of Western-style Chinese physicians, trained at institutions such as the Peking Union Medical College, which, in 1951, was nationalized to become the Union Medical College of China. Initially, their power base remained undisturbed. "Since the liberation," announced an early and optimistic editorial in the *China Medical*

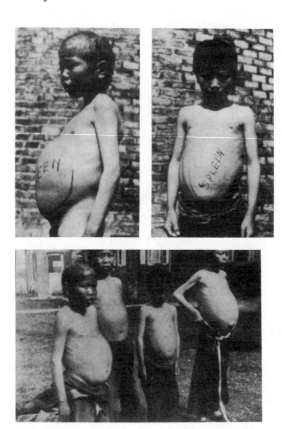

Figure 12.1. Bilharzia victims in China (Courtesy of the Chinese Medical Association)

Journal, the official English-language journal of the Chinese Medical Association and mouthpiece of these physicians, "the journal has not met the fate predicted by many." As in the past, the urban-based Association continued to support quality over quantity, to stress the value of disinterested medical research, and to oppose traditional Chinese medicine. Likewise, according to the editorial, the Chinese Medical Association remained a free organization, and existed independent of Party influences. Science had, according to the editor, "no national boundary especially the science of medicine."[3]

Nevertheless, the same issue of the journal contained a warning. "Schistosomiasis japonica," an author from the National Medical College of Shanghai concluded, "poses before the medical profession in China the important problems of prevention and treatment of a devastating disease undermining the very health and existence of our nation which depends chiefly on agriculture for her national resources";[4] But, at that time, Chinese physicians had paid little heed to problems of rural health. But this state of affairs was not to last.

THE POLITICIZATION OF HEALTH

At the First National Health Conference in 1950, three major policy decisions were made that clearly threatened the status quo. In the future the conference resolved, attention must be paid to the health of workers, peasants, and soldiers; there must be an emphasis on preventive medicine; and traditional and modern medicine must be combined. The head office of the Chinese Medical Association moved from Shanghai to Peking, and, at the same time, the *Chinese Medical Journal* announced that all papers were to be written in Chinese, with the editor selecting those that would be translated into English. Medical workers were urged also to "cultivate interests outside their specialization" and to learn "political and social sciences, for this is only way through which science can develop along the right track."

Only when working among the people and for the people can science grow and flourish. The previous Chinese political system would not allow science to develop among the people. The political system of New China . . . is aimed at promoting science among the people and to assist and foster our scientists to become scientific workers of the people and for the people.[5]

By the mid-1950s the Party had gained control of the Ministry of Health and of the profession. In 1953, Lien-chang, President of the Chinese Medical Association and a leading figure in the Red Army hospital system, announced that members of the medical profession had been "called to duty." According to him, they were working in factories and mines and in border regions beyond the lure of big cities. They were involved also in practical research, working jointly with practitioners of traditional medicine. "The ideology of service to the people is taking root among medical workers," Lien-chang declared, and they have "freed themselves from the narrow confines of self-interest and prestige." But, he warned, although the level of political consciousness had been raised, the Association was weak in ideological leadership, and too few articles were being published on preventive medicine, factory and village hygiene, and advanced Soviet medicine. Instead, he complained, many still emphasized curative Western-style medicine, and, with their distrust of native physicians, were "lacking in the mass standpoint."[6]

Members of the medical profession were urged also to follow the guidelines of dialectical materialism. According to Lien-chang, Soviet medicine was the most advanced in the world, and only by mastering dialectical materialism could the Chinese understand physiological phenomena, investigate causes of disease, and carry out correct preventive measures. "Disease is related to both the body and the environment," he wrote, in obvious homage to Pavlovian thinking, but medicine in the old days "was founded on idealism and mechanical materialism and was, therefore, in many respects, unscientific and divorced from the needs of the people."[7]

Further undermining of the influence of Western-style medical professionals occurred with the formation of special health committees answering only to the Party. In 1955, for example, a so-called Nine-Man Subcommittee on Schistosomiasis was set up under the leadership of two politicians, K'O Ch'ing-shih and Wei Wen-po. Nevertheless, according to Lampton, the actual medical policies changed very little; the Party was still dependent on the skills of those trained in Western ways. Even though Party membership had been opened to these "higher intellectuals" in the hope of transforming their ideologies, most members of the Chinese medical profession retained their urban base and still supported the Western approach to medical problems.

Nevertheless, according to Chinese sources, changes were beginning to take place in the rural health field. At the 1953 meeting of the Pakistan Association for the Advancement of Science, Kung Nai-chuan, Vice-President of the Chinese Medical Association was nothing but enthusiastic. "Under the inspiring leadership of Chairman Mao Tse-tung," he began, "New China has made brilliant achievements in public medical service." Urban and rural health-care facilities had increased enormously, he reported, and many infectious diseases have been brought under control.[8] By the mid-1950s, according to the Chinese delegates at a joint session with Soviet scientists, thousands of health personnel had been trained to work in campaigns against bilharzia, "the most serious parasitic disease in China." Numerous stations, substations, and field units had been established, and 60 percent of the over 50,000 cases treated in 1953 had been "restored to health." In the four years since the revolution, the delegates reported, the number of research papers on the disease had almost doubled over what it had been in the previous 40 years.[9]

Some of this research was of the standard fare: testing various molluscicides, from copper sulfate to Paris green and DDT; testing various antimony drugs for their therapeutic effects; surveying reservoir hosts; and searching for more reliable diagnostic methods. But other aspects of this research such as finding methods of killing schistosome eggs in feces stored for fertilizers, and testing native herbal drugs for their therapeutic and molluscicidal effects, had a uniquely Chinese flavor. Croton oil emulsion, for example, a powerful purgative drug, was found to kill snails. Platycodon, the balloon flower with a bitter-tasting latex; Piper, the pepper plant, containing a powerful stimulant and irritant; Gleditschia, with poisonous alkaloids in the leaves and bark; Chrysanthemum and Stephania, the moonseed with bitter-tasting roots – all were found to have therapeutic effects. Many labor-intensive physical methods, such as grass burning, burial in soil, and reclamation of low and flooded land by dike building, were found effective in rendering areas free from the amphibious snail host, *Oncomelania*.

The Chinese snail host of the schistosomes, being amphibious, favors poorly drained swamps and marshes. Thus, they cannot survive well in drained and cultivated land with steep-sided drainage canals and ditches. In this they are very different from the snail hosts of the other two schistosome species that thrive in irrigated areas. One can overemphasize the difference between China and elsewhere, however. The contents of a Chinese handbook dealing with the prevention and treatment of bilharzia, published by the Shanghai Municipal Institute for Prevention and Treatment of Schistosomiasis, does not differ significantly from one that might have been written in any other country. It gives advice on many methods of snail elimination, on the proper treatment of manure, and on treatment. It recommends the use of tartar emetic and two oral antimony drugs – antischistosome-846 and antimony-273. Where it differs is the recommended use of acupuncture and herbal medicines to counter the side effects of the antimony drugs, and in the audience for whom the book is intended; this is a field guide, not a book aimed only at experts.[10]

In 1956, at the end of the first five-year plan following the initial National Health Conference, Lien-chang announced even more ambitious plans. In that year, the Central Committee of the Party put forward its program for agricultural development, which aimed to eradicate the most dangerous diseases in 12 years. But 12 years proved to be too long a wait. In 1958, to revitalize agriculture and to accelerate agricultural production which had been lagging behind, the Party initiated the Great Leap Forward. The anticipated rise in agricultural productivity resulting from this plan would provide, they predicted, the finances for massive rural health campaigns, in which the treasurehouse of traditional Chinese medical wisdom would play a vital role.

THE MASS CAMPAIGN

Among these health campaigns none was more famous than the mass campaign against bilharzia, initiated by the Nine-Man Schistosomiasis Subcommittee, and carried out by Party committees at the local level, dominated by nonprofessional cadres of middle-level health workers. Seventeen thousand specialized workers in 1,282 prevention and treatment units, working out of 197 centers and 42 research institutes, carried out the antibilharzia campaign "according to the principle of science integrated with mass movement and prevention and treatment integrated with production."[11] The traditional three-week to one-month treatment with antimony tartrate was cut to two or three days, with a cure rate reported to be over 85 percent. Logistical improvements were reported to have speeded up the examination and diagnostic procedures to such an extent that health teams claimed to have examined 2,800,000 Chinese in the first nine months of 1958. One health inspection team stretched credulity to the breaking point by claiming to have examined 1,200 patients in a single day! In these same nine months, the Chinese claimed to have reduced the contamination of soil by schistosome eggs with the construction or repair of 67,270,000 latrines. But, most impressive of all, thousands of peasants reclaimed swamp land, dug new drainage ditches, buried snails under the earth, burned grass, and applied chemicals. By these means, the snail host was reported to have been eliminated from 3,000 million square meters of land (Figures 12.2 and 12.3).

"Thanks to these effective measures," Ch'ien Hsin-chung announced at the end of 1958, "schistosomiasis has been basically wiped out in more than half the endemic areas in the country (167 counties and cities, including the whole of Kiangsu and Fukien provinces, and Shanghai). The day is not far off when schistosomiasis will be basically or completely wiped out in the whole country."[12]

Yukiang County in Kiangsu Province was the first to claim total elimination of the disease, while, in adjacent Anhwei, 10 million peasants cleared snails from 11 counties.[13] In Fukien Province, where an antibilharzia campaign was launched "simultaneously with their efforts to develop production and their struggle against the traitorous Chiang Kai-shek clique entrenched in Quemoy and Matsu Islands," 96 percent of 45,000 patients with the disease were reported cured, and 13 million square meters cleared of snails.[14] There was once a lake in Hupei Province, Wei Pen-po reported, that was flooded in summer and full of weeds and snails in winter. Those who used the lake to grow crops died. But in the past two years the lake bed had been ploughed three times, the snails buried, and the land reclaimed for cotton (Figure 12.4). By this integration of a mass movement with science and technology, he argued, "the Party can cure what the powers above have failed to do." With political guidance, he reported, 120,000–150,000 peasants in Kiangsu Province, working day and night, buried snails, drained water, improved irrigation, and increased the amount of arable land.

> Welcome the sunrise, come under the stars, work from dusk to daybreak
>
> Our strength is boundless, our enthusiasm is redder than fire . . .
> Be the river like a sea, drained clean it shall be . . .
>
> Empty the rivers to wipe out the snails, resolutely fight the big belly disease.[15]

When Mao Tse-tung read that bilharzia had been wiped out in Yukiang County, he penned his famous lines:

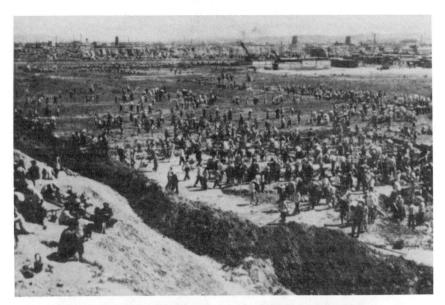

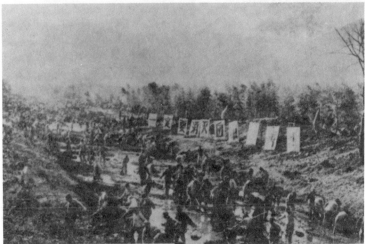

Figure 12.2. The mass campaign against bilharzia in China, I: dredging the river bed, ditch digging, paring the soil, and snail burying. The posters read "Perish the Snail Fever." (Courtesy of the Chinese Medical Association)

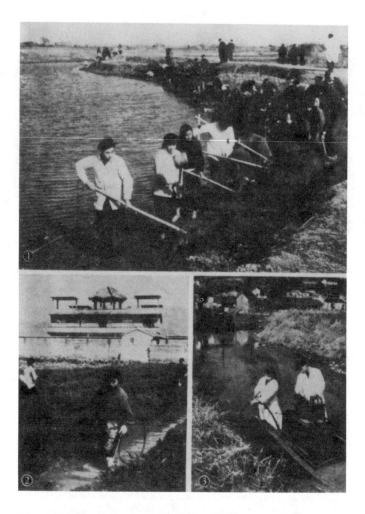

Figure 12.3. The mass campaign against bilharzia in China, II: paring the soil and applying sodium pentachlorophenate (Courtesy of the Chinese Medical Association)

Farewell to the God of Plague

So many green streams and blue hills, but to what avail?
This tiny creature left even Hua To powerless!
Hundreds of villages choked with weeds, men wasted away;
Thousands of homes deserted, ghosts chanted mournfully.
Motionless, by earth I travel eighty thousand li a day,
Surveying the sky I see a myriad milky ways from afar.

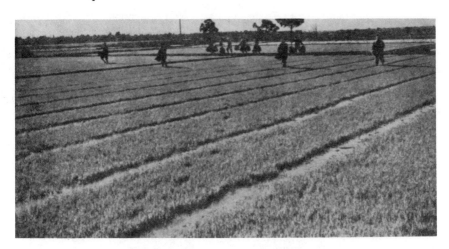

Figure 12.4. The mass campaign against bilharzia in China, III: land reclamation (Courtesy of the Chinese Medical Association)

Should the Cowherd ask tidings of the God of Plague,
Say the same griefs flow down the stream of time.

The spring wind blows amid profuse willow wands,
Six hundred million in this land all equal Yao and Shun.
Crimson rain swirls in waves under our will,
Green mountains turn to bridges at our wish.
Gleaming mattocks fall on the Five Ridges heaven-high;
Mighty arms move to rock the earth round the Triple River.
We ask the God of Plague: "Where are you bound?"
Paper barges aflame and candlelight illuminate the sky.[16]

Enthusiasm reached new heights when delegates to an All-China Conference on Parasitic Diseases, in November 1958, resolved to eradicate the five major parasitic diseases (malaria, bilharzia, filariasis, hookworm, and kala-azur) in one year to honor the forthcoming tenth anniversary of the People's Republic of China. To reach this objective, it was necessary to:

1. Determinedly carry through the absolute leadership of the Communist Party in science and technology, continue to do away with the influences of bourgeois scientific views, carry out the policy [to] "let all schools of thought contend and let all flowers bloom," foster the democratic spirit in science, overcome rightist conservatism and blind reverence for established rules, and advance the development of science.
2. Follow the mass line, keep in close contact with the masses, integrate theory with practice, do away with the mysterious notions about science, combine scientific research with the mass technical revolution and the mass campaign

to wipe out the four pests and improve sanitary conditions. . . . carry out the combination of Western medicine and traditional Chinese medicine and the use of both native and foreign methods.

3. Centre research work around the improvement of the six hundred million people's health . . .

4. Develop the communist spirit of full cooperation, overcome localism, group egoism, individualism, and all those erroneous ideas based on personal inclination of working alone without cooperation with others, learn from each other, promote exchange of experiences and mutual help, and develop the noble communist virtue of "one for all and all for one."[17]

That same year the *Chinese Medical Journal* announced that a campaign against the four pests was also under way: 1,240,000,000 rats and 1,206,000 grain-eating sparrows had already been destroyed, they announced, while 61,682,800 kg of dead flies had been weighed, and – once again stretching credulity to the breaking point – 6,285,000 kg of mosquitos were reported to have been laboriously caught, collected, and weighed![18]

The Party provided the driving force for the campaign, while the "experts and intelligentsia" came in for some well-aimed barbs. They preach the superiority of foreign ways, noted an editorial in *Renmin Ribao*, and "were loud in their own praises, making a mystery of science and treating it as something esoteric meant only for the initiated few. In this way they tried to fool people into believing that all technical innovations, discoveries and inventions could be made only by well-known experts and no one else." The message was clear: Let the movement "maintain its spirit of vigorous enthusiasm and continue to progress"; let us "take the initiative in the struggle against nature"; let us "wipe out the four pests, improve sanitary conditions, promote sports, eliminate the principal diseases, break down superstitions, reform customs and change habits, and invigorate the national spirit."[19]

The tenth anniversary of the revolution witnessed a host of self-congratulatory messages. Progress in public health has been rapid, reported the Minister of Public Health. Under the inspiration of "getting all out, aiming higher and getting greater, quicker, better, and more economical results to build socialism," he claimed that bilharzia had been cleared from 65.4 percent of previously affected areas.[20] Under the reactionary Kuomintang, reported a member of the Nine-Man Schistosomiasis Subcommittee, "this beautiful land was literally turned into a hell on earth." But today, in contrast, "desolate villages are filled with children and laughter." The antischistosomiasis campaign had "invigorated the national spirit," he argued, and raised "political consciousness":

What the Gods failed to cure is not insurmountable to the Communist Party. With the Communist Party and the people's communes there is nothing on earth that cannot be done. . . . It is our firm belief that if we resolutely oppose rightist deviation and exert all our efforts, a decisive victory will soon be won.[21]

The victory over bilharzia is a victory of the socialist road to public health, argued Hsu Yun-pei, Vice-Minister of Public Health. It is a victory over "the dictatorship of experts, supremacy of technique, disregard of patients' needs and interests, and neglect of preventive work." We have discarded "the bourgeois policy of letting professors and experts run schools," who, he claimed, by "disregarding the masses and training students to be proficient professionally but devoid of proletarian ideology," divorced medical education from "politics, the masses and reality."[22]

But, as David Lampton so accurately noted: "Like a leading character in a Greek tragedy, this mobilization system had a tragic flaw; there were no individuals charged with objectively evaluating the progress which was, or was not, being made."[23] Nobody, including the Chinese themselves, can really know the results of that extraordinary campaign.

In the early 1960s, as agricultural and industrial production started to fall, these mass public health activities began to collapse. Mao Tse-tung's influence eroded, commune sizes were cut, and, with depleted resources, the health-unit teams decreased in size. In famous Yukiang County, Kiangsu Province, for example, the number of health workers decreased from 3,900 in 1960 to only 300 five years later. Medical educators emphasized quality again, as longer curricula of higher standards came into vogue. There were no short cuts to better health, the Vice-Minister of Public Health warned, rather a "long term persistent effort" is needed.[24] The Nine-Man Subcommittee, meeting in 1964 after four years of inactivity, turned again to expert advice, rejected a return to mass campaigns, and reported on bilharzia in words that indicate just how much their position had changed since the 1950s: "Schistosomiasis affects wide areas, and the factors for its outbreak are very complicated. Those who have been cured of this disease may be affected by it again. It is impossible to wipe out all snails within a short time."[25] Chinese medicine had returned to an urban base.

THE GREAT PROLETARIAN CULTURAL REVOLUTION

On June 26, 1965, Mao Tse-tung began his counterattack. In a devastating speech he told the Ministry of Public Health

that it only works for fifteen percent of the total population of the country and that this fifteen percent is mainly composed of gentlemen, while the broad masses of the peasants do not get any medical treatment. . . . The Ministry of Public Health is not a Ministry of Public Health for the people, so why not change its name to the Ministry of Urban Health, the Ministry of Gentlemen's Health, or even to Ministry of Urban Gentlemen's Health?

Medical education, Mao Tse-tung argued, needed to be simplified and shortened. Three years post-primary education should be enough, he wrote, because these medical workers would then raise their standards through experience. Such doctors, he believed, would serve the villages better than the medical elite; at least the villages could afford to pay for their services. This elite, he complained with much justification, spend their energies studying rare and difficult diseases "at the so-called pinnacle of science," yet ignore "commonly seen, frequently occurring and widespread diseases." All medical doctors should be sent to work in the countryside, he concluded.[26]

A year later, Mao Tse-tung launched the Great Proletarian Cultural Revolution attacking the "capitalist road." Not surprisingly, urban-based, elitist health-care systems came under attack in the pages of the *Chinese Medical Journal*, whose editorial announced that "a nationwide upsurge to go to the countryside to serve the peasants has started."[27] According to articles in the *Chinese Medical Journal*, rural production teams were to include "politically progressive" volunteer health workers who would require two to three months' training in first aid and simple preventive methods. Each production team would, in turn, be part of a production brigade, staffed by a few part-time "barefoot" doctors, trained for three to six months in country hospitals to diagnose, treat, and prevent common diseases, and to provide leadership in health education. The largest unit, the commune, on the other hand, would have three to five fully qualified, full-time physicians, trained for three years in a medical college.[28] By 1968, there were reported to be 4,500 "barefoot doctors" and 29,000 "health workers" in the rural areas of Shanghai Province alone.[29]

But the rural peasant was not to be a passive recipient of medical wisdom. They were expected to revolutionize their urban teachers. "We cured the physical diseases of the peasants," wrote the Minister of Health, and "the peasants cured our ideological diseases." Each health team became "a revolutionized fighting force," and in the course of their work each comrade was expected also to accept responsibility for indoctrinating others in the political and ideological struggle.[30] After one such struggle, Ts'ao Feng-kang announced he had become a rural doctor. He learned of the crimes of the exploiting classes, he admitted, only after his medical tours in the rural areas. He discovered, as many professionals in the Third World have yet to discover, that peasants cannot afford the time or money to attend medical clinics that open only during a professional's working day usually in or close to urban centers. His life as an urban doctor had been wasted, he realized, so this 42-year-old physician settled in a rural area as "a red revolutionary seed."[31]

The 1966 volume of the *Chinese Medical Journal* unleashed an extraordinary avalanche of passionate comment in support of Mao and his Cultural Revolution, and in opposition to experts and their ways.

Although the "scholars," "specialists," and "professors" who oppose the Party and socialism don all sorts of cloaks, strike grand poses, and deliberately turn simple things into mysteries, they can neither daunt nor mislead us. We have the all-conquering weapon of Mao Tse-tung's thought. Truth is with us. Let us hold ever higher the great red banner of Mao Tse-tung's thought, resolutely destroy the black anti-Party and anti-socialist line of the bourgeoisie and the revisionists and carry out the great socialist Cultural Revolution through to the end.[32]

After the chaos of the Cultural Revolution, rural campaigns against diseases got underway again. "The cooperative medical service is blossoming," announced an editorial in the *Chinese Medical Journal* on the tenth anniversary of the Cultural Revolution, "and a million-strong barefoot doctors are maturing."[33] On the death of Mao, in 1976, spokespersons from Yukiang County announced that they had "persisted in the struggle against capitalism, revisionism, and schistosomiasis." We have turned, they announced, "snail-infested swamps, into 'rivers of happiness.' We must forever uphold the first red banner on the schistosomiasis control front . . . repulse the rightist deviationists . . . and carry through the proletarian revolutionary cause."[34]

The victory over bilharzia, according to another article, was "a victory of Chairman Mao's revolutionary line, and a powerful rebuff to the reactionary nonsense that 'schistosomiasis cannot be wiped out.'"[35]

AN ASSESSMENT

Can we now answer John Grant's question of 1949? Was China, a totalitarian country, the first to provide adequate health care, and, more particularly, was China the first country to successfully eliminate bilharzia?

The answer to the first of these questions now seems reasonably clear. One can no longer claim, as was done in 1948, that "China presents perhaps the greatest and most intractable public health problem of any nation in the world."[36] China is no longer "the sick man of Asia." But the answer to the second question is far more controversial. Some of the Chinese claims are clearly outlandish, and much of their data unsubstantiated. In addition, the rhetoric and politicization of the process are so foreign to the majority of us, who have little understanding of China and its history, that we automatically draw back from accepting their claims. Nevertheless, there now seems little doubt that the Chinese have had more success combating bilharzia than any other country of comparable wealth. "The degree of Chinese success," Sandbach wrote in 1977, "is in any case extremely significant when one considers that throughout the world the disease remains largely uncontrolled and its prevalence is increasing."[37] Many experts on the disease agree with his assessment.

In 1984, Paul Basch of Stanford University School of Medicine traveled to China to examine the status of bilharzia. He reported that although there were still about 2.4 million cases of bilharzia in China, most were light, and in some areas where the snail host had been drastically reduced or even eliminated, there had sometimes been a 90 percent reduction in the number of diseased patients. Even in the Great Lakes Region, where the problem of bilharzia can be compared to that in the Nile Delta, great improvements had taken place. Cattle, Basch concluded "provide 90% of the total fecal contamination of the environment," and human carriers no longer acted as the main source of schistosome eggs.[38] But, as Dr. Jordan pointed out to me, Basch's statement is somewhat misleading; in China cattle and domestic animals have always provided the bulk of fecal contamination.

But that was not Basch's first visit to China. In 1975, he participated in the American Schistosomiasis Delegation, which was invited to review the bilharzia problem in China at that time. By 1975, profound changes had taken place in American–Chinese relations, which began, four years earlier, with the China tour of the U.S. table-tennis team. The delegates spent most of their time in the major rice-growing areas of the Yangtze Delta, close to Shanghai, where, they reported, "the record of success in suppressing the disease was dramatically evident." Although frustrated by their inability to visit many important sites of the disease, they felt able to conclude their report on a positive note:

Complete eradication may still remain elusive in the Yangtze River delta, and even more so in other areas, but this does not negate the very considerable advances made in the control of schistosomiasis. At a time when, with the exception of Japan, the disease is on the increase in virtually every other country in the world where it has been endemic, there can be no doubt that great progress has been achieved and that both incidence and prevalence of the infection are markedly declining in the People's Republic of China.[39]

Perhaps, given the great advances in public health, Tien Hsi-cheng concluded "outside observers should not be inordinately surprised to find, in another decade or so, that schistosomiasis, like cholera and bubonic plague, has ceased to be a menace to the millions of Chinese."[40]

The contrast between the situation in China and that in Egypt is striking; optimism and hope in one, pessimism and worsening conditions in the other. There seems to be one paramount reason for this: the superior primary health care system of China. Joshua Horn, a British surgeon who worked in China, expressed this well when he praised "the conviction that the ordinary people possess great strength and wisdom and that when their initiative is given full play they can accomplish miracles."[41] What China had demonstrated in the area of health care, James Grant (the son of John Grant) so correctly pointed out, was that "primary health care must involve popular participation to be successful, and a vertical medical system cannot be truly effective, or even stand by itself, unless it is integrated with other activities in a joint attack on the problems of development and social reconstruction."[42]

But before World War II, the medical approach taken by Britain and the United States denied the potential of ordinary people at home and abroad to become involved in the formulation of their own health care policies. They had unquestioned faith in Western, technical superiority.

PART III

The professional approach (1950–1970s)

13

The new British Empire: Finding the experts

Whatever success the Chinese had had in their campaigns against bilharzia was achieved by the Chinese themselves; no foreign experts were brought in to impose their solutions. In addition, their success was achieved by utilizing a broad range of health workers, some of whom had very minimal training. In postwar British Africa, however, neither of these possibilities existed. Very few Africans had been trained in either medicine or public health, and the possibility of building a health service based on a cadre of lower-level "barefoot doctors" was rejected by both the African elite and members of the British medical profession. By the 1950s, the African colonies, who were shortly to gain their independence, had opted for a health system that was, as much as possible, a replica of that in Britain. In addition, a great deal of emphasis was directed toward fundamental medical research. But there were so few fully trained Africans capable of doing this research, and such negative opinions on their abilities, that the researchers were recruited directly from Britain.

These foreign experts, scientific to the core, continued to believe that the solution to health problems in the British Empire required a step-by-step elimination of each tropical disease. This, they assumed, could best be attained by the "technological fix," which would succeed irrespective of the cultural setting in which it was to be applied. What worked in the relatively affluent setting of Britain would necessarily work also in tropical Africa. Arguments advocating a more cultural and socioeconomic approach must have seemed reminiscent of the era before the germ theory, when disease was attributed to a multitude of human and environmental factors. The scientific way was the narrow way; to broaden out now into the social field must have seemed a step back in time to the era of prescientific medicine. The British Empire was not about to step backwards.

AFRICAN PHYSICIANS

Before World War II, British educational policy in Africa buttressed their Empire of trusteeship. Africans were not to be treated in the British manner;

they were to receive "native education on native lines."[1] Emphasis was placed on general literacy and practical agricultural training. Christian moral and religious teachings were stressed, while, at the same time, the "desirable" parts of the Africans' cultural background were to be retained. For example, the famous 1925 report of the Advisory Committee on Native Education, chaired by Ormsby-Gore, had taken a strong stand in favor of "adaptation." Education, the report noted, should be adapted to the Africans' way of life, "conserving all sound and healthy elements in the fabric of their social life." To retain what is beneficial and to replace the defective, the report argued, religious and moral teaching should be placed on equal footing with secular subjects. Africans should be taught "discipline of work, habits of industry, manliness"; boarding schools, field games and boy scout activities should be encouraged; and "it should be the aim of the educational system to instill into pupils the view that vocational careers are no less honourable than the clerical."[2] British views on medical education paralleled those on general education. Africans were not to be trained as physicians, but as subordinate, intermediate, and lower-level health workers.

The few African physicians who did exist, all trained in Britain after schooling in British missionary schools, were segregated from their European colleagues, listed separately in all reports, and placed on a level of the medical hierarchy immediately above European nurses and below European medical officers, however junior. In 1911, for example, there were four such African doctors in Southern Nigeria, working in dispensaries and asylums where few British were prepared to tread. Job security was nonexistent; Drs. Lumkin and Adeniyi-Jones were fired sometime during 1911 or 1912 for complaining about their inferior status, leaving only two Nigerian doctors in service.[3]

In Uganda of the 1920s, the majority of intermediate-level health workers were Indian subassistant surgeons. But in 1923, the Mulago Hospital in Kampala, built originally as a venereal disease hospital for Africans, was converted to a general hospital and used to train African ward attendants and dressers. In addition, newly arrived British medical officers were posted there for six months "to familiarize them with natives and native diseases."[4] Three years later, as part of a general reorganization of medical services in Uganda in response to the call for a "native medical service," the African assistants in Uganda were reorganized into an extraordinary nine-tiered medical African hierarchy (see Table 13.1), all except the top two levels receiving their training in the Mulago Hospital.[5] The top two tiers, the medical assistants, passed through a two-year basic science program at Makerere College, before completing their training at a new medical school built in 1928 adjacent to the Mulago Hospital. The aim of this five-year program, Dr. H. B. Owen, the Medical School's first Principal reported, was "not to produce a doctor, but an assistant capable of diagnosing and treating intelligently the common and less difficult diseases of the country and of realizing when to call a doctor."[6]

Table 13.1. *Hierarchy of medical personnel in Uganda, 1926*

European	
Medical officers	
Nursing sisters	
Asiatic	
Subassistant surgeons	
African	
Level 1.	Senior medical assistants
Level 2.	Medical assistants
Level 3.	Senior medical attendants
Level 4.	Medical attendants, Class A
Level 5.	Medical attendants, Class B
Level 6.	Learners (male)
Level 7.	Ward mistresses
Level 8.	Native nurses
Level 9.	Learners (female)

This scheme was one part of a general plan to introduce an "adapted" form of higher education to East Africa. The technical school at Makerere, opened in 1922, was transformed into a central training college in which students were given preparatory training in medicine, agriculture, and veterinary medicine. Future clerks, chiefs, and teachers, on the other hand, were recipients of a general liberal education. For the present, the Government of Uganda noted, "the aim should be rather to provide in the country such higher education as will fit students for careers in it than to base the instruction on the subjects required for entrance examinations to foreign schools and universities."[7] The desire to produce medical assistants was clearly part of this scheme. By 1935, although only 29 students had passed through the medical assistants' training course, Owen felt well satisfied. "We have succeeded in our aim to produce an Assistant capable of replacing the sub-Assistant Surgeon," he wrote, and no plans were afoot to advance the standards any higher.[8]

Similar events were unfolding in West Africa. As early as 1928, a committee set up to examine the possibility of a West African medical school concluded, as expected, that "the provision of an auxiliary medical staff is a more immediate necessity than that of fully qualified practitioners." Although, somewhat surprisingly, the committee did recommend the establishment of a small six-year medical school with British standards, geared to graduate about 30 physicians per year, their major concern was the establishment of a separate four-year training school needed to handle a yearly quota of about 150 medical assistants. But, after the governments of Nigeria, Gold Coast, and Sierra Leone failed to agree on the scheme, Nigeria acted alone. In 1930, a four-year medical assistants' training college was opened at Yaba, a few miles from

Lagos. By 1934, the total student body had reached only 36, and the authorities were complaining about the "poor tone" of the students, who were said to lack intelligence, ability, and discipline.[9]

Thus, paradoxically, the British Empire of indirect rule and trusteeship had put in place the nucleus of a medical system that could have provided an adequate rural health-care delivery system. But, unlike the situation in China, these Africans were subservient to foreigners, not African physicians. From the Africans' point of view the system was inherently racist.

Members of the African medical elite, who had slipped through the system by passing from missionary schools to British medical schools, were naturally opposed to all of these plans that limited Africans to subordinate positions within the health service. Their own status in African society was threatened by the presence of a "lesser-elite" immediately beneath them, and they were only too well aware that many who favored the training of an African medical auxiliary were often those who felt Africans to be intellectually incapable of a total medical training. Dr. H. B. Owen, for example, noted in 1933 that Africans can assimilate scientific ideas provided only that pains are taken to simplify the data and stimulate their minds. "The need for stimulus," he explained, "is to be expected when it is remembered that the students' immediate forebears concerned themselves with little beyond stock, crops, sexual matters, and intertribal warfare."[10] "Africanization," however justified within an African context, carried racial overtones. As Ashby wrote in the context of higher education in general: "The African intellectual, educated in London or Cambridge or Manchester, would have been indignant at any softening of standards, and substitution of easier options, any cheapened version of higher education. The African wanted a replica of the British university at its best."[11]

Yaba College, in particular, was attacked by members of the West African elite. They were opposed to its inferior status and to a diploma that was recognized only in West Africa, and that restricted its holders to positions of permanent subordination to British medical officers. Out of this conflict was forged the Lagos Youth Movement, one of the first nationalist organizations in West Africa, which, in 1936, expanded its base to become the National Youth Movement.[12]

This then was the background faced by Worthington and Hailey in their African survey of the late 1930s. How could the health needs of Africans best be met, and who was to staff this African medical service, they asked? Since it was highly unlikely that enough British physicians would condescend to serve in such communities, only two other possibilities remained. Priority could be given to the training of fully qualified African physicians, who would attend African medical schools modeled after those in Britain. Or, on the other hand, quality could be sacrificed to quantity, and the medical service could be run by lesser qualified, but "adapted," African medical assistants.

Worthington, using the model of the French colonial medical system, opted for the latter approach. In French West Africa, Worthington explained, the central hospitals staffed by European doctors "are regarded essentially as the Headquarters for a large number of field stations in rural areas, rather than as centres to which sick people should come for expert treatment." These field stations consisted of a ring of *infirmeries* and dispensaries, staffed respectively by African auxiliary doctors and African nurses, both of whom were trained at the Dakar Medical School. "This type of medical attention," Worthington concluded, "though greater in quantity, is probably inferior in quality compared with the British." But, as he went on to state, "The latter system may be described as seeking to persuade the native to appreciate the high standards of European medicine; the former as lowering the standard to meet the current native ideas."[13]

In an empire that should now be concerned, as never before, with the needs of the African population, trained African assistants were required, according to Worthington; a health service predominantly set up to care for British officials was no longer adequate. The new medical service "can be envisaged in the form of a pyramid," Worthington wrote, "in which the base is formed by a large number of nurses, dispensers, etc., the apex by the European medical officers, and the central part by auxiliary doctors or medical aids."[14] British Africa, Worthington stressed, urgently needed special medical schools to train this middle layer of the pyramid.

Not surprisingly, given that the scientific and medical aspects of the *African Survey* were taken almost word for word from Worthington's report, Hailey agreed with these views. The new medical services must, he agreed, share responsibility for "the improvement of African conditions of life." Intensive medical campaigns against disease should replace "perfecting of the hospital system," and to carry out these goals it was vital "to expand the cadre of locally trained medical assistants," and to expend limited resources training fully qualified Africans. In all fields, medicine included, the new Empire required training at the "middle-manpower" level.

In regard to the employment of Africans, experience shows that it is in what has been described as the "intermediate" rather than in the purely subordinate cadres that the most pressing problems arise. It is to the existence of the former class, with an adequate technical training, and with the standards of conduct necessary for the exercise of responsibility, that administrations must in future look for the means of expanding the operations of their ancillary services.[15]

But the problem remained. However much a medical policy based on the recommendations of the *African Survey* could have provided a basic first step toward answering the health needs of African societies, the medical auxiliaries were still subservient to Europeans. Europeans occupied the apex of the pyramid, Africans the middle and the base. Hailey's *African Survey* had restated the adaptive creed, and was out of date even before it was published.

By the time of the *African Survey*, the two centers for training African assistants at Makerere and Yaba were both coming under mounting criticism from African leaders and others, anxious for them to move toward true medical-school status. By then these two medical schools were being prepared to train and graduate fully qualified physicians, not members of a middle-manpower cadre. The situation in Africa was moving rapidly toward the situation that then existed in India. There, "by 1939, the idea that only one type of medical education was relevant to Indian conditions, namely as close an approximation as possible to medical education in Britain, had become firmly established."[16]

The first crack in the British armor had appeared in 1932. A conference of East African educationalists placed the issue of higher education in the hands of a committee, chaired by Sir James Currie. "The only real policy for the Government," the report concluded, "is to think out ahead a scheme of developing selected institutions in Africa up to a real University standard." In this report, the concept of adaptiveness was turned on its head. Whereas before it had been used as a justification to discourage Africans from attending universities, now it was used to justify indigenous rather than European-styled universities, which had been "designed with no regard whatever to the social and intellectual background of African students."[17] Africa, according to this report, needed specifically African universities. But, paradoxically, the route to that goal was to be achieved by a university college status, affiliated with London or another British university. And, to "clear the native mind of any suspicion," the report continued, the degrees of such universities must eventually rank equally with European universities. But suspicions existed. Within the context of educational adaptation, any Africanized university was in danger of being stigmatized as second class. Such suspicions seemed justified when another commission, set up specifically to examine the future of Makerere College, reiterated its belief in educational adaptation and the necessity for a university rooted in African soil. In this context they approved of the medical assistants who were regarded by the commission as physicians adapted to an African situation. They were, the report noted, "gratified to note that every attention has been paid to bringing the course into close relation with the actual conditions in East Africa."[18] As a result, a small vocal group of the British-trained African elite began to turn against the idea of Africanized universities. What was needed, they argued, was not adapted universities, but universities offering the highest levels of academic qualifications. African universities had to become replicas of British universities.[19]

Both Makerere and Yaba were moving in that direction. In 1936, with Makerere College and Mulago Hospital now acting as a training center for the whole of British East Africa, the newly formed Joint East African Examination Board recommended an additional year of clinical training for the medical assistants. Also, in those years, many arguments were made in favor of converting Makerere College into a university college and eventually a university. At the same time, hope was expressed that "Mulago may continue to produce in increasing numbers medical men with drive and initiative to solve the problems of rural sanitation, tropical diseases, and preventive medicine amongst an African population." Finally, in 1936, the assistants were renamed African Assistant Medical Officers, and one of them appointed Assistant Medical Officer of Health in Buganda. Clearly, "registrable qualifications" were not far away.[20] Likewise in West Africa; as early as 1936, despite numerous complaints over the "general tone," intelligence, ability, and discipline of the Yaba students, the "substandard course of training" was upgraded to a five-year program, and those graduating received a Diploma in Medicine and Surgery allowing them to practice in Nigeria.[21]

Thus, by World War II, in both West and East Africa, medical education was rapidly moving away from the "adaptive" model toward a British-styled training. No one, including the prospective African medical student, seemed much concerned with the massive problems of rural health if that meant being trained at a lower level and being subservient to the European physician. The African elite, taught the basics in African mission schools and trained in British medical schools, were uncompromisingly hostile to any lowering of medical standards. Their opinions had been molded by the British medical profession. They had no sympathy with the argument that to meet the peculiar health needs of Africa, large numbers of medical auxiliaries were a more important priority than necessarily small numbers of scientifically trained, European-style physicians.

THE NEW EMPIRE

Education became a key component in the new-style British Empire which developed after the passage of the Colonial Development and Welfare Acts in 1940, 1945, and 1950. In this new Empire of African development and long-term preparation for self-government, leaders were required. No longer was educational policy to be directed toward the supply of middle manpower for a British-controlled establishment. High-grade universities were essential, and however much rhetoric was expended on the ideals of Africanization, the goal was to be quality and the model was to be British. In such an empire, fully trained physicians, not medical assistants, were to be produced.

Beginning even before the war ended, the British Government appointed four commissions to look into higher education in the colonies.[22] They all agreed that the new British Empire demanded universities, "as an inescapable corollary of any policy which aims at the achievement of Colonial self-government," and that university colleges should be set up immediately as halfway stages to degree-granting status. Likewise, they argued, the centers of medical education must aim to attain British standards, with qualifications recognized by the British General Medical Council. Medical assistants were still required, but they must be given a totally different training and should receive "no title that could imply claims for consideration as a qualified doctor."[23]

By that time, only about 30 students per year were enrolling for the Diploma in Medicine and Surgery at Yaba; it no longer met the aspirations of Africans who required more than a low-prestige qualification that allowed the recipient to practice as an assistant medical officer only in West Africa and that was not recognized in Britain. In its place, the Elliot Commission recommended a Medical College of West Africa to be built alongside a new university college at Ibadan, not at Yaba, and whose facilities would be such that its diploma would gain recognition by the General Medical Council "at the earliest possible moment."

Quality, not relevance, was the new key. Thus, far from advocating Africanized universities, the Commission was now recommending nothing but trivial modifications of the British pattern. Similarly, African medical students were to be trained also in the British way, with very little recognition of the special social conditions that influenced health in the areas in which many of them would practice. The African elite were to receive what they desired: "a replica of the British University at its best."

To reach this desired plateau, however, the African medical degree had to gain recognition from the General Medical Council in London. But the authorities in Nigeria and Uganda differed from each other in the way they chose to gain this recognition. Dr. K. Mellanby, the first Principal of the University of Ibadan, chose immediately to press for the London medical degree, the M.B. Ch.B, whereas at Makerere the authorities pressed for recognition of their own Diploma in Medicine.

Beginning from scratch, as it were, with new buildings in a completely new location, Ibadan faced a major hurdle. The Higher College of Yaba had been transferred to the new University of Ibadan on its opening in February 1948, but the medical school was forced to remain behind in Lagos. Later that year, the premedical years were transferred to Ibadan, but the Lagos Native Hospital was still required for the clinical years. Naturally, the clinical facilities at Lagos did not meet the requirements of the British General Medical Council, whose inspection team visited the new medical school in 1950 and 1951. Only in 1957, with the opening of an elaborate and expensive British-style hospital at the university, was the long-awaited recognition received. Until that year, West African medical students were required to spend their clinical years in Britain. In Makerere, meanwhile, a similar inspection team recommended that holders of the Licentiate of Medicine and Surgery (East Africa) be recognized for local service only, full recognition being received only in 1956. With recognition, the Interuniversity Council for Higher Education in the Colonies, set up to foster the advance of African colleges through university-college status to fully-fledged universities, could report having reached "a critical point in the story, 'the end of the beginning.'"[24]

But the training these African medical students received was so British in character that to receive instruction in tropical medicine it was necessary for them to spend time at the London School of Hygiene and Tropical Medicine. Thus as the new British Empire developed after World War II, the number of African students attending the School increased dramatically (Figure 13.1).

IMPERIAL RESEARCH

The new universities and medical schools were designed to be "seats of learning" and centers of fundamental, not utilitarian, research. In the context of countries faced by serious social, medical, and economic problems, the Asquith Commission reported: "It is not the function of universities directly to provide this type of help [utilitarian]. . . . To expect them to do so would indicate a fundamental misapprehension of the place of research in universities." As Ashby points out, "The Commission's idea of the place of research in the university was in the pure line of nineteenth-century German tradition."[25] Indeed, medical research seems to have become a major priority in British Africa after World War II. It formed one of the main foci of Lord Hailey's *African Survey* and Worthington's *Science in Africa*. "That Africa has problems of its own, which require intensive study, needs perhaps no demonstration," wrote Lord Hailey, "the development of Africa is not a process of gradual evolution: it assumes . . . something of the character of a transformation, and its achievement inevitably demands more than the routine application of existing knowledge."[26]

Research is needed in all areas, Hailey argued, and Worthington, in the opening chapter of his book, entitled "Some problems of research," pointed out that African development had so far been uninfluenced by the results of scientific research. "A development based on a real understanding of Africa's potentialities has hardly yet begun," he concluded, "and will be impossible until the necessity of scientific knowledge is recognized."[27]

If the importance of research led Worthington to begin his study with the topic; equally it led Hailey to conclude his lengthy treatise with a section entitled "The future of African Studies."

We see before us now the most formative period of African history, and much that is done today will have a decisive effect on the future of the African peoples. The task of guiding the social and material development of Africa gives rise to problems which cannot be solved by the application of routine knowledge; they require a

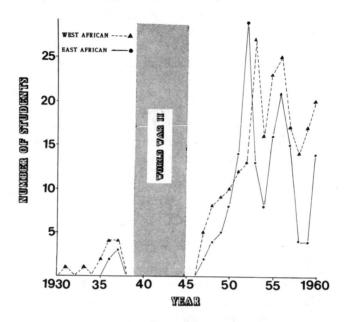

Figure 13.1. The number of East and West African students attending the London School of Hygiene and Tropical Medicine each year between 1930 and 1960

special knowledge, which can only be gained by an intensive study of the unusual conditions. This study must be pursued in the field of the social as well as in that of the physical sciences. But for this purpose assistance is required from the Imperial Government. . . .[28]

The necessity of pursuing more scientific research was also one of the major conclusions reached by the Economic Advisory Council's Committee on Nutrition in the Colonial Empire, which had published its final report in 1939 after the discovery of malnutrition in the Empire. "The problem of nutrition is still to a considerable degree," they wrote, "a scientific problem," and one role of the Imperial Government should be to stimulate research in the area.[29] It was as if, in the words of Worboys, they believed that "if people knew what to grow, how to grow it, what to eat and how to cook it, then there would be less poverty and hence less disease."[30]

This report is significant, I believe, in illustrating how difficult it was for the British medical and political elite to comprehend what malnutrition and poverty really entailed, and enabled them to dismiss so easily the arguments of those pressing for a more social approach to health problems. It also helps to explain Grant's frustration over the lack of action in the field of social medicine. The medical elite recognized that malnutrition produced ill health and lowered resistance to disease; yet they saw malnutrition as basically a problem of agriculture and ignorance. They recognized that the root cause of malnutrition was the low standard of living, but believed this could be ameliorated by simply decreeing that "as many people as possible should grow at least part of their foodstuffs they themselves consume," and by assuring that people grew crops of nutritive value. Those who worked on estates and plantations, they argued, should be given allotments, while the landless should be given plots of land – a quite extraordinary and naive suggestion, given the economic situation under which these people existed. But the real hopelessness and human decay that flow from poverty escaped them. High infant mortality, they noted, stems in part from poverty, but "when due allowance has been made for these causes there can be no doubt that sheer ignorance is one of the chief factors." This ignorance, they believed, was responsible for what they assumed to be an absence of parental responsibility for the welfare of children. Single mothers in the West Indies, they noted, "will often for instance be unable to breast-feed her babies for to do so would interfere with her power to earn money for their upkeep." But this problem was not blamed on the economic system in which these mothers worked. The solution, they concluded, rested with the West Indian Government who "should educate their people in the duties of parenthood."

In addition, what was believed to constitute malnutrition had changed over the years. Instead of a lack of food and calories, the new science of nutrition now defined malnutrition in terms of vitamin deficiencies and the absence of some essential but minute amounts of specific foodstuffs. As a result, biochemical intervention was deemed to play an essential role in the solution to any problems of colonial malnutrition; as with disease the economic and social conditions in which people lived and worked retreated into the background.

The Committee on Nutrition believed that a nucleus of full-time scientists funded by the Medical Research Council would suffice to carry out research and offer advice. But Hailey had a broader perspective. A coordinated plan of action was needed in all areas of science, Hailey urged, that would be organized from research institutes in Britain but with a central body in charge of research funding. Experts could perhaps, he suggested, establish careers for themselves in colonial research by membership in a Metropolitan Research Institution.[31]

But these experts were to be British; there was no other choice. There were, as yet, few if any African experts available who would have qualified as research scientists. But more than that, Africans were often considered as unsuitable candidates. In 1960, at the last meeting of the East African Medical Research Scientific Advisory Committee, Africans were castigated as "technically poor," capable, in the long run, of training only to the level of laboratory assistant. "The African," they concluded "is not naturally dexterous or accurate in observation."[32]

By the end of 1944, despite the war, a bureaucracy had been set up in London to manage research funding, and £26,218 out of a total research budget of £414,128 had been allocated for medical research. The major committee, the Colonial Development and Welfare Advisory Committee, had been set up in 1941, and the following June, Harold MacMillan, Parliamentary Under-Secretary of State for the Colonies, announced the formation of the Colonial Research Advisory Committee. Chaired by Lord Hailey, it included Edward Appleton of the Department of Scientific and Industrial Research, A. V. Hill of the Royal Society, Edward Mellenby of the Medical Research Council, and W. Topky of the Agricultural Research Council. Realizing that medical research was to be a priority, they requested the long established Colonial Advisory Medical Committee to review the situation.

"There is a great need for more central guidance and control of research," this Committee advised. We need, they urged, "to raise the prestige of medical research work in the Colonies and to give those engaged in this work a proper status and security of employment," This would ensure, they argued, that "the best class of worker is attracted to the Colonies." They recommended that medical researchers be formed into a separate Colonial Medical Service, and a new central body established in London to formulate plans, and to advise and coordinate medical research.[33]

This central medical body, the Colonial Medical Research Committee, chaired by Edward Mellenby, held its first meeting in May 1945. "The way is now clear," reported the Colonial Research Advisory Committee, "for a rapid and systematic attack on the major medical problems of the Colonies."[34] Thus, as formally reported in 1945, "with the establishment of specialist research committees, the main work of organization in this country for Colonial research may be said to be well advanced."[35]

By the time the new medical committee had met, a second Colonial Development and Welfare Bill had received Royal Assent. A total of £120 million were made available for the ten-year period between 1946 and 1956, with a maximum of £17.5 million earmarked for research. Again, members were nothing but enthusiastic toward the change. Conscious, as always, of America's call for colonial liberation, Creech-Jones assured the House:

It is significant that the purpose of this Bill is to achieve these very purposes. I doubt if any Imperial Power has ever before embarked upon a policy of deliberately disintegrating its Empire. This is the effect of the Bill in the long run. It will contribute to training the Colonial people for complete and responsible self-government fitting them, socially and economically, to discharge their responsibility in the world.[36]

But many Tories, more paternalistic in approach, were not prepared to watch passively the liquidation of the British Empire. They viewed the bill as a new attempt to "consolidate the 60 million people in the Colonial Empire."[37] According to Lord Hailey, however, the new philosophy of empire attempted to accommodate the views of paternalists and liberals alike. "We realise," he informed the House of Lords, "that self-government cannot be a reality unless it is based upon a substantial foundation of improved standards of life and an adequate social structure."[38] Self-government would come one day; for the present, however, the Empire was years away from any liquidation.

Curiously, for the first time during these debates, members became aware of bilharzia. Pethick-Lawrence, in supporting the second reading of the bill, urged that colonial troops, returning home after wartime service, must find health conditions in their home countries as they were in the army. "The tsetse fly must be wiped out," he urged, "hookworm and bilharzia must be abolished."[39] Members unaware of the disease would not have been helped, however, by Viscount Bledisloe's vagueness. Stressing the necessity of medical research, he paid particular attention to bilharzia. "I am told," he remarked, "that this wretched disease, the germ of which spends half its time in some moisture-loving animal, is a good deal more rampant than they were some years ago."[40]

The need to recruit the "right men" to undertake the necessary research in some kind of colonial research service dominated early deliberations of the Colonial Medical Research Committee. Research fellowships for those wishing to make their careers in a Colonial Medical Research Service, they decided, should be offered for recent British graduates in the social and natural sciences, who were under 35 years of age.[41] "Until this service has been instituted," the Committee reported, "much of the work of the committee is made impossible; recruitment of men to carry out research is prevented and men, now being demobilized, are taking up other posts and will not be available later."[42]

But setting up the research service proved to be a difficult and prolonged process; bureaucratic delays and professional jealousies came into operation. With so much delay, Hamilton Fairley began "to doubt whether the committee were even wasting their time in making recommendations which seemed to lead to so little action."[43] But the Colonial Office's proposals for the service, presented two months later, met with disapproval by the Committee, who desired a separate Medical Research Service under their control rather than a unified Colonial Research Service under the control of the Colonial Office. "Medical science," they argued, "was somewhat different from the other sciences."[44]

The Colonial Office responded hastily to the Committee's complaints. Since the funding for medical research, they pointed out, comes from the Colonial Development and Welfare Act, the Colonial Secretary can hardly divest himself from responsibility. "A maximum possible degree of central organization and oversight" is needed, they claimed, adding that since the colonial people themselves provided some money for the research and since they will in time provide the researchers, "this implies that they should in

Table 13.2. *Priority research items presented to the first meeting of the Colonial Medical Research Committee, May 29, 1945*

1. DDT	11. Cholera
2. Nutrition	12. Bacillary dysentery
3. Malaria	13. Tuberculosis
4. Trypanosomiasis	14. Leprosy
5. Relapsing fever	15. Filariasis/onchocerciasis
6. Yaws	16. Bilharzia/hookworm
7. Amoebic dysentery	17. Viruses
8. Plague	18. Tropical ulcer
9. Brucellosis	19. Physiology of hot climates
10. Enteric fevers	20. Mental affections

Source: "Colonial Medical Research Committee notes on future plans for Colonial Medical Research." Memo C.M.R. (45) 6, *Miscellaneous Papers*, CO 913/1.

some manner be associated with the running of it. It cannot therefore be directed altogether arbitrarily from London."[45] The Committee was forced to climb down, and a unified Colonial Research Service was established shortly afterward. However, they managed to procure additional pay for medical researchers.

A list of priority problems was presented to the first meeting of the Committee (Table 13.2), although clearly the academic viewpoint ("Select the right man, and he will select his own research topics") was favored.[46] Nevertheless, the list of priority items is of interest. The biochemistry of nutrition ranked high, but, basically their ideas were once again fixed on specific diseases and their elimination, with top funding directed toward the newly produced wonder-insecticide DDT.

Clearly money had now been made available for experts in the medical and natural sciences to begin a serious study of disease in the new British Empire. But in this disease-centered approach to the problems of colonial health, bilharzia had been ranked down toward the bottom of their list of priority concerns.

14

South Africa (1950–1960): Social medicine versus scientific research

The switch from a socioeconomic approach to health to a parasite- and disease-oriented approach, in which specific diseases rather than malnutrition and socioeconomic conditions took precedence, and where fundamental biological research came to occupy a central role, was nowhere better illustrated than in South Africa. There, as those carrying the diseases were relocated in the so-called *Bantustans* (or "homelands") and "townships" with their health ignored, the diseases they carried became the focus of an intensive research effort.

THE COLLAPSE OF THE NATIONAL HEALTH SERVICE

By 1950, the bright future that had been predicted earlier for the much vaunted South African National Health Service had dissipated. It no longer enjoyed the support of the Medical Association of South Africa, and dark political clouds had gathered when the apartheid election of 1948 resulted in the election of the *Herenigde Nasionale* Party under D. F. Malan.

Second thoughts about the service had begun to pervade the medical profession almost as soon as the scheme had been proposed in the Gluckmann report of 1945, *The Health of the Nation*.[1] Editorials in the *South African Medical Journal* advocating an end to private medical practice drew the ire of many private practitioners.[2] Some writers to the journal expressed support for the idea that the state should limit itself to the promotion of health, while the medical profession should retain control over preventive and curative services. But, as one physician noted: "If the state in meeting this demand attempts to substitute the part for the whole by instituting and organising only a medical service for the cure and alleviation of "sickness" alone, then the determined and united resistance of the medical profession is to be anticipated."[3]

By 1945, the Medical Association was beginning to realize the dangers the new health service presented to their own professional needs. Coining their remarks in the spotless language typical of any professional group deeming itself threatened, they began to back away from their initial enthusiastic support for the scheme. They were able to achieve this by arguing that whereas they would be willing to accept the scheme as outlined in the original report, they were not willing to become "socialized" as part of any decentralized, watered-down version of the National Health Service. Their response was "all or nothing." "If we are to be asked to sacrifice our liberty we must be satisfied that the cause is a worthy one, unreservedly to the good of the nation," urged Dr A. Sweetapple in an address to the Natal Branch of the Association, "but we are not prepared to sacrifice our freedom "for some makeshift scheme in which the original ideal has been sacrificed to considerations of political expediency."[4]

But one must doubt whether the medical profession would have been able to accept the fully developed scheme, whatever their public utterances were. This was indicated by their overwhelmingly hostile reaction to the decision of the Transvaal Government to introduce free universal hospitalization, a major component of the original scheme. This was not the time, they argued; without more hospital space, free service should be provided gradually, beginning with the poor. "To allow all persons to compete on an equal footing for the limited accommodation and facilities available in public hospitals," the Federal Council noted, "is, under existing conditions, a gross injustice to the poor." With a free system and without a massive increase in hospital facilities, they argued, the middle and upper classes would receive priority treatment over the poor. Thus, without a means test, "it appears inevitable that the scheme of free hospitalization will perpetuate and aggravate the unbalanced and uncoordinated patchwork of health services in South Africa without achieving any appreciable improvement in the health of the people." But, in reality, their primary concern was not with the poor, and certainly not with poor Africans. Their opposition to free hospitalization was based on the objections that such a system would transform all health professionals into civil servants, and that fee-paying patients would seek free medical advice from the staff of these hospitals. Such staff, some members noted with horror, "will be graded, classified, paid, promoted, transferred, disciplined, given hours of duty and leaves, by hospital administrators."[5] In an address entitled "Civil servants with a bedside manner," Dr. Sweetapple wondered, "Would it not be more logical to provide free food, or free housing, or free justice – or any of the many other commodities more essential to human health and happiness than free doctoring?"[6]

Dr. Gluckmann tried to placate the profession in his address to the 1946 Medical Congress in Durban. The health centers, he pointed out, will not clash with the vested interests of local medical practitioners. They were to be placed only in the poorest areas where few could afford to pay private practitioners, although, he admitted, a decision will have to be made shortly whether the centers would be restricted to "the subeconomic groups" or extended to the whole population.[7] Following the Congress, a referendum was held among members; 88 percent of the 54 percent who bothered to respond expressed dissatisfaction with any attempt to share authority for the Health Service between the Union and provincial governments, and also with the ordinances of the Transvaal and Cape governments in favor of free hospitalization.[8]

But to the horror of many branches, the Federal Council decided they had no option but to support the Government's watered-down version of the National Health Scheme. Since only 54 percent voted, they argued, "3000 approximately who apparently are willing to accept or are not averse to accepting appointments or are indifferent in their attitudes" leaves no option but to cooperate.[9]

In 1948, the President of the Medical Association of South Africa issued a press statement. The Government's action, he noted, came as a rude shock to members of the Association, the only group that "had voluntarily offered to socialize their services." Neither, he continued, does the Association oppose free hospitalization as long as the poor are not penalized. But, he wrote:

The Association cannot accept the proposition that a service, into which only a limited number of medical men would be absorbed, should enter into competition with the rest of the medical profession. The medical profession has always given its services free to the poor, but if the provincial governments have now decided to pay, from public money, for the services, and to give them equally also to the middle income group and the rich, then surely no private practitioner would be able to survive such competition.[10]

A "contented medical personnel," the President concluded, is conditional upon a "means test."

Thus, in the final analysis, the Medical Association came out in favor of a two-tiered medical system: one for fee-paying whites and the other for poverty-stricken Africans. The health centers would cater only to the latter, and in this way "there is no encroachment upon private practice." In addition, the centers would become centers of preventive medicine, and "an endeavor will be made to persuade persons requiring curative treatment to seek it from private practitioners." All this, Dr. G. W. Gale, the Secretary of Health argued, would serve the interests of the medical profession. Health centers would increase demand for curative services, and private practitioners could serve part-time in the centers and receive payment for services "rendered by them to persons to whom, formerly, if they served them at all, they gave *pro deo* services or services for which they were poorly remunerated by reason of the partial waiving of fees and the accumulation of bad debts."[11]

THE APARTHEID STATE

While the medical profession argued among themselves over the merits of the National Health Service, the Nationalist Government began to establish the apartheid state. *Apartheid*, the Afrikaans word for "separation," led to the social and geographical separation of the major so-called racial groups. The Government planned to relocate the Africans, who made up approximately 70 percent of the population, into "homelands" or *Bantustans*, which constituted 13 percent of the area of South Africa, and were grouped in a crescent around South Africa's major industrial regions (Figure 14.1). Each homeland was to become the base of one of the ten "racial" groups (Xhosas, Tsongas, etc.) into which all nonwhites were allocated in the 1950s – a process which created the illusion that whites, also classified as a single racial group, were not a minority. Eventually, according to the South African Government, each homeland was to become an independent political state, leaving a totally white Republic of South Africa.

But the nationalists were not united over the degree to which they were prepared to establish apartheid. The "visionaries," as represented in the massive Tomlinson report of 1955, were prepared to separate the races entirely, whereas the "pragmatists" were more realistic in their approach. The Tomlinson Commission, set up to examine the economics of establishing African reserves, was concerned over the impact of increasing industrialization in the cities of the Union. While recognizing that "the Bantu are particularly suited to the performance of monotonous work in which the actions are purely repetitive" ("In other words, they are good machine operators in the semi-skilled category"), the Commission was concerned that the move to the cities would urbanize, Westernize, and detribalize Africans leading to assimilation and "a new biological entity." But since Europeans, the report continued, were not willing "to sacrifice their right of existence as a separate national and racial entity," then "the only alternative is to promote the establishment of separate communities in their own, separate territories where each will have the fullest opportunity for self-expression and development."[12]

According to the Tomlinson Commission, in order to absorb the increasing African population the homeland areas needed to be developed. This would require increased agricultural efficiency, the development of white-controlled industries on the borders of the homelands to which the Africans could easily travel for work, and an annual investment of £104 million. Health problems in the homelands also needed to be addressed that would, according to the dictates of this "pure" apartheid, be controlled eventually by Africans outside the jurisdiction of the provincial and Union health departments.

But, by 1955, the South African economy was no longer based entirely on the primary industries of mining and agriculture. New urban secondary industries were increasing, which also needed cheap black labor. Thus, to separate the races as the visionaries wished would threaten the profitability of these industries by denying them access to a cheap labor force, and undermine the well-being of the white population. In such a country, the whites could no

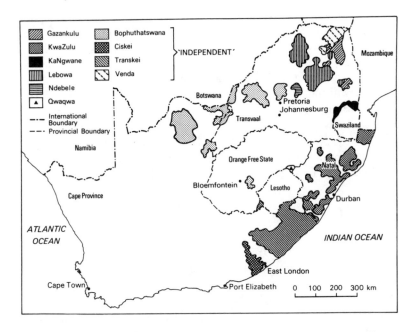

Figure 14.1. The South African "homelands" (Reprinted with permission from D. Smith, *UPDATE: Apartheid in South Africa*, Cambridge: Cambridge University Press, 1987)

longer expect to enjoy the fruits of cheap black labor in perpetuity and would therefore be required to make economic sacrifices in order to set up an apartheid system. The pragmatists, realizing this, were not prepared to pay that price for a political ideology. Their view of apartheid was such as to retain the cheap labor force. As one of their members noted:

Segregation is the policy of pushing the Black man out of the way of the White man, in order that the European can preserve his own racial purity, and keep it free from the so-called impure colour of the Native. But since the cheap labour of the Native would be needed in the European industries, segregation would ensure that this labour would always be available. When the Natives had served their purpose, however, they would be sent back to the locations and left to look after themselves. The Reserves would only exist as a source of even more of this cheap labour, and a dumping-ground for the used-up labour from the cities.[13]

The argument was won by the pragmatists; the white South Africans continued to use cheap black labor. Thus, the government moved very slowly toward the consolidation of the homelands and rejected the idea of spending £104 million which Tomlinson had estimated to be the cost of developing them. The modified apartheid that evolved retained parts of the African labor force by segregating Africans in "townships," setup on the periphery of the cities by a process called "orderly urbanization." As one minister remarked in 1954, "Total territorial separation of the races can be a wonderful ideal, but to embark on it immediately would, in my opinion, be as impossible and disastrous as a bicycle ride to the moon."[14]

By permitting white South Africans the continued use of cheap African labor, this modified apartheid allowed the South African economy to flourish. Labor costs were reduced, not only because of low wages but also because part of the cost was transferred to the homelands, to the foreign countries of Lesotho, Swaziland, and others, or finally, to the "independent states" of Bophuthatswana, Ciskei, Transkei, and Venda.[15]

Medical education

If, as was argued, the homelands were to become independent states, then it would be necessary to train some of the Africans for future roles in these societies as well as within the white society. Thus, in 1949, "to prepare Natives more effectively for their future occupations," the Nationalist Government appointed a Commission on Native Education. There was need, the Commission argued in their report of 1951, to develop a "modern Bantu culture," to prepare them for their role in society while at the same time satisfying their aspirations as members of Bantu nations. In that way, they noted, "the fullest application of Bantu brains and brawn" would be realized. Thus, the Commission reasoned, African children not only needed instruction in the language, literature, and religions of their own societies, but also needed knowledge of hygiene, agricultural and technical trade skills, English, and Afrikaans. They also needed to be taught the social values of punctuality, initiative, duty, neatness, and reliability, to make them useful members of society. Only by such means, they argued, would a "progressive, modern, and self-respecting Bantu order of life" arise in the homelands.[16] In 1957, following a series of other commissions dealing specifically with higher education, the Government introduced its Separate University Education Bill, in which a separate university was planned for each ethnic group on the grounds that open universities would make Africans aliens to their own cultures. These universities were required to train African professionals for service in the new homelands. Financed eventually by the Africans themselves, these universities were predicted to be able to "take their place among the best in the world."[17] Under this system the college in Durban, site of the African medical school, was to be reserved for Indians only. Thus the Minister of Education informed Dr. Malherbe, the Principal of the Medical School, that in 1957 the School would be required to move out of the University of Natal.[18]

This announcement came as a morale-shattering blow to the staff of the medical school, who, from the very beginning, had had severe financial problems. Even before the school opened, the authorities at the university of Natal had tried again to tap the resources of the Rockefeller Foundation. Dr. E. Malherbe had visited the Foundation in New York in 1949, and, a year later, Dr. R. Morrison of the Foundation traveled to South Africa to meet with the committee concerned with the new school. Well aware of the previous Rockefeller experience with the South African Government, Morrison was now even more hesitant with the election of an Afrikaner government, and a medical school committee of English-speaking South Africans who seemed incapable of taking the new government seriously. Until the government intentions over the issue became clear, Morrison announced, the Rockefeller Foundation would not move.

A few months later, the Government approved a capital and equipment grant of £224,760 and 15 student bursaries of £150. But the Rockefeller Foundation remained unimpressed. No provision had been made in the budget, they observed, for accommodation, staff, or even research – this latter oversight being of most concern to the Foundation. They were also concerned lest support for the new school would be construed as support for apartheid. So, in the end, they agreed merely to supplement the low salary of the Dean, Dr. Gale, by £660 for each of three years.[19] The school opened in 1951, but, under the rules of apartheid, only non-Europeans from the Union, Swaziland, and Basutoland were eligible for entrance; it was no longer to be a school for students of any race who wished to work in the African health centers. As D. F. Malan remarked to the House of Assembly in 1948, "We do not want to withhold higher education from the non-Europeans and will take every possible step to give both the Natives and the Coloured peoples university training as soon as we can, but in their own sphere, in other words in separate institutions."[20]

Despite these setbacks the Medical School planned to integrate the Institute of Family and Community Health, founded in the 1940s, into the Medical School as the Department of Family Practice to deal mainly with the problems of African rural health. The Department, they hoped, would not only train nurses, midwives, social workers, health educators and statisticians, but would also introduce the medical student to health care practice – the processes in family and community living that promoted health. It was to be a training school in "social medicine."[21] Faced with the Government's continued indifference, however, they were forced to turn again to the Rockefeller Foundation, requesting, in 1954, an annual three-year grant of £26,150 to assist in establishing the new department.[22] Please hurry, Gale urged, "those of us who are liberal in matters of Bantu advancement are fighting a desperate battle against reaction in various forms."[23] Finally, after receiving a guarded assurance of support from a young and inexperienced Minister of Health, the Rockefeller Foundation agreed to grant £42,400 for the new Department over a five-year period.[24] The grant was announced in a 1954 press release:

The Durban Medical School will be the first medical school in South Africa to make provision . . . for training in clinical practice in the consulting room and the home, and among perhaps only a dozen in the world which do so, although such a step is in accordance with the recommendations which medical educationalists have been making for many years.[25]

After considerable delay, the Department of Social, Preventive and Family Medicine was finally opened in 1956, only one year before the decision was taken to close the medical school. Naturally, with that decision, the morale of the staff collapsed. Our hopes are "shattered," Dr. S. L. Kark, Head of the Department, informed Malherbe; we "feel there is no place or situation here in which we could develop with reasonable freedom from autocratic and ideological interference." By then, after the Rockefeller Foundation had refused to continue to supplement the Dean's salary, Dr. Gale had left South Africa for the security of Makerere College, knowing that the "cause of non-European higher education is not popular in South Africa, and I am in any case suspect as a liberal and a man with progressive ideas about the natives."[26] Thus, in 1958, "with the sword of Damocles hanging over their heads," Kark, too, left South Africa, to take up a temporary position in the School of Public Health, University of North Carolina.[27]

Naturally, with its grant to the Department due to expire in 1960, the Rockefeller Foundation began to question the desirability of continuing the support, even though the Government was stalling over its plans to include separate medical schools as part of its plans to separate the universities. Clearly it was financially impractical to open separate medical schools for each African "race." Thus the Separate University Education Bill of 1957 was revised to exclude the medical school before its final passage in 1959.[28] Nevertheless, in 1960, the Rockefeller Foundation sent out its troubleshooter, and once again Dr. John Weir was asked to report on the situation.

In what he described to me as one of the worst experiences of his life, Weir reported back that the future of the school looked very bleak. The situation was not helped, he added, by its first graduates, who acted as house officers in Durban, taking strike action over their pay scale (two-thirds that of whites), and attempting to set up practices near Durban rather than in the rural reserves. Even more alarming, Weir reported that unbeknown to the Government (a statement that I find hard to believe), 88 of the 207-strong student body were Indian, and the failure rate for African students was alarmingly high. Thus, of the 45 students who had graduated from the school by 1960, only 25 were African; half the Africans had failed. The Indians do much better work, Weir concluded, the Africans were not measuring up.[29] In 1960, on Weir's recommendation, the Rockefeller Foundation withdrew its support from South Africa, and without support, the Department of Social, Preventive and Family Medicine collapsed.

Health

The provision of medical care to the African population was of little concern to the South African Government. The unemployed, unemployable, and sick African had become a "surplus appendage," to be deposited in the homelands. By these means, the government was able to solve partially a chronic unemployment problem created by increased levels of mechanization and decreased foreign investment, and also solve any medical problems, by exporting them. These ideas were made crystal clear in a government circular of 1967.

> General Circular No. 25, 1967
> SETTLING OF NON-PRODUCTIVE BANTU RESIDENT IN EUROPEAN AREAS, IN THE HOME LANDS
>
> 1. It is accepted Government policy that the Bantu are only temporarily resident in the European areas of the Republic, for as long as they offer their labour there. As soon as they become, for some reason or another, no longer fit for work or superfluous in the labour market, they are expected to return to their country of origin or the territory of the national unit where they fit in ethnically if they were not born and bred in the homeland.
> 2. The Bantu in the European areas who are normally regarded as non-productive and as such have to be resettled in the homelands, are conveniently classified as follows:
>   (i) the aged, the unfit, widows, women with dependent children and also families who do not qualify . . . for family accommodation in the European urban areas;
>   (ii) Bantu on European farms who become superfluous as a result of age, disability. . . .
>   (iii) Professional Bantu such as doctors, attorneys, agents, traders, industrialists, etc. Also such persons are not regarded as essential for the European labour market, and as such they must also be settled in the homelands, in so far as they are not essential for serving their compatriots in the European areas.[30]

But except for those who lived in the border areas of some of the homelands and which were, in reality, working-class appendages to white industry, few services were offered to these people. Whereas the former lived in fully serviced houses with water, sewerage, and laid-out roads (Figure 14.2a), most lived under conditions that created serious health problems (Figure 14.2b). There were, for example, towns "developed for families of which the breadwinners are usually employed as migrant labourers," in which water was obtained from street pumps and cesspits were used as much as possible. But most lived in temporaray settlements where rivers, small dams, and boreholes provided the only services.[31]

Naturally, moving this surplus African labor into increasingly overcrowded, unsanitary, and economically nonviable homelands had a devastating impact on their health; people literally starved to death in homelands that could not

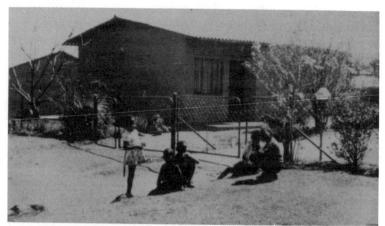

a

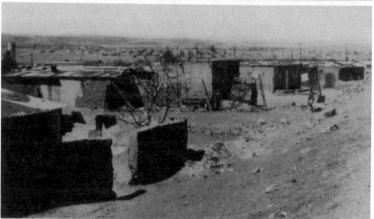

b

Figure 14.2. The "homelands": (a) home of Bophuthatswana factory worker in a modern sector; (b) squatter huts in the interior of Bophuthatswana (Reprinted with permission from D. Smith, *UPDATE: Apartheid in South Africa*, Cambridge: Cambridge University Press, 1987)

support the population. But, because these people had become residents of what the South African Government saw as foreign or near-foreign countries, provision of health care for them was thus no longer a concern of South Africa, and health statistics from these areas were excluded from any government publications. The "diseased natives" no longer existed.

A sickening picture emerges from what few health statistics are available from the "homelands." Perhaps 50,000 African children die of malnutrition every year; enteritis and pneumonia account for 60–80 percent of deaths in

African children compared to less than 10 percent in whites; in the Lovedale hospital of Ciskei, gastroenteritis has increased by 1,500 percent since the end of World War II; 65,000 Africans come down with kwashiorkor every year; tuberculosis has increased by 425 percent; and in Bophuthatswana, tuberculosis is said to be "like a common cold." If figures from the homelands are included, South Africa provides a glaring exception to the general rule that as the GNP increases, there is a corresponding decrease in infant mortality (see Table 14.1).

"The risk of infectious disease is constantly maintained at high levels by the squalor and overcrowding in the official 'townships' for Africans," noted a WHO report; the result is that typhoid, cholera, diphtheria, and bilharzia are now endemic to these areas.[32] But as long as these diseases could be safely contained in the black areas, as can be done when the basic causes are overcrowding and a lack of sanitation, the South African Government took little action. On the other hand, the South African authorities were greatly exercised by diseases, such as malaria, which are carried by vectors and thus know no color bar.[33] Bilharzia was included among such diseases.

And thus the tragic scenario of South Africa unfolded: As the health centers, the Durban medical school, and its Department of Social, Preventive, and Family Medicine faded away, and as the "diseased natives" were exported and ignored, some of the diseases they carried became increasingly important – the focus of a substantial research effort. Whereas the South African Government ignored the health problems of most of its African population, they could not ignore the diseases that could threaten their own society; social inactivity was counterbalanced by medical research activity. This activity was supported by the South Africa Council of Scientific and Industrial Research, set up in 1945 to build national laboratories and to fund research in the universities and industrial laboratories.

Bilharzia research

Bilharzia, endemic to the homelands and large areas of the Transvaal and a constant threat to white farmers, white suburbanites, and white mineowners, was among the diseases to benefit from this new research interest. The discovery that the disease was "running a completely unchecked course," and assuming "gigantic proportions" in the Transvaal, because "for all practical purposes the whole native population is suffering from bilharziasis,"[34] stimulated the Medical Research Committee of the Council of Scientific and Industrial Research to set up the Bilharziasis and Tropical Disease Unit in 1948, stationed at the South African Institute for Medical Research. In addition, a subsidiary Bilharzia Natural History Unit was established one year later to work on the confusing problem of snail systematics. Thus, by 1950, bilharzia had once again become a disease of concern in South Africa. The

Table 14.1. *Relationship between infant mortality and the Gross National Product*

Country	GNP ($U.S.)	Infant mortality (per 1000)
Botswana	41	97
Guyana	630	40
Malaysia	860	75
South Africa	1340	117

Source: *Apartheid and Health* (Geneva: WHO, 1983).

Federal Council of the Medical Association of South Africa urged, in a memorandum to the Minister of Health,

that bilharzia is the cause of considerable morbidity in the populace of the Union; that all conditions are favourable for the spread of this disease; that the attention of the Minister of Health to be drawn to these facts; and that he be requested, through the Union Health Department, to institute and conduct a campaign against this disease.[35]

This concern was related clearly to the spread of irrigation schemes, and the potential threat of spreading bilharzia to the white farming community. As R. J. Pitchford, leader of the Bilharzia Natural History Unit noted, "With the dams, canals, and pumps will come ideal homes for snails and with labour will come faeces, urine and some bilharzia. With time will come a disease-ridden population unable to work the land they tilled a few years before."[36]

The threat of labor efficiency was also a major impetus for the renewed interest in bilharzia. At the 1951 meeting of the South African Mine Medical Officers Association, which was devoted to bilharzia, a question was posed as to whether research on the disease was justified since it could probably be suppressed by adequate nutrition and hygiene in the mines. By way of an answer, the meeting was warned that bilharzia threatened the efficiency of the workforce because of a possible link between the disease and mental retardation.[37]

But bilharzia also threatened white suburbanites. "Since tropical natives," Botha de Meillon, Director of the Bilharzia and Tropical Disease Unit noted, "are banned from urban centres they settle on small farms in close proximity to towns and cities, and thereby present a real threat to our periurban centres as well as to town dwellers, who wish to escape to the country during the weekends."[38]

Apart from the usual and much overworked concern with the taxonomy, bionomics, and distribution of the susceptible snails, the South Africans were particularly concerned with the pathology of the disease and the question whether it in any way diminished the effectiveness of the African worker.

A warning that bilharzia may lead to decreased efficiency had come from the Chief Medical Inspector of the Transvaal schools. From a few case studies, without any controls, the inspector had announced that "the mental symptoms are so monotonously uniform in character that a diagnosis of schistosomiasis could almost be made on these alone." These alarming symptoms, to which, he warned, adults may be subjected, included forgetfulness, indifference to punishment, laziness, disinclination to mental exertion, nervous irritability, obstreperousness, and mental fatigue. He also reported that after treatment for bilharzia, a dull, listless schoolboy had been transformed into a bright, active, industrious, child.[39] This notion of mental deterioration also gained support from a Southern Rhodesian study in which European schoolboys from a "modern" school were discovered to have more presumed (diagnosed by a skin test) and more proven (diagnosed by detection of schistosome eggs in the urine and/or feces) cases of bilharzia than boys from an "academic" school. Thus, the authors concluded, "schistosomiasis may have prevented boys in the primary school from attaining a high enough academic standing to enter the academic school."[40]

But among African schoolboys, the opposite seemed to hold. "On balance," they reported, "the infected children have a better record than those free from the disease." They argued that less than half of those with the disease failed examinations and were graded in the lower half of the class, whereas if bilharzia had been detrimental to the health of the child, one would expect more than half of those infected to do poorly at school. But whereas the authors had stressed the number of *presumed* cases in their argument that less than half those infected were in the lower half of the class (46.9%), they had stressed the number of *proven* cases (48%) in their claim that less than half had also failed the examinations. Had they been consistent, then they should also have noted that 63 percent, more than half, of those presumed infected had failed the examinations. But the real problem lay with the data. The authors assumed that children who did well or poorly in their survey differed only in the presence or absence of bilharzia. Worm loads were ignored, as were also the social factors that are so significant in school achievement. What the conclusions to these tests suggested, of course, was that the disease had a greater impact on whites than on Africans. Similar results became apparent from research on the pathology of the disease in laboratory animals.

This laboratory approach enabled studies to be made on the chronic form of the disease under conditions that appeared similar to that of the African population; laboratory monkeys, mice, and rats could be substituted for malnourished Africans. They examined, for example, the pathology of the disease in mice subjected to repeated infections and to a low-protein diet. In the context of apartheid South Africa, some of these experiments carried ominous implications.

One such experiment on the disease in white mice was used to cast doubt on the validity of any attempt at mass treatment. Mice, injected with an initial dose of 50 and a subsequent dose of 200 cercariae, seemed to present a less serious disease picture than mice given one dose of 250 cercariae, or one dose of 50 cercariae. In addition, the pathological changes after a single dose of cercariae were not repeated after subsequent doses unless the mice were cured between the two doses. "In light of these findings," de Meillon concluded, "the advisability of administering curative doses of antibilharzia drugs to infected populations constantly at risk of reinfection merits serious thought."[41] In addition, another set of experiments revealed that fewer worms were recovered from mice given repeated weekly injections of cercariae than from mice given only a single injection.[42] These experiments, and negative results obtained with Miracil D probably helped to convince Pitchford that "with [the] present drugs available, mass treatment is of doubtful value in attempting to control bilharziasis in South Africa."[43]

The social implications of these laboratory experiments were also made abundantly clear in one of the very few papers ever published on the impact of malnutrition on the disease. They discovered that a low-protein diet led to a striking increase in mortality, which was particularly marked in those infected with bilharzia: After 30 weeks, 89 percent of infected mice on a low-protein diet had died, compared with 48 percent of noninfected mice (see Table 14.2).[44]

But, what caught the attention of the experimenters was not this enhanced mortality but the discovery that the schistosome worms in those few poorly fed mice that did survive were smaller, showed abnormal reproductive systems, and passed fewer eggs. This "we never suspected," they wrote, "because we were looking for graver pathology and not for crippled schistosomes." Indeed, they were so surprised by what they clearly saw as an advantage possessed by malnourished Africans, that they withheld publication until after W. B. DeWitt in the United States had published similar findings. DeWitt found that mice, fed on a yeast diet lacking vitamin E and the essential amino acid cystine, contained worms that, like those in the South African experiments, developed abnormally and failed to produce viable eggs.[45] In an extraordinary conclusion, which must be viewed against the background of an apartheid state, de Meillon and Patterson ignored the increased mortality to state that "the action on the surviving mice was not more drastic as a result of the protein deficiency." But only 11 percent survived!

In the 12th Annual Report of the South African Council of Scientific and Industrial Research, these findings were succinctly summarized. In Egypt, the report noted, the constant reinfection of the *fellaheen* breaks down their resistance and immunity and leads to a severe pathology. But, they reported, the assumption that increased use of irrigation in South Africa will lead to the same result has not been supported by experiments.

Table 14.2. *Effect of bilharzia on mortality in mice fed a low-protein diet*

Weeks after infection	Mortality, infected mice (%)	Mortality, noninfected mice (%)
Normal diet		
9	1	0
17	23	1
30	N.D.[a]	N.D.[a]
Low protein diet		
9	22	11
17	46	25
30	89	48

[a]N.D. = no data.
Source: Adapted from B. de Meillon and S. Patterson, *South African Medical Journal* 32 (1958): 1086–8.

A first infection produces a definite pattern of disease which is not repeated on subsequent infections unless the monkey is first cured by drugs. Secondly, repeated weekly reinfection of monkeys and mice over the course of a year or more has not produced a pathology as assessed by liver histology any more severe than that following a single infection. . . . The first infection is all important. It can be so heavy as to kill an animal in a day or so, or it can be mild, producing a pattern of disease which is characteristic for almost each species of animal but which cannot be aggravated by further infections.

In addition, they noted, a low-protein diet does not aggravate the lesions of bilharzia. Thus, they optimistically concluded, there should be no fear of severe bilharzia in South Africa, and the handicap of bilharzia to African schoolchildren may be less than usually believed.[46]

Attention was also paid to the acute form of bilharzia with which Europeans were usually inflicted after a weekend swim. From the experimental infection of laboratory animals, they were able to investigate the pathology and diagnosis of early bilharzia before the appearance of the eggs. In this way, they hoped, the white population could be diagnosed and treated before the eggs appeared some two months after infection – a possibility of little help to the African population suffering from the chronic form of the disease.[47] There was also a possibility that drugs could be developed that would prevent infection after one of these careless casual weekend contacts. In 1956, for example, the Hoechst Company developed the drug S 616, which, after testing in South Africa, seemed to act as a prophylactic when administered up to four days after contact with the cercariae and before the young stages of the worms reached the liver.[48]

And so the appalling contrast. South Africa has become a leader in medical research, their laboratories are among the very best in the world, and their physicians and scientists rank among the very best of those working on bilharzia. But these affluent laboratories and magnificient hospitals exist in a society of "homelands" into which "misfits in the profit system are thrown without pity or shame," and in which bilharzia and other diseases flourish.[49]

15

Bilharzia: Second to only one

In the immediate postwar years, few experts would have ranked bilharzia among the world's most serious tropical diseases. It was clearly a major problem in Egypt, China, Brazil, and, to some extent, in South Africa and Southern Rhodesia, but the Colonial Medical Research Committee in London was probably accurate in ranking bilharzia below malaria, dysentery, yaws, leprosy, filariasis, and others.

Bilharzia certainly did not rank high among members of the newly created World Health Organization, despite valiant efforts by the Egyptian delegates to increase awareness of the disease. In the summer of 1946, at an international health conference in New York, an Interim Commission was set up to prepare the agenda for the first formal meeting of the WHO. This Commission formed a Committe on Programme to define what WHO's priorities were to be. The Committee, while agreeing to the immediate formation of expert committees on malaria and tuberculosis (a sign of high priority), agreed only to examine further the claims of smallpox, cancer, alcoholism, and bilharzia for equal status.

In an attempt to have an expert committee on bilharzia formed, the Egyptian delegate, Aly Tewfik Shousha Pasha, submitted a document to the Committee entitled "On the inclusion of schistosomiasis on the agenda of the World Health Assembly," in which he argued that the disease was "of very urgent public health importance."[1] Four months later, he presented a more detailed report entitled "Schistosomiasis: A world problem," and moved that the Executive Board of the first assembly of WHO establish a committee of experts on the disease.[2]

We have met Aly Shousha before. He had graduated in medicine from Berlin in 1915 and had postgraduate experience in bacteriology from the University of Zurich. He was the undersecretary of State for the Ministry of Health, and a supporter of Barlow's Snail Destruction Section. His second report was as much directed against Khalil as toward the WHO. He maintained not only that the disease was an international problem which irrigation had rendered second only to malaria in importance and which demanded the attention of an expert committee, but also that bilharzia could best be controlled by killing the snail hosts, as was being done successfully in Egypt by the Bilharzia Snail Destruction Section.

That an expert committee on the disease should be formed was supported also by the Food and Agricultural Organization of the United Nations (FAO), and by a group of 25 experts, including Bang, Brackett, Faust, Meleney, W. H. Wright, and others, most of whom had been involved in the Leyte campaign, who met to consider the matter during the Fourth International Conference on Tropical Medicine which was held in Washington, D.C. in 1948.[3]

But members from the Soviet Union, Czechoslovakia, Poland, and Rumania opposed Shousha's motion. The disease, they argued, was only of localized importance and should be studied by "regional organizations"; expert committees, they believed, should address only generalized problems.[4] After some debate, the Eastern bloc countries had their way: Bilharzia was not included either among the 11 expert committees formed in 1948, or in the six others established the following year.[5] The Egyptian delegate had to be satisfied instead with a joint study group of the Office International d'Hygiene Publique (OIHP) and of the WHO.[6]

But then, quite suddenly, the scene changed. In 1950, only one year after the study group had been formed, members of the American Society of Parasitology were informed by their President, Dr. W. H. Wright, that next to malaria, bilharzia is "the most important tropical disease in the world today." In that year also, the Director General of the WHO warned delegates of the increasingly serious problem of bilharzia, and, a few months later, a report to the British Colonial Medical Research Committee announced also that bilharzia was "next in importance to malaria."[7] In a very few years, bilharzia had climbed from almost total obscurity and was poised to become second to only one. But there was little data to support such a dramatic claim. Norman Stoll's figures, for example, showed that bilharzia was not even the most prevalent helminth disease in the world.[8] In addition, virtually nothing was known about its impact on any community in terms of mortality or morbidity. Why, then, was the claim made at the same time in the United States, the WHO, and Britain? In this chapter I shall examine numerous issues that played a role in raising the visibility of the disease.

PROFESSIONAL NEEDS

The question of bilharzia cannot be considered in isolation; it must be seen against a background of professional concern that was being expressed most vehemently by Americans working in tropical medicine and parasitology. In

1942, for example, the American Society of Tropical Medicine, not for a moment believing that the war could be lost, established a Committee on War and Postwar Problems to promote graduate and undergraduate research and education in tropical medicine. Tropical medicine, must, they resolved in 1943, be "energetically promoted now and in the future."[9] By the end of the war, members of the American Society of Tropical Medicine, although acutely aware that the war had brought money, increased membership, and an enhanced status to themselves and their discipline, nevertheless felt insecure. Would this happy state of affairs last, they wondered? Those involved were not sure. "We are concerned lest tropical medicine be allowed to deteriorate to its pre-war level," explained the Society in a 1945 resolution to President Truman. Present training and research, they informed the President, were "woefully inadequate." As a result, they reminded the President, the U.S. Army and Navy both had to establish emergency educational programs in tropical diseases at the beginning of the war. "We therefore recommend," they concluded in the telegram, "immediate and active development of this important phase of American medicine."[10]

During the late 1940s and early 1950s, the minutes of the American Society, Academy, and Foundation of Tropical Medicine, and their colleagues in parasitology, showed an overriding concern with promoting and enhancing their disciplines. Committees were formed to "activate the provisions of the constitution of the Academy with respect to education and research," and to "awaken the interest of the general public through publicity." Proposals were also made to strengthen these efforts by the formation of various federations within the biological and medical sciences.

In 1946, for example, the National Research Council proposed that an insitute of American biologists be formed to further the interests of biology and the profession. In the past, they noted, biologists had been concerned almost exclusively with teaching, but "now biological research and practice is emerging as a profession in itself." The proposed institute, would, they hoped, "safeguard the professional interests of biologists, and assist in providing the material means for the promotion of biological research."[11] The following year, the parasitologists were invited to become charter members of the institute, and in 1948, with 12 chartered societies, the American Institute of Biological Sciences was formed for "the advancement of the biological societies and their application to human welfare."[12]

Strength through unity was also achieved by those in tropical medicine. In 1951, for example, with the elimination of malaria from North America, the National Malarial Society was amalgamated with the Society of Tropical Medicine and renamed the American Society of Tropical Medicine and Hygiene. Two years later, the American Academy of Tropical Medicine was also amalgamated with it.

INTERNATIONAL COMMUNISM

Political events in the postwar world also helped to enhance the status of those engaged in tropical medicine and parasitology. The resolution to amalgamate the American Academy of Tropical Medicine with the American Society of Tropical Medicine and Hygiene drew attention to some of these:

The importance of tropical medicine to the U.S.A. is greater today than at any time previously in its history, because of current defense commitments in tropical lands, because of increasing dependence on basic metals or other strategic materials from tropical areas, because of the importance of an expanding export trade with tropical countries and because of the need to assist the development of tropical peoples in the interests of international peace and stability.[13]

The phrase "international peace and stability" had, by the 1950s, become synonymous with containing communism and preserving the "free world" for capitalistic development. By then the American Government and the American public had become convinced that a Moscow-centered international communist conspiracy existed. According to this view, the communist monolith was intent on overcoming the "free world," and had, very recently, tested international waters by initiating an attack on South Korea. Containment of the communist menace, through the Marshall Plan, NATO, and the Truman Declaration of U.S. intervention to prevent the spread of communism, became the dominant theme of U.S. foreign policy; the Cold War had begun.

Tropical medicine became an important component of these policies. People, it was argued, who were healthy and free of tropical diseases were less likely to fall prey to communist propaganda. Thus, for the Americans, the encouragement of research into the cause, treatment, and prevention of tropical diseases became another arm in their stand against "communist imperialism."

Harry Truman, in his inaugural address of January 20, 1949, announced such a program for stability and "peace and freedom." Four courses of action were laid down during the address, including point four: "We must embark on a bold program for making the benefits of our scientific advances and industrial progress available for the improvement and growth of underdeveloped countries." According to this plan, "free" and "peace-loving peoples" must be aided so as to achieve "peace, plenty and freedom." Thus, according to Samual Hayes, long-range programs in basic education, health, sanitation, and food will lead to a "revolutionary improvement in the material and social well-being of the world's peoples," and thereby ensure a final victory over communism.[14]

An Act for International Development (the so-called Point IV program) was approved in 1950, and an International Development Advisory Board, under the chairmanship of Nelson Rockefeller, set up later that year. Its first priority was to attack hunger and ill health, and by 1951, 350 Point IV technicians were operating 108 projects in 27 countries. Naturally those involved in tropical medicine were only too anxious to benefit from this program. The American Foundation of Tropical Medicine applied for funding, and in 1950, a Tropical Medicine and World Health Committee urged the President "to constantly utilize and be guided by the training, the practical competence, the experience of the U.S. Public Health Service."[15]

"Operation Bootstrap" in Puerto Rico, which included an important campaign against bilharzia, was thought to be a particularly fine example of "the best counterpropaganda the United States can use to deflect Communist aims." By this program, Puerto Rico was reported to have become "a signpost pointing the way to security with freedom, to hope with dignity."[16] "Operation bootstrap" was a massive industrialization program initiated by Luis Marin, leader of the Puerto Rican Popular Democratic Party who, in 1944, had been elected to the head of the Puerto Rican Senate. It began by the Puerto Rican government opening a small nucleus of factories, backed by a central planning agency and a central bank. Naturally, U.S. business leaders saw this as a "socialist experiment," totally unsuitable for an attack against the communist menace. It was, announced one business leader in the *New York Herald Tribune*, "a Utopian–Marxist–Soviet dream," which would frighten away American capital. Thus the island government was forced to switch to private enterprise, and by the use of U.S. capital and technology, industry gradually replaced agriculture as the major income producer on the island: Beggars could not be choosers.[17] This policy, begun under President Roosevelt and continued under Truman, Eisenhower, Kennedy, and Johnson, poured U.S. money into the island in the form of government aid and private investment, and, as a result, the average yearly income per capita increased from $122 in 1940 to $677 in 1960.[18]

Whether one accepts the glowing rhetoric of U.S. governments, and such publications as Earl Hanson's *Puerto Rico: Land of Wonders*, or whether one believes that this policy once again favored the United States at the expense of the people of Puerto Rico,[19] there can be little doubt that by shifting the economic base away from agriculture, the prevalence of a rural disease like bilharzia would necessarily change. As I shall discuss in the next chapter, such a change indeed occurred.

The U.S. Government was not alone in using medicine as a weapon in the fight for stability and against the communist menace. The United Fruit Company, fresh from its victory over the Nazis in Latin America, was only too willing to enter the moral crusade in defense of freedom and free enterprise. They were able to convince the U.S. Government, for example, that a Guatemalan attempt to expropriate land owned by the Company, was, in fact, an example of "a Moscow-directed Communist conspiracy in Central America," and, as a result, they and the CIA cooperated to overthrow the elected government of Jacabo Arbenz and impose a new leader, Castillo Armas, with whom the United Fruit Company concluded a new pact, regained control of land expropriated by the previous government, and banned all union activity. They flooded members of the U.S. Congress with highly colored accounts of these and other events in Latin America, and its public relations office in New York became the source of news for the U.S. press, including a film entitled "Why the Kremlin hates bananas."[20] In 1955, Edmund Whitman, the Company's Director of Public Relations, delivered an address to the International Advertising Association, at the Hotel Roosevelt in New York, entitled "How an American company, through advertising and public relations, has combatted communism in Latin America." He told the audience how Guatemala, with the help of his Company, had become the first nation "to throw back the red surge of international communism." The Company had, he pointed out, virtually eliminated yellow fever, smallpox, and malaria from the country, and had set up a huge medical service costing $4.5 million per year, which employed 2,000 health workers in 15 hospitals and 120 dispensaries. These and other actions, Whitman continued, "are some of the 'good deeds' that make up our corporate character" and "represent a way of life that the Communists fear, and cannot match." The Kremlin not only "hates bananas," he concluded, but "gags" on them:

> Why is it that [the] United Fruit Company symbolizes all that the Soviet fears and hates in its relentless propaganda line directed to the Western Hemisphere? Well, the answer should not be too difficult to find. In the first place, the Company has demonstrated that the private enterprise system provides the free world with personnel, heart and technology capable of running far-flung operations. It has demonstrated that it is capable of wiping out disease, of producing strategic crops; capable of operating an extensive, efficient Merchant Marine; capable of giving employment and improving living standards in areas where otherwise the soil would be ripe for the Soviet seeds of discontent. Is it any wonder that the Soviet gags on the banana?[21]

Pablo Neruda, the Chilean poet and member of the Allende government before it, too, was disposed by the CIA, expressed his views on this medically benevolent Company in his 1950 poem entitled "La United Fruit Co."

> When the trumpets had sounded and all
> was in readiness on the face of the earth,
> Jehovah divided his universe:
> Anaconda, Ford Motors,
> Coca Cola Inc., and similar entities:
> the most succulent item of all,
> The United Fruit Company Incorporated
> reserved for itself: the heartland
> and coasts of my country,
> the delectable waist of America.
> They rechristened their properties:

the "Banana Republics" –
and over the languishing dead,
the uneasy repose of the heroes
who harried that greatness,
their flags and their freedoms,
they established an *opera bouffe* . . .

The United Fruit Company Incorporated
sailed off with a booty of coffee and fruits
brimming its cargo boats, gliding
like trays with the spoils
of our drowning dominions.

And all the while, somewhere, in the sugary
hells of our seaports,
smothered by gases, an Indian
fell in the morning:
a body spun off, an anonymous
chattel, some numeral tumbling,
a branch with its death running out of it
in the vat of the carrion, fruit laden and foul.[22]

THE RISE OF BILHARZIA

As the professionals in tropical medicine and parasitology moved to assert their important role in a communist-threatened world, bilharzia steadily grew in importance. As mentioned previously, Andrew Warren, Chairman of the Committee on War and Postwar Problems, listed it among the six most important diseases of the tropical world, but, by 1950, W. H. Wright had given it the number two billing. In 1947, Norman Stoll, of the Rockefeller Institute of Medical Research and President of the American Society of Parasitology, delivered his famous presidential address. Entitled "This wormy world," it set out to answer the question, "How much helminthiasis is there in the world?"[23]

Doing the best that he could with the data available, Stoll concluded that from a total human population of 2,166.8 million, there were 2,257.1 million helminth infections. Nematodes, such as *Ascaris*, hookworm, and *Trichuris*, were judged to be the most common helminths, with the schistosomes being by far the most widespread of the trematodes (see Table 15.1).

But the purpose of the article was not simply to draw attention to the prevalence of helminth diseases in the world, but rather to suggest ways in which "parasitologists can help reduce the prospect of having the world forge ahead to more than 3,000 million human helminthiases by the year 2000." To do that, he argued, parasitologists needed to strengthen the teaching of medical parasitology in the medical schools, aid in the more rapid dissemina-

Table 15.1. *The number of human helminth infections, in millions*

Parasite	Total number of cases
Ascaris	644.4
Hookworm	456.8
Trichuris	355.1
Pinworm	208.8
Wuchereria	189.0
Schistosoma (3 species)	114.4
japonicum	46.0
haematobium	39.2
mansoni	29.2
Guinea worm	48.3
Taenia	41.4

Source: Data from Norman Stoll, *Journal of Parasitology* 33 (1947): 1–18.

tion of ideas, and finally and most important, begin to address the basic problems that still needed to be solved.

Bilharzia quickly emerged as one of these basic problems. Unlike hookworm, bilharzia seemed to be a particularly complex disease about which little was known. Thus, in order to combat this disease, it was first necessary to support a research program on it.

Bilharzia had become a disease that answered the professional needs of academics working in the fields of tropical medicine and parasitology.

Bilharzia in North America

The importance of bilharzia was considerably enhanced by the potential threat it posed to the American mainland as one of the diseases that could conceivably be introduced by troops returning from the tropics. Americans of course had always expressed concern that returning troops could introduce tropical diseases into the United States. This fear had surfaced during the 1898 clash with Spain, after World War I, and, with increasing vigor, after World War II. But, in 1945, unlike previous wars and with Leyte fresh in American minds, bilharzia was named as a likely candidate. Stoll became quite emotional about the problem:

One cannot have experienced the war without having been impressed anew, and depressed, by the amount of parasitism in the world. Speaking helminthologically, it may be referred to as the grave host role which the lives of men play in the lives of worms. Or, think of it the other way about, for there is likewise the great parasitic role the lives of worms play in the lives of men. Back from the Pacific come a thousand-odd Americans with schistosomiasis, and a few times that many with filariasis, and several multiples more with ancylostomiasis (hookworm). To homes widely dispersed throughout the land go these ex-service men, to live a lifetime in familiarity with the strangely sounding names of their distantly-acquired helminthiases.[24]

Andrew Warren also remarked in 1944 that returning troops were in danger of being misdiagnosed by physicians ignorant of tropical diseases. "It is not beyond reason to expect," he wrote, "that *S. mansoni* cases might have operations for cancer and hemorrhoids, [and] *S. haematobium* cases have kidneys removed."[25]

But, as was of course recognized in 1945, there needed to be snails in North America susceptible to the larval stages of human schistosomes if the disease was to become endemic. The possibility that there may be such snails in the United States became a concern even before the war ended.

The schistosome worms are not unknown in North America. They are abundant in the blood vessels of migratory birds, and, as Cort discovered, their larval stages are a cause of an irritating rash, swimmer's itch, which is widespread in the lakes of the northern states and Canada. More ominously – or so it appeared after the war – there were at least two North American schistosome species known to occur in mammals: *Heterobilharzia americana* from Florida, Texas, and North Carolina; and *Schistosomatium douthitti* from the northern states, Ontario, and Manitoba. Such mammalian forms could perhaps present a greater problem than any other North American schistosomes. But the real issue was whether North American snails could become infected with the miracidia of the human schistosome species. Between 1943 and 1946, the Office of Scientific Research and the Office of the Surgeon General supported research to answer that question. Most of this research was carried out in the laboratories of the U.S. Public Health Service. Colonies of snails infected with the three human schistosome species were set up in these laboratories, and individual snails representing 103 species were collected from 31 States in the Union. In 1945, testing of these snails for susceptibility to the larvae of the human schistosomes began.[26]

Major interest was focused on the possible susceptibility of *Tropicorbis havanensis* from Louisiana and southern Texas to the larval stages of *S. mansoni*. Preliminary studies had shown that the miracidia of *S. mansoni* were attracted to it, and other members of the genus were known to carry the parasite in South America. Considerable excitement was generated, therefore, when Eloise Cram and her co-workers reported a successful infection of a few specimens of *Tropicorbis*, which had been collected from a pond on the campus of Louisiana State University in Baton Rouge. Basically, two from 21 snails taken directly from the pond and exposed to the miracidia released cercariae, which in turn produced the mature worms in laboratory animals, and seven from 88 laboratory snails reared from these pond snails likewise proved to be susceptible. However, repeated attempts to infect 750 other *Tropicorbis* snails from other areas of Louisiana were unsuccessful.[27]

Although none of the American amnicolid snails (the family to which the snail host of *S. japonicum* belongs) proved susceptible to the miracidia of *S. japonicum*, six individuals of the genus *Pomatiopsis* from Michigan and Virginia developed sporocysts that seemed indistinguishable from those of *S. japonicum*. None of them released cercariae, but nevertheless the authors felt able to conclude that "the possibility of *S. japonicum* developing in an American snail may not be discounted entirely."[28] Experiments with the miracidia of *S. haematobium* were utterly inconclusive. No American snails proved susceptible, but neither would the miracidia obtained from infected laboratory animals infect the control snails from Africa.[29] A series of similar experiments by Harold Stunkard were negative for all the tested snails, a fact, he warned, that should not "lead to a false sense of security." Nevertheless, he was honest enough to admit, "the failure hitherto of the parasites to become established in the United States is a significant and heartening epidemiological fact," an obviously sound observation that no other person made.[30]

During this activity, Dr. W. H. Wright of the U.S. Public Health Department wrote a note to Barlow in Egypt. There was concern, Wright explained, that returning troops carrying schistosome worms might enable bilharzia to become established in the United States. Thus, domestic snails were being exposed to the miracidia of *S. mansoni* to ascertain whether these snails could act as a possible intermediate host. Wishing also to make similar tests with *S. haematobium*, Wright asked Barlow to ship some infected bulinid snails from Egypt. This Barlow appears to have done, but few snails survived the journey, and, as Wright noted in a succeeding letter, U.S. immigration regulations would prohibit the "shipping" of an infected Egyptian. "I should not like to advise that you infect yourself with *S. haematobium* for the sake of bringing material to this country," Wright was careful to state, "this would seem to me to be too severe a sacrifice to ask of anyone."[31] But the die was cast. On July 4, 1944, with his contract with the Egyptian Government expired, Barlow left for the United States for a well-earned leave carrying over 200 worms of *S. haematobium* inside him.

By December, Barlow was desperately ill. On December 14, he noted in his "Diary of self-infliction," 4,630 eggs were passed in a seminal discharge and over 200 eggs in his urine. A month earlier, a biopsy of some itching scrotal nodules, which had been oozing bloody serum for two weeks, revealed the presence of worms and eggs. Christmas was spent in a "torture of fever, pain, tenesmus, and constant urination." But all treatment was refused, because, as he wrote, "I still had hope that I would be asked to do an environmental survey of the snails of the U.S. and I could not jeopardize it all by losing the only human source of eggs in America." Night and day throughout his ordeal, Barlow kept his diary up to date: temperature, pulse, egg count, frequency of urination. By February 1945, Barlow was passing an average of 23,063 eggs every 24 hours![32]

But all to no avail; he was never asked to provide these eggs for the survey. On March 21, 1945, he received the final word from the Office of Scientific Research and Development: It would be impossible to obtain permission to infect U.S. snails in the field, as Barlow wished to do, and the number of U.S. personnel infected with *S. haematobium* was too low to justify research of that nature.[33] On April 13, a bitterly disillusioned Barlow began Fouadin treatment which reduced his egg output to 3,046 on April 23 and 307 on April 25. In May, this 69-year-old man with chronic bilharzia returned to Egypt for further treatment – in his own eyes rejected, betrayed, and ignored by his own country and by the Rockefeller Foundation which never lifted a finger on his behalf. In November, with eggs still present in his urine, Barlow received another two-week series of injections, this time with tartar emetic. At last, in April 1946, almost two years after his initial infection, he was pronounced cured; no further eggs appeared in his urine. "Along with my own injection of Potassium Antimony Tartrate," he noted, "a deeper and more sympathetic understanding of the treatment was injected into my veins."[34] Unfortunately such sympathy never osmosed through to the U.S. bureaucracy. The only reaction he received during this ordeal was a cold-blooded note from the Division of Parasitology of the Army Medical School asking for some of the schistosome eggs he was passing.[35] Perhaps the award of the President's Certificate of Merit, on July 16, 1947, was thought sufficient to recompense Barlow for the agonies he went through.

Although the potential danger of bilharzia in mainland United States, the career needs of professionals, and the menace of international communism were all significant factors in the increased postwar visibility of bilharzia, none compared in importance to the association of the disease with the food crisis of the 1950s.

The food crisis

Before World War II, the Western world had not been troubled by the specter of famine, although, as explained earlier, by the end of the 1930s the authorities at the British Colonial Office had become conscious of serious malnutrition in many colonies of the British Empire. The experts at that time were guided by an optimistic model which predicted that, in the long run, populations would reach an equilibrium between death rate and birth rate, and any overpopulation was necessarily short-lived. This model was derived from what had presumably happened during the Industrial Revolution in Europe. Then, the argument went, more and better food and a higher standard of living had led to a decline in the death rate. The population began to increase, but, as more children survived, there was less economic necessity to give birth to large numbers of them. As a result, there was a voluntary decline in the birth rate, and the population stabilized once again. According to this model, the population of the world had been increasing over time, but only by moving up from one equilibrium to a slightly higher one, each in balance with the living standards of the population at that time. Overpopulation occurred only in relatively short bursts, as the population went through what was called a "demographic transition." Nature, according to this model, was benevolent. There would be no massive population increase and no threat of famine in the tropical world until they, too, had passed through an industrial-type revolution, and their standard of living had begun to increase. And even then, such an overpopulation would be short-lived, as they moved through their own demographic transition.[36]

By the 1950s, however, this model had been superseded by a decidedly pessimistic one. According to this new view, what happened in Europe during the Industrial Revolution was not applicable to the tropical countries. In these countries, there had been a fall in the death rate without any corresponding improvement in the social conditions. And, without any such social improvement, the birth rates remained unchanged at a high level, and the populations had begun to explode. This decline in the death rate was assumed to be the result of "a rapid cultural diffusion of death-control techniques which did not depend on the diffusion of other cultural elements or basic changes in the institutions and customs of the people affected." Modern Western scientific medicine was held responsible. It had, by introducing new methods of treatment and control, brought about an unanticipated drop in the death rate.[37] The major weapon that was assumed to have led to this decline was the new wonder chemical DDT, through its use as a residual spray in the control of malaria, but the widespread postwar use of penicillin and the sulfonamides was equally significant.[38]

This sudden postwar increase in population led to a corresponding alarm about food supplies and the dangers of famine. As early as 1945, the First World Food Survey of the FAO reported that over half the world's population was malnourished or undernourished. A Second World Food Survey, seven years later, was equally pessimistic.[39] But pessimism reached new heights with the publication of Paul Ehrlich's widely acclaimed *The Population Bomb*, and the cold-blooded *Famine 1975!* by William Paddock. According to the latter, the world faced certain famine.[40] To avoid such a catastrophe, he argued, the United States must divide the nations into three groups: first, those who cannot be saved and whose citizens must be left to starve; second, those nations described as "the walking wounded," who could survive without food aid from the United States; and finally, those nations who could be saved by emergency food aid, and in which birth control measures and agricultural re-search would eventually solve the problem. The choice depended also on "political, economic, and psychological factors," but clearly the one that mattered most was whether a country helped "maintain the economic viability and prosperity of the U.S.A."

In the less developed tropical countries, the U.S. Department of Agriculture reported in 1961, "population is expanding rapidly, malnutrition is widespread and persistent, and there is no likelihood that the food problem soon will be solved."[41] This pessimism was not only an expression of concern for the welfare of those living in these malnourished countries, but also of a deeply felt fear that, with famine, would come revolutions and social instability, which might even threaten the fabric of Western societies. There seemed to be only two ways by which the impending catastrophe could be averted: the implementation of birth control measures in these tropical countries, and a massive increase in food production.

The world food supply needed to be doubled during the next 25 years, warned W. H. Wright, in his presidential address of 1950 to the American Society of Parasitology. Africa, he thought, with its cheap labor and long growing season, seemed to offer the best possibilities for such an increase. Wright, like most agriculturalists of that era, was unaware that the seemingly rich tropical forests hid a demineralized soil leached by torrential rains, and thus believed Africa to be an untapped source of agricultural bounty. But, to reap this bounty, Wright pointed out, the parasitic diseases needed to be controlled.

Wright saw Africa in imperialistic terms. Parasites needed to be controlled in order to improve Africa's productivity and serve the needs of the United States. Bilharzia, he believed, had reduced productivity in Egypt by 33 percent; in contrast, a malarial control project on a rubber estate in the Malay States had reduced the number of man-days lost per year from 862 to 186. With diseases controlled, he stated, "we may expect an improved economy, greater production and an expanded trade with these countries which are rich in raw materials which this country lacks and acutely needs." Diseases, he continued, will affect the supplies and costs of these raw materials, and thus, for the benefit of the United States, these diseases must be controlled. He acknowledged the past health work of the United Fruit Company, whose bananas, he noted, could not have been produced at the right price "without a medical department noted for its conquests of . . . tropical diseases."[42]

But, as Wright also realized, to increase food productivity in the tropical world would inevitably lead to an increased prevalence of many of those diseases that had to be controlled. Bilharzia was one of them; to increase food production on a grand scale necessarily required an increased use of irrigation. And with irrigation comes bilharzia.

Irrigation and bilharzia

Much of the increased food production that took place over the ensuing years was based on the so-called Green Revolution. This revolution rested on the production of high-yield varieties of wheat (and later of rice), which had been first developed at the Rockefeller Foundation's research institute in Mexico. Their plant-breeding program, begun in 1945, achieved its greatest success when these varieties were introduced into India and Pakistan in 1967. But the potential of these high-yield varieties could be achieved only by the use of Western technology; pesticides, fungicides, herbicides, fertilizers, and finally, irrigation. Hence many critics have argued that the Green Revolution has favored only the multinational corporations, who supply these technologies, and the large landowners who can afford them.[43]

The use of irrigation schemes in the growth of these new varieties has taken place mainly in the Indian subcontinent and the rest of Asia, and has as yet had little impact on bilharzia there: India is free of the disease, and *S. japonicum* in Asia has fewer foci than do the other schistosome species. In Africa, however, the demand for greater food production has created large numbers of smaller irrigation schemes (Figure 15.1), which provide ideal environments for the snail hosts. In one Kenyan province, for example, 50,000 small dams were constructed between 1957 and 1960.[44] But, as far as I know, no health measures were included in any of these small dam projects. Most health concerns in

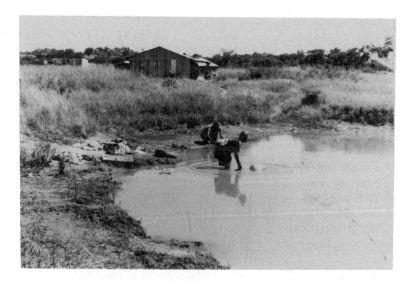

Figure 15.1. How bilharzia spreads: East Africa, 1960s (Courtesy of the Rockefeller Archive Center)

Africa have focused on the huge irrigation and hydroelectric dams (see Table 15.2) which have created large man-made lakes and perfect environments for the snail hosts of the two schistosome species.

The Akosombo Dam on the River Volta in Ghana provides a good example of the impact of such large dams on bilharzia. Built to provide power for the manufacture of aluminum, it was finally completed in 1965. From the beginning, the possibility that bilharzia would become a problem in Volta Lake was realized. Bilharzia was known to be endemic on the lower reaches of the river as well as in some of the upper river villages where swamps, small streams, and ponds were common. George Macdonald, of the London School of Hygiene and Tropical Medicine, and a medical consultant for the project, had warned of the danger. "The creation of the lake," he wrote,

will provide a suitable medium for their [the snail's] implantation and multiplication, and if no precautions were to be taken it could rationally be expected that schistosomiasis might be freely transmitted along the lake border. The risks are exaggerated by the fact that the fisherfolk who normally migrate along the river are permanently domiciled in an endemic zone where *Physopsis africanus* and *Schistosoma haematobium* are common and so constitute the greatest risk to health inherent in the scheme.[45]

By 1966, the snail hosts of *S. haematobium* had appeared, living among the dense aquatic vegetation that was beginning to accumulate in the bays and inlets of the rising lake. Nevertheless, the author of the report concluded, "it is too early to predict the future of the Volta Lake as a focus of schistosomiasis transmission."[46] Two short years later, bilharzia had appeared. By 1968, approximately 50 percent of the population in two lakeside villages had become infected with *S. haematobium*.[47] This example, Hunter and his co-authors noted, "provides irrefutable evidence of a major hazard of the rapid spread of urinary schistosomiasis at an explosive level and on a large scale resulting from a water resources development."[48]

The claims of the 1950s, that bilharzia had become a worldwide scourge, was primarily a reaction to the fear of overpopulation and famine and the widespread concern that irrigation and hydroelectric schemes would cause the disease to grow into an international menace. But there are those who believe

Table 15.2. *Some major dams in Africa*

Dam	Country	Date of completion
Sennar	Sudan	1924
Owen Falls	Uganda	1954
Kariba	Zambia	1959
Akosombo	Ghana	1965
Aswan High Dam	Egypt	1970

that the most serious menace came from the smaller irrigation schemes which, unlike the larger and more publicized dams, were built without much recognition of the problems that could ensue.

The WHO

No organization was more concerned with the health dangers of hydroelectric and irrigation schemes than the WHO. "The introduction or development of irrigation schemes, as well as the change from basin to perennial irrigation, has always resulted in a considerable increase in the incidence and intensity of bilharziasis," noted the members of the joint OIHP/WHO Study Group in 1949.[49] This Committee, which included Azim Bey and Aly Shousha from Egypt, Blair from Southern Rhodesia, and W. H. Wright from the United States, visited Egypt for five days in 1949, where it spent its time interviewing various Egyptian officials concerned with public health, including Barlow, and three other members of the Bilharzia Snail Destruction Section. Their recommendations to avoid the unavoidable were basically administrative: Every potential irrigation scheme, they argued, must be considered by public health authorities and should proceed only with their approval. Furthermore, they added, these public health authorities should be represented on the governing body of the irrigation scheme. They also urged the WHO to draw the attention of the United Nations to the danger of introducing irrigation schemes without proper sanitary and snail control. Whatever the cost of doing this, the Committee concluded, "it would be amply compensated by the maintenance of health and of the productive power of the labourers and of their families in the irrigated areas."

In 1950, the Director General of the WHO also added his voice to these concerns by pointing out the dangers that irrigation schemes posed in areas subject to bilharzia. A year later, the Fourth World Assembly recommended that although arid lands must be developed, the irrigation must be done in such a way as to prevent the introduction or aggravation of bilharzia.[50] In addition, a series of surveys during the 1950s revealed that indeed bilharzia was more widespread than previously assumed.[51]

Finally, this irrigation threat must have acted as the major stimulus to the formation of a seven-member Expert Committee on Bilharzia, which held its first meeting in Puerto Rico in the autumn of 1952.[52] Their report of the following year provided an excellent summary of what was known about the disease at that time and followed the standard view that "the control of molluscan intermediate hosts is the most important single method of preventing bilharziasis." But its major thrust was to urge for a massive research effort into the disease: Surveys were needed; laboratory studies on immunity were required; malacologists should address the vexing problem of snail systematics;

and the possible impact of bilharzia on productive efficiency should be investigated.[53]

The British

The British, at this time, also became aware of the threat of bilharzia inherent in the construction of irrigation schemes. Dr. E. D. Pridie, Chief Medical Officer to the Colonial Office and member of the Medical Research Advisory Committee, was astonished, he wrote, "by the lack of appreciation in some parts of tropical Africa and the Middle East of the menace bilharziasis can be to public health in irrigation schemes being started without any true appreciation of this very grave risk by the authorities concerned." The disease, he warned, may take ten years or more to become established in these areas, "but when it gets a hold, it is almost impossible to get rid of." When this occurs, he continued, "the inhabitants, with their health ruined, will live to curse the day the scheme was ever started!"[54]

But British interest in bilharzia was initially stimulated by a chance remark made by Ernest Bevan, the British Foreign Secretary in the newly elected British Labour Government. On May 24, 1946, Bevan, replying to a fairly vitriolic debate over the Government's decision to remove its troops from the Suez Canal and grant Egypt its independence, took issue with the opposition's "Poona mentality," and brought up the issue of bilharzia. "We have never gained the gratitude and thankfulness of the masses of the people of Egypt," he complained, and the great wealth added to the country by British policy "has never flowed down to the *fellaheen*." But, he added: "If we had spent one-tenth of the money that we have spent on defence, in grappling with that awful disease that weakens the whole fibre, due to impure water in Egypt, we should have earned the eternal gratitude of the Egyptians."[55]

The Colonial Medical Research Committee reacted with alacrity. A memo entitled "Proposals for research in helminthic diseases" was hastily prepared and presented to the August meeting of the Committee. Denying the validity of Bevan's accusation, the report nevertheless proposed the establishment of a Helminth Subcommittee to "promote research on helminthiasis."[56] The Subcommittee was formed immediately, with Hamilton Fairley in the Chair. The new British Colonial Empire was about to enter the fight against bilharzia.

In May 1949, Creech Jones, the Labour Government's new Colonial Secretary, presented yet another Colonial Development and Welfare Bill to Parliament. Progress has been insufficient, he told members, and the annual ceiling needed to be increased to £20 million and the research ceiling to £2.5 million.[57] By 1950, £7.7 million of the Colonial Development and Welfare Fund had been allotted to colonial research, almost two million or 24.9 percent of which

Table 15.3. *List of British medical research projects in order of money allocated, 1940–50*

1. Trypanosomiasis	£605,468
2. Virus research	483,409
3. Nutrition	184,188
4. Malaria	183,595
5. Physiology	70,969
6. Filariasis	47,000
7. Scrub typhus	31,949
8. Loasis	24,675
9. Relapsing fever	9,710
10. Leprosy	7,250
11. Bilharzia	1,100
12. Flies/ticks	700
13. Cancer/diabetes	470

Source: Colonial Research Reports: Cmd 6486 (1942–3); Cmd 6535 (1943–4); Cmd 6663 (1944–5); Col 208 (1945–6); Cmd 7151 (1946–7); Cmd 7493 (1947–8); Cmd 7739 (1948–9); Cmd 8063 (1949–50).

was assigned to medical research. Bilharzia, however, was still very low on the priority list (Table 15.3).

Funding for bilharzia was not simply low; by 1950, a decision was reached to terminate what little research had been done on the disease. The Helminth Subcommittee recognized the serious nature of bilharzia, it noted in 1951, but could not recommend any new research projects. Nevertheless, they concluded, the disease is "next in importance to malaria."[58]

16

Bilharzia (1950–1970s): A strategic change

With bilharzia elevated to the number two position among the world's tropical diseases, the resources of the U.S. military, the Rockefeller Foundation, and the British Colonial Office were once again thrown into the battle. But by then, a new recruit had been added to these old campaigners: the World Health Organization.

In 1953, the WHO set up the Qaliubiya Health Demonstration Area, which was, more or less, an expansion of the earlier Sindbis project of the Rockefeller Foundation. The scheme, set up in part by Claude Barlow, was but one example of the "new outlook" in the WHO. Such demonstration areas were to be centers from which simultaneous attacks on many diseases and the environment were to be directed, and in which an active interest in "health promotion" would be taken.[1] The goal of the Qaliubiya Centre was in line with these new directives. Occupying 5,000 acres with a population of 32,000 people, it was set up, the WHO grandly announced, "to correlate medical services with services for social and economic development and to evaluate results in terms of the effect on health and social and economic status of the population."[2] But the project ran into difficulties, and the WHO was forced back into believing that the parasites could best be eliminated by killing the snail hosts. But as these snail destruction campaigns unfolded, it became apparent that this seemingly simple procedure was, once again, doomed to failure; new strategies were needed. By the late 1960s, what this new strategy was to be had become apparent.

How ineffective the WHO's Qaliubiya project had become was made obvious when, in 1956, with the preliminary engineering studies of the Aswan High Dam completed, the Rockefeller Foundation was again invited by the Egyptian Government to assist in planning for the changes that would accrue when the dam began operating. John Weir was sent out again to review the changes that had taken place since the Egyptian Revolution and the withdrawal of the Rockefeller Foundation four years previously. After meeting with various officials of the Ministry of Health, the Point IV Training Centre, the Qaliubiya WHO Health Demonstration Centre, and numerous foreign advisers, and, after visiting the sites of their work, Weir reported back to the Rockefeller officials. His report was totally damning.[3]

Although pleased to note that Egyptians were now "free men on their way to a new life in a regenerated Egypt," he was less enthusiastic to find government officials functioning "at about the same level of dreaming and inactivity as they did before the revolution." The only way the promised economic, social, and physical changes would be brought to the Egyptian village, Weir wrote in his usual blunt way, would be "to boot the bureaucrats out of their offices in Cairo and put them to work in the villages." The Point IV Training Centre was, not surprisingly, described by Weir as an "ivory tower" – totally unsuitable for the Egyptian situation. But the most damning remarks pertained to the Qaliubiya project. Given that it was following the plan outlined by Weir many years before, the program itself was regarded as "ideal." But its execution was another matter. The program, according to Weir, was lacking in "discipline and energy." The WHO "managed to send some singularly impotent, and in several instances, incompetent, individuals to advise." Many of them were relatives and cronies of Dr. Aly Shousha Pasha, the Egyptian delegate to the WHO,[4] and many were also lazy, arriving for work at 10.00 A.M. and departing for the day two hours later. No wells and only four latrines had been built in two years, according to Weir, and almost no one had been trained. Cairo-based officials, he reported, showed him "fancy lighted charts showing all villages having water piped to them from the old water tanks," but, when he arrived in these villages, "there was no evidence that water was there and indeed, faced with the evidence, everyone exclaimed that of course it was not yet available but would be shortly, *enshallah.*" But the most chilling statistic revealed by Weir concerned the agricultural farms that had been set up to educate the *fellaheen* in modern farming methods. They were being used, Weir reported, to grow lovely flowers for the dining tables of Cairo politicians and the Qaliubiya directors of the WHO.[5]

Similar disasters seemed to surround the Egypt-10 project of the WHO, set up as part of the Qaliubiya project, but directed specifically at bilharzia. Initially planned as a program to demonstrate the impact of a coordinated attack on the disease, using the tools of education, sanitation, snail destruction, and treatment, it, too, soon ran into trouble. Coordination became a pipe dream; each of these four lines of attack was controlled by a different section of the Egyptian Government, each headed by a politician unwilling to lose face by surrendering control of any branch of his domain. If that were not enough, there were also difficulties in the villages. Because of the high water table, latrines soon degenerated into open, putrified, fly-infested cesspools, and the poverty in the villages was such that few could afford to suffer through the tarter emetic treatment routine that usually incapacitated a *fellah* for almost three weeks.[6]

Thus, once again, there seemed no other option but to kill snails; all other general lines of attack seemed to have failed. Humans could be treated by worm-killing drugs; the pollution of freshwater by schistosome eggs could be reduced or, in theory, even abolished by the provision of latrines and by education in hygienic sanitary habits; or contact between infected humans and water could be reduced by the provision of adequate safe water for all domestic needs. But there were no effective therapeutic drugs; people failed to accept and use filthy fly-attracting common latrines; and contact with water was inevitable, given its use for bathing, drinking, and household use. Thus, killing snails seemed to be the only alternative, and the WHO perhaps conditioned by their early experiences in Egypt, came to accept the Western creed that there were major advantages in imposing solutions that did not require the cooperation of the people involved.[7]

But killing snails did not plan out as expected. Effective molluscicides were lacking at that time, and most of the experts lacked necessary skills and knowledge in such new fields as epidemiology and quantitative animal ecology. Many of them were parasitologists who, in those years, had been trained only to describe new species and to uncover their life cycles. None, as far as I can tell, was in any way familiar with the logistic growth curve of density-dependent animal populations, and, as a result, seemed to believe that as molluscicides were applied and snail populations declined in numbers their potential for increase would necessarily decline also. In reality, they do the exact opposite, increasing almost exponentially when numbers are very low, and leveling off to an equilibrium as numbers increase. But there seemed no other practical way, and so once again another field project to ascertain the impact of copper sulfate on snail populations was designed – this time by the directors of the Egypt-10 project.

MOLLUSCICIDES: THE FIRST STRATEGY

In the summer of 1953, after discovering that 34 percent of the 1,420 drains and canals surveyed contained snails susceptible to the schistosome parasites, 17 metric tons of copper sulfate were deposited. The results were encouraging, according to the author of the report.[8] Not only was the paucity of snail-inhabited canals in the autumn and early winter following treatment attributed to the effect of copper sulfate, but the author claimed also that the number of snails that were present had decreased considerably, and that, again, this drop was due to the treatment.

But these claims were highly suspect. There were no controls, that is to say, no surveyed canals in which copper sulfate was not added, and although, by the spring of 1954, the number of susceptible snails had increased again, the author, again without any justification, claimed that their numbers had been held in check by the sulfation. However, after claiming that "the normal and known rise of infectivity during the summer to high levels in autumn and winter was arrested quite effectively by the various sulfations of the year 1953," the author was forced to admit that "it was impossible to keep the vectors away from the area for long. After one year of thorough sulfation the snails were again abundant . . . and infection once more found to be widespread." Treatment with copper sulfate alone, the report concluded, was too costly and would not completely eliminate the snails.

The Egyptian Government had also signed an agreement with the U.S. Government to test the effectiveness of the new molluscicide, sodium pentachlorophenate in the village of Warraq El-Arab. But this time, in contrast to the Egypt-10 conclusions, the leaders of the project decided that control by mollusciciding alone did seem feasible. The tests seemed successful; the prevalence of the parasite among children of the area was reported to have decreased between 1954 and 1958.[9]

But the statistical basis for this conclusion appeared to be in doubt, and, understandably confused and concerned by what was happening in the Nile Delta, the WHO sent out advisory teams to report on the situation. These assessments were uniformly pessimistic in tone. Without government interest and coordination between departments, the hopelessly ambitious Qaliubiya project should be abandoned, they concluded, and there was little point either in continuing the Warraq project.[10]

Neither did the 29 experts who attended the 1956 African conference on the disease help to resolve the problem. According to one of its participants, Dr. P. L. Le Roux of the London School of Hygiene and Tropical Medicine, all the working documents had been published previously, and some of the participants were not even familiar with already published material.[11] Le Roux seemed to have been right; the conference report merely published what everyone involved with the disease already knew (or should have known). Molluscicide application, they noted, to the surprise of no one, required knowledge of "snail ecology, type of terrain, pH, temperature, chemistry of dissolved solids, aquatic vegetation and streamflow," and "irrigation projects must pose a new problem in bilharziasis control." A joint meeting between experts of the FAO and the WHO should be convened, they argued, "with a view to joint action to lessen the dangers inherent in the opening up of Africa."[12]

But what could such experts achieve in 1956 in the fight against bilharzia? What were their joint actions to be? Were they still to put their faith in copper sulfate or other molluscicides? Were they correct in believing that the parasite could be eliminated by these methods? The answers were appearing more and more contradictory.

One set of answers appeared out of Japan, where, following U.S. occupation, the U.S. Army had set up the 406th Medical General Laboratory to provide backup laboratory services for the Medical Corps and to carry out research into diseases that affected the health of their military personnel and, curiously, their animals. Bilharzia, or schistosomiasis as the Americans always called the disease, became an important research area for the Medical Zoology Section, under the command of Lt.-Col. George Hunter, III.

In those years bilharzia was known to be endemic in four separate foci in Japan: the Kofu, Katayama, Chikugo, and Tone River areas (see Figure 4.7). The prevalence of the disease had increased during the war, but nevertheless it could hardly have been construed as a major threat to military health in Japan. But with wide strategic interests in Southeast Asia and communist-controlled China, the U.S. military was greatly concerned over the threat of *Schistosoma japonicum*, the least understood of all the schistosomes.

In 1950, the 406th Laboratory began "Operation Santobrite," a large-scale field trial of the molluscicide sodium pentachlorophenate, in a 150-acre site of the Fukuoka Prefecture, with a population of over 1,000 people, 73 percent of whom carried the schistosome worms. Immediately after the initial application, only 3 percent of the 1433 snails collected remained alive, but six months later, the number of living snails had increased by a factor of 13. Thus, although the laboratory reported a 90.2 percent reduction of living snails after two applications of the chemical, they also expressed disappointment over the manner in which the snail population recovered, but not sufficient disappointment, however, to stop them from expressing an opinion "that complete eradication of the snails in this area may be approached by the end of 1951."[13]

By the following year, after another two rounds of chemical application, they realized that the summer rise in the snail population was due to the propagation of those snails that had survived the spring application. "It appears then," they were surprised to learn (showing no awareness of density-dependent population growth), "that the propagation potential remains high even when the population level approaches extinction." But, they still insisted, with that optimism that research projects bring out in everyone, that the snails' ability to recover after treatment could be countered by a change in tactics. An initial large-scale chemical treatment, they argued, followed by "spot treatments" for several years, might "terminate schistosomiasis as a major public health problem."[14]

By 1954, following what was termed "fundamental studies in snail biology" and the discovery that before becoming amphibious the juvenile snails remained aquatic for the first three years of their lives, the mollusciciding team changed tactics again. In this new approach, the initial treatments were given in the form of sprays directed at the adult snails, whereas the "spot treatments" were applied to irrigated water in order to kill the juveniles.[15]

Initially, all went well. In 1955, they again predicted the virtual elimination of the snails in three years. But, by the end of the decade, the snail population had reached a plateau, below which it seemed impossible to move. A four-year chemical application that ended in 1956, for example, still enabled field workers to collect, on the average, 41 snails per hour, and this number had increased to 67 three years later. By 1963, severe pessimism had set in. "The awesome population build-up following the cessation of molluscicide activities must be overcome," they wrote, "before eventual control of the disease can be achieved."[16] Barely hanging on by the thinnest of threads, they once again urged for the continuation of molluscicides, but this time directed only at the loci of infected snails. Such a method, they pointed out, would be more effective and less costly than attempts to eliminate all the snails. But this was easier said than done; labor-intensive hard work was required to find these loci. A survey of 40,837 acres near Kofu, for example, led to the discovery of 4,447 sites. But it took 14,548 helpers 44 days to do this.[17]

But there was better news elsewhere. Those who continued to believe in the effectiveness of snail killing received a boost in 1958, when the Bayer Company produced a new molluscicide, Bayluscide or Bayer 73. The chemical was, the Second African Conference on Bilharzia reported, effective at much lower concentrations than any other chemical.[18] A British team formed to investigate bilharzia in Tanganyika at that time also reported success with the new Bayer chemical.

The British attack

Renewed British interest in bilharzia can be traced to the infamous Groundnut (or peanuts) Scheme.[19] In 1946, Frank Samuel, Managing Director of the United Africa Company, a subsidiary of the giant Unilever, and R. Miller, Director of Agriculture in Tanganyika, suggested that Britain's postwar fat shortages could be overcome by the mechanical production of groundnuts on the wastelands of Tanganyika. After a successful brief to the British Labour Government, a mission was sent out under the leadership of John Wakefield, an experienced agriculturalist and early critic of the old-style British Empire. As George Hall, the Colonial Secretary, announced in Parliament:

There is everywhere in the Colonies a determination to send more food to Britain, and with the cooperation of my colleague, the Minister of Food, I am doing everything possible to help them to fulfil this task. A bumper crop of groundnuts has just been harvested in Nigeria. Supplies of this valuable source of fat are, however, so short, and are likely to be for some years to come, that the Government have decided to make a special investigation of a project for large scale new production of groundnuts in East Africa.[20]

The mission recommended three sites in Tanganyika where the soil was sandy, where there were few inhabitants, and where, unknown to them, the rainfall was disastrously low. They proposed to establish 80 mechanized units, each of 30,000 acres, and estimated that by 1950, a minimum of 600,000 tons of groundnuts would have been produced with an eventual annual production of

800,000 tons. By 1947, a vast armada of mechanized transport, much of it left over from the North African and Philippine military campaigns, began arriving at Dar-es-Salam, which, without suitable rail-links to the sites, quickly became a bottleneck. The first swathes were cut in June 1947, but breakages and shortages of spare parts soon began to take their toll. As Wood wrote, "The Groundnut Army, was, in fact, in very much the same position as an army which had gone into action in a fit of absentmindedness, and forgotten to take any RASC [Royal Army Service Corps] with it."

The scheme was, as the opposition spokesman Oliver Stanley correctly noted, "primarily for the benefit of the consumers of this country." Indeed the African laborers, gathered at the opening ceremonies, must have been puzzled at the Minister of Food's remark that "on your success depends more than on any other single factor whether the harassed housewives of Great Britain get more margarine, cooking fats and soap."[21] But, as befitted the new Empire, the scheme was also planned to bring about progressive health, nutritional, housing, welfare, and labor policies so as to raise the Africans' standard of life. By introducing what they fondly regarded as a revolution in agricultural techniques, the British Government hoped to break the cycle of rising population and malnutrition. They also believed that the tsetse fly could be eliminated and stock farming introduced by using the fodder of the groundnuts and grassleys (the crop with which the groundnuts were rotated) for animal feed.[22]

The Groundnut Scheme also had a medical component to it. An East African Medical Survey, proposed in 1946, "to elicit information as to the relative incidence and importance of diseases and their causes in East Africa," was included among the plans for African betterment associated with the Groundnut Scheme.[23] But it seems to have become dissociated from the Scheme rather early. The initial medical and sanitary survey of the area was planned to be centered at Malya, south of Lake Victoria, but got off to a very unpromising beginning. The first Director, a Dr. Davidson, after a shipboard romance, resigned almost immediately after taking up his appointment. The survey was then transferred to Mwanza, on the east coast of Lake Victoria, where it joined the already existing Filariasis Research Unit under the direction of Col. W. Lurie, a former member of the Indian Medical Service. Thus, in effect, the medical work was never coordinated with the Groundnut Scheme at all; dealing with East African villagers began to seem more logical than surveying a heterogeneous labor force drawn in from a large area. Nevertheless, the idea of setting up a medical survey project in Tanganyika was part of the groundnut affair.

By 1954, when Lurie resigned, the survey, like its cousin the Groundnut Scheme, was in total disarray. Like many surveys before and since, it had become an end to itself, and not a means to uncover future research problems. Worse, the data collecting had continued without being analyzed. According to George Macdonald, the survey lacked "scientific precision" and personnel knowledgeable in statistics. Accordingly the survey was discontinued, re-named the East Africa Medical Survey and Research Institute, and placed under the direction of Professor E. G. Holmes, Chairman of Physiology at Makerere College. It had become a laboratory-based, academic research institute.[24]

To compound the problems of the Mwanza-based institute, the political situation in British Africa had entered a period of rapid change and instability which created great uncertainty in medical circles. Harold MacMillan had taken over from Anthony Eden, following the last fling of British imperialism in the Suez Canal fiasco. Unlike his predecessor, MacMillan believed that the future prosperity of Britain lay more with Europe than with the old empire, and that it was now in Britain's interest to withdraw from Africa as quickly and quietly as possible. Thus the end came, as first Ghana and then country after country obtained their independence, surrounded by a rhetoric extolling the benefits of a British Commonwealth of Nations, designed to appease both old Tory imperialists and Labour Party "developers."

By 1960, the British, through their Colonial Development and Welfare Acts, had spent nearly £6.5 million on medical research, representing 26.6 percent of the total colonial research budget; £1.8 million of this had been allocated to trypanosomiasis and the tsetse fly, whereas malaria garnered approximately £572,000 to stand in third place (see Table 16.1). Bilharzia, said to be the second most serious tropical disease in the world, ranked a very distant 13th, behind filariasis, trachoma, leprosy, scrub typhus, relapsing fever, and loasis, with a total budget of £48,828. Indeed, not until these last years of empire, did the British finally take a serious interest in the disease; it became a priority item in the Mwanza-based institute. In this institute a team of investigators gathered who were to become the British experts on bilharzia, and some of whom today are on the staff of the London School of Hygiene and Tropical Medicine.

Back in London, the members of the Medical Research Committee and its subsidiary, the Helminth Subcommittee, had become aware that any serious work on bilharzia needed the services of expert malacologists, and, given the threat of the disease in a postwar world of irrigation schemes, there existed prospects for "a career in field malacology." What was needed, they argued, were colonial research scholarships in malacology. Such malacologists would be appointed to help clarify the confusion over the identification of African snail hosts and to provide information on their anatomy and ecology.

Snails are, perhaps, one of the most difficult groups of organisms to identify, particularly if their keys are based on shell characteristics alone. Those engaged in bilharzia were always concerned with this problem. In any given location, they wanted to know which snail species or variety was acting as the major intermediate host. This concern seemed justified by what had happened to malaria. This "disappearing disease" had been attacked by what was called

Table 16.1. *Colonial Development and Welfare Act budget allocations, 1940–60*

1. Trypanosomes/tsetse	£1,811,662
2. Viruses	762,129
3. Malaria	571,791
4. Nutrition	427,947
5. Physiology of hot climates	193,094
6. Filariasis	136,666
7. Trachoma	114,959
8. Immunity	110,995
9. Leprosy	56,429
10. Scrub typhus	56,257
11. Relapsing fever	49,390
12. Loasis	49,315
13. Bilharzia	48,828
14. Leishmania/kala azar	42,383
15. Typhoid	38,750
16. Tuberculosis	23,610
17. Flies/ticks	15,838
18. Guinea worm	7,167
19. Onchocerciasis	2,486
20. Trichinella	600

Source: Colonial Research Reports: 1940–1950 (see Table 15.3): Cmd 8303 (1950–1); Cmd 8665 (1951–2); Cmd 8971 (1952–3); Cmd 9303 (1953–4); Cmd 9626 (1954–5); Cmnd 52 (1955–6); Cmnd 321 (1956–7); Cmnd 591 (1957–8); Cmnd 938 (1958–9); Cmnd 1215 (1959–60).

"species sanitation." Malaria was transmitted by a limited number of *Anopheles* species, each with a specific breeding site. Thus, by attacking the breeding site of the known mosquito vector in any area, the vectors could be destroyed and malaria controlled, without attempting the futile task of killing all mosquitoes in the region. Malacologists were required, therefore, to set in motion the same sequence of events for bilharzia, even though there seems to me to be little parallel between the breeding sites of mosquitoes and those of aquatic snails; molluscicides were never designed or applied to kill only one variety of snail, breeding in one isolated area. But the connection was made, and a great deal of unnecessary energy (and a great deal of intense backbiting) was expended on the systematics of schistosome-susceptible snails. As members of the Helminth Subcommittee noted in 1955, "Medical malacology today was in much the same position as medical entomology in the days of Ross, when the vectors of malaria were recognized as "dappled-wing mosquitoes."[25]

In order to enter into this "new line of research," the Committee wanted to employ two medical malacologists. Each would be required to spend two years at the British Museum or abroad, and two years with Professor Graham at Reading University or Professor Yonge at Glasgow University, before finally studying the medical or veterinary aspects at London or Liverpool. The advertisement was published in 1955, long after India had departed and only two years before Ghana became autonomous:

The Medical Research Council have a vacancy (possibly two) on their staff for a young man with a good honours degree in zoology, or others suitably qualified, and willing to make a career in the systematic and ecological study of fresh water molluscs, with special reference to the snail vectors of helminth infections in the tropics.[26]

Meanwhile, however, a few malacologists, who had not received the training suggested, were posted to Africa. In 1955, for example, W. F. McClelland, who had worked previously in the Gezira Scheme in the Sudan, arrived in Mwanza on a two-year appointment to work on the dynamics of transmission with a view to future molluscicide trials. But, working alone with little support from London, he was not the first nor the last to find great difficulty identifying the various *Bulinus* species. In addition, he found very few infected snails in a region with a high prevalence of *S. haematobium*.

George Macdonald (Figure 16.1), back from a tour of East Africa, was scathing in his criticisms of work that had been done on bilharzia. "The

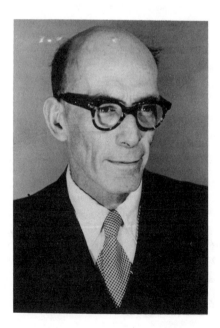

Figure 16.1. George Macdonald (Courtesy David Bradley)

astonishing thing about schistosomiasis," he wrote, "is the number of people in Africa who are working on it and have a special interest in it." But, he continued, "the work is characterized by a lack of coordination; everybody we met seemed to be doing a minor variation of the work done by everybody else without relation to any general scheme."[27] In 1958, Macdonald reported that discussions about bilharzia in East Africa had been "a waste of time." If any conclusions had been reached, he wrote, "it was not the business of anybody in particular to take these conclusions up after the meeting ended." Furthermore, he complained, only the Tanganyikan health authorities considered bilharzia to be "of serious economic importance."[28]

Born in Sheffield, a medical graduate of Liverpool and its school of tropical medicine, Macdonald, after working in Sierra Leone, India, and Assam, had become one of the world's most dominant malariologists and an important medical consultant to the British forces in World War II. In 1947, he had become Professor of Tropical Hygiene at the London School, and began to work on quantitative malariology, which climaxed in 1957 with the publication of *The Epidemiology and Control of Malaria*. Then, believing the contol of malaria to be in sight, and believing, like many others, that bilharzia was about to assume great importance, he turned his considerable talents to the disease.[29]

The appointment of Macdonald to the Chair of a new committee, the Mollusc-Borne Diseases Subcommittee, set fire to the British campaign against bilharzia. This committee put together a bilharzia team in Mwanza, under the directorship of Peter Jordan. Peter Jordan had graduated in medicine from St. Bartholomew's Hospital in 1946, and, after naval service and training at the London School of Hygiene and Tropical Medicine, had joined the Colonial Medical Research Service in 1950. He was immediately posted to Mwanza, where he remained for the next 15 years, working initially on filariasis before turning to bilharzia.

By 1961, the team was in place. Apart from Jordan, it consisted of Gerald Webbe, who arrived first, David Bradley, D. M. Forsyth, and R. F. Sturrock (Figure 16.2). They were a mixed group. Webbe, a graduate in chemistry and zoology from Sheffield University, had initially worked on malaria and larvicides, but switched to bilharzia in Mwanza, after spending a leave in Copenhagen with the malacologist, Mandahl-Barth, author of the 1958 text, *Intermediate Hosts of Schistosoma*. The other three arrived in 1961: Forsyth, an experienced ex-oil company medical officer from Saudi Arabia; Bradley, a recent medical graduate of Cambridge; and Sturrock, a parasitologist with a doctorate from Imperial College, who, although more familiar with nematodes, worked on schistosomes after posting to Mwanza. With the team in place, one of the members told me, bilharzia became "George's new disease."

Mwanza did for the British what Leyte had done many years before for the Americans; it placed the disease solidly on the British map. In a very short time, they gathered together an extraordinary amount of information on the

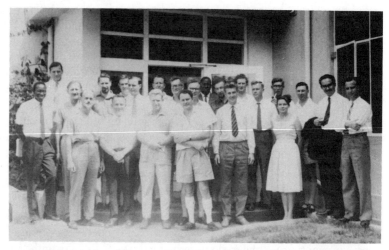

a

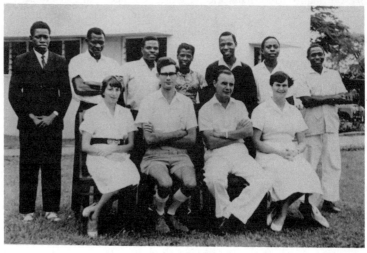

b

Figure 16.2. The British team at Mwanza: (a) the Bilharzia Coordinating Committee, 1962 (D. M. Forsyth – rear, sixth from left; Peter Jordan – rear, seventh from left; Gerald Webbe – front, middle with shorts; R. F. Sturrock – rear, sixth from right); (b) David Bradley (left front), D. M. Forsyth, and staff of the Ross Institute research team. (a, Courtesy of Peter Jordan; b, courtesy of David Bradley)

epidemiology of the disease in Tanganyika. By the end of 1961, for example, "the question 'where and when' the people of Sukumaland get infected with *S. haematobium* has been answered."[30] Also, with a radiological examination of 100 schoolchildren came the first real information that severe pathologies could occur with *S. haematobium*. Forsyth and Bradley reported that severe pathological changes, including bladder calcification and hydronephrosis, occurred in about 20 percent of the schoolchildren tested.[31] "Those who are apathetic about the necessity of control measures for *S. haematobium*," the institute's report noted, "must surely think twice when they see Dr. Forsyth's findings."[32]

In addition, the possibilities of control seemed brighter than ever before, according to Webbe. Not only was Bayer 73 an effective molluscicide, but knowledge gained of the breeding habits, growth, and period of maximum infectivity had convinced Webbe that the chemical should be applied twice per year, before and after the rainy season. A field test, using Bayer 73 against the snail host of *S. mansoni* in the Mirongo River, seemed to achieve, according to Webbe, "a very satisfactory degree of control of *S. mansoni* transmission in the river."[33]

The Egypt-49 project

By the 1960s, positive results with molluscicides were appearing also in Egypt, where, as in Tanganyika, Bayer 73 was proving its worth. The WHO and UNICEF had formally agreed to collaborate on a pilot control project with the chemical, and were pressed by the Egyptian authorities to set up the project in Egypt. But the WHO, somewhat soured by their previous experiences in Egypt and deeply suspicious that any promised support by the government would materialize, were reluctant to acquiesce to the Egyptian Government's wishes. Nevertheless, with deep misgivings they agreed, and in 1961 the pilot project began on a site a few miles from Alexandria (Figure 16.3).[34]

The Egypt-49 program was an extremely important one; it represented the first time that the impact of a control program was measured with the use of a new statistical tool – "incidence" rather than "prevalence." Until that time, those engaged in designing control programs were hindered by an insensitive statistical test. They measured the "prevalence" of the parasite – that is, the number of individuals in a population infected with the worms. Prevalence is a static concept that fails to indicate, in the short term, whether the transmission cycle of the parasite is being broken. For this, one needs to measure "incidence" – that is, the number of persons who become infected during a certain known time period. Obviously, in testing drugs or molluscicides, incidence is a more significant statistic than prevalence, since it measures the rate at which new cases appear.

American epidemiologists began calculating incidence values in the 1940s, and it had become a common practice among them by the 1950s. The first use in tropical medicine seems to have occurred with leprosy studies in the Philippines, and curiously, it was there, 16 years later, that the statistic was first applied to bilharzia.[35]

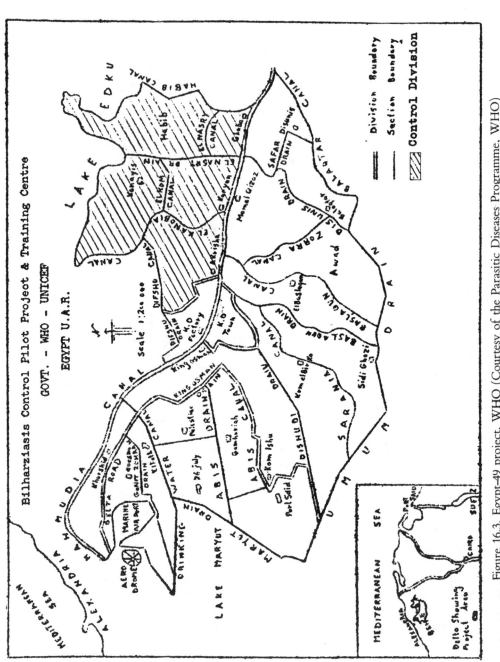

Figure 16.3. Egypt-49 project, WHO (Courtesy of the Parasitic Diseases Programme, WHO)

In 1951, the Philippine Government, which had three years earlier inaugurated a bilharzia research program, approached the WHO with a request to study the problem on the islands (Figure 16.4). The WHO team that was sent out to investigate recommended that a pilot project be set up in Leyte which would completely survey the island and, if feasible, apply environmental controls.[36] The project, called Philippines-9, began in June 1953. They found that of 200 children aged 5–9 years, who had been negative for bilharzia in 1953 and 1954, 70 had become positive 22 months later. With necessary statistical corrections to account for unequal sampling techniques, that gave an incidence of 20.4 percent.[37]

Pesigan and his co-workers, including Dr. M. Farooq, viewed bilharzia in the Philippines as a "biosocial problem" in which the standard snail-killing approach was of little use. It was not, they argued, a medical problem, but an engineering one that required drainage, ponding, earth filling, improved agricultural practices, and perhaps molluscicides as well, but never latrines. Thus, they never set about testing the effect of a control project on the incidence of the parasite; that occurred in Egypt where two men who had been associated with Pesigan – M. Farooq and N. Hairston – became WHO advisers to the project. As they so clearly wrote:

Direct observation of the rate at which negative children become positive is the most useful and economical method of measuring the incidence of bilharziasis, and is obviously the method of choice for the determination of the success of control operations. . . . It is the rates of becoming positive and negative that determine the number of people infected at any given time, and it is through changing these rates that control of the disease will become possible.[38]

They tested the new Bayer molluscicide, and reported, in 1963, that the *incidence* of both *S. haematobium* and *S. mansoni* in 171 children aged 1–6 years had dropped to about one-third of what it had been before molluscicide application (Figure 16.5). Regarding *S. haematobium*, for example, the incidence in one village was reported to have dropped from 22.8 percent in 1963 to 7.1 percent in 1964, 8.3 percent in 1965, and 8.5 percent in 1966, whereas the incidence in the control area had increased during that period from 18.0 to 26.6 percent. "We believe," Farooq and his team reported, "that the present experiment represents the first satisfactory demonstration of the interruption of transmission of *S. haematobium* and *S. mansoni* in the Nile valley and delta."[39]

But there were dark clouds gathering on the horizon. The 1967 report by Farooq's successors continued in the same positive vein, but was heavily edited by some unknown official in Geneva who admitted "minimizing gain and exaggerating shortcomings."[40] The major shortcomings were, as always, sampling techniques. By the following year, the new team announced that the previous techniques were indeed invalid and that new measurements for incidence and prevalence had to be made. The problems were, according to

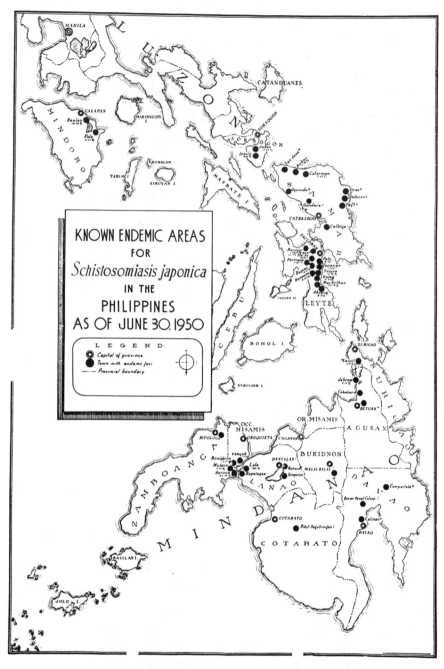

Figure 16.4. Distribution of *S. japonicum* in the Philippines, prior to the Philippine-9 project. Black circles indicate towns with endemic foci; dot-dashed lines indicate provincial boundaries, and open-circles the provincial capitals. (Courtesy of the Parasitic Diseases Programme, WHO)

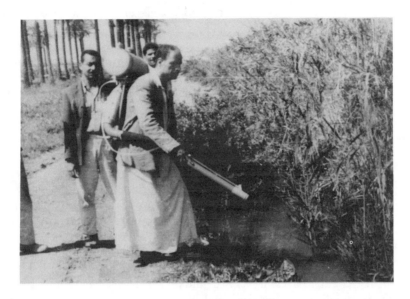

Figure 16.5. Spraying with Bayer 73, Egypt-49 project (Courtesy of the Parasitic Diseases Programme, WHO)

the report, that the villages from which the major incidence data had been gathered were not typical of the area in general, and that the sites within the villages were not typical of those villages. Thus, for example, whereas the sample from sites in the Kom Ishu village used by Farooq gave a prevalence of 11.7 percent, a mass sample from the entire village gave a prevalence twice as high: 22.9 percent. In addition, in four of the ten areas examined, the incidence of infection had actually increased.[41] The 1969 report was even more pessimistic. An experienced microscopist had reexamined some of the 1962 material and obtained results that differed from the original in 144 of the 551 urine and feces samples examined. Thus, he concluded, the data gathered during the Egypt-49 project had to be rejected as inaccurate and unreliable.[42]

In 1970, the WHO called in an independent assessor, Dr. H. M. Giles from the Liverpool School of Tropical Medicine, who reported that because 80.1 percent of the children who had been negative in 1962–3 now carried the parasite, "the overall interruption of transmission over the 7 year period of the project was unsatisfactory and that as a single method of control molluscicid-ing is not to be recommended."[43] But as Peter Jordan explained a year later, Gilles had misread Farooq's incidence data, and that indeed there had been a drop in incidence between 1962 and 1966, although the control had broken down in later years.[44] The Regional Director of WHO's Middle East Region was not at all happy with Gilles's damning assessment, believing Farooq's results and data to be "rather good," and certainly adequate enough to conclude that indeed "molluscicides used alone can have a useful impact on transmission."[45] But this reaction was only to be expected, and given the confusion that is always generated by arguments over sampling techniques, a comment made in 1971 seems more appropriate: "For outsiders the general feeling is that the project failed and a huge amount of money has been spent in vain."[46]

Puerto Rico

A similar degree of confusion over the value of mollusciciding was generated in Puerto Rico. The problem of bilharzia had reemerged on the island in 1945, when the U.S. Army Medical Corps discovered that nearly 10 percent of 19,139 Selective Service recruits, aged 18–38, were infected with *S. mansoni*. The survey also indicated that bilharzia was widespread on the island among members of varied socioeconomic groups, and occurred in both irrigated and nonirrigated areas.[47] Thus, in 1952, the Puerto Rico Department of Health and the U.S. Public Health Service initiated a 14-year program designed to eliminate bilharzia from the island.

The initial fecal examinations of 10,000 schoolchildren showed the disease picture on the island to be the same as previously reported by Faust and Weller. Then, after ten years of mollusciciding with sodium pentachlorophenate, the disease was reported to be no longer a public health problem in Patillas, in Guayama, or on Viegas Island.[48] But, as the workers noted, the value of the work had been "obscured" by a parallel decline in Caguas where no molluscicides had been applied. Thus, for example, while the prevalence of the parasite in Patillas had declined from 7.4 to 0.4 percent between 1954 and 1963, the parasite had also declined from 11.3 to 1.3 percent in Caguas. "It cannot be concluded," they wrote, "that the success of the program was due to snail control alone, since improvements in sanitation and economic development undoubtedly played a part in the decline of the disease." But, as they went on to state, "the experiment proved that the disease could be controlled by simple methods." This implied, of course, that the simple method of mollusciciding was responsible for the decline, and, thus, that an island-wide campaign against bilharzia should begin.

This large program, which began in 1968, was aided by a much easier monitoring system: the intradermal skin test, the development of which had been a major research priority in the late 1950s and into the 1960s.[49] The ease of diagnosis allowed by this test, even if not as infallible as finding eggs in the feces, allowed 10,000 children to be tested three times – in 1963, in 1969, and again in 1976. Over this period, in areas where sodium pentachlorophenate and then Bayer 73 were used, the prevalence of positive skin tests dropped 36 percent. But again, the prevalence dropped by 24 percent in the control areas, where no molluscicides had been applied.[50]

A NEW STRATEGY

The evidence that chemicals which killed snails in the laboratory in low dilutions would not only continue to do so in the field, but would also lead to a decline in the incidence and the prevalence of the disease remained tantalizingly inconclusive. Although the possibility of entirely eliminating snails from an area no longer appeared to be a viable proposition, many believed that the cycle of transmission could be broken if the number of snails was reduced sufficiently. But by how much? The answer came in 1965. While Farooq and his co-workers in Egypt were enjoying seeming success with the new molluscicide, Dr. George Macdonald had concluded pessimistically that it would take 20 years to reduce sufficiently the number of snails by mollusciciding before the parasite would disappear, even if, as was highly unlikely, their application could be carried out effectively over such a long period.

Macdonald arrived at this conclusion after setting up a computer model for the parasite's transmission, in which different values for the "contamination factor," the "snail factor," the "exposure factor," and the "longevity factor" were applied. In any given situation, he concluded, there was a "break point" or a worm load "below which the infection is unable to maintain itself."

For any given environment there is a critical number of worms; the presence of more will lead to multiplication till equilibrium is reached, or of less to progressive diminuation. This is represented in terms of the mean worm load for the community concerned and is termed the "break point," the significant of this term being that this number of worms is not only critical in preventing or allowing introduction of the infection, but also . . . in causing an abrupt break between maintained transmission and eradication when control measures are introduced.[51]

What then, Macdonald asked, was the best method of lowering the worm load to the breakpoint? As Barlow and Scott had discovered earlier in Egypt, the computer model indicated to Macdonald that "sanitation produced no measurable effect." The "common supposition," he wrote, "that 'sanitation diseases' are best controlled by provision of latrines finds very little support." Even more surprising, the model predicted that it would take 20 years for the worm load to decrease to the breakpoint, using snail control as the only weapon. The effect of reducing snail numbers, Macdonald wrote, is "so slow as to be almost despairing." But the breakpoint would be reached in five years, he predicted, if treatment became the major weapon combined with either a reduction of exposure by the provision of safe water, or snail control. Thus, Macdonald concluded, the major research effort in the future should concentrate on finding a better drug with no side effects, for henceforth therapy, not molluscicides, had to become the main line of attack.

But this was a conclusion based on a mathematical model. What would happen in nature? Would therapy achieve better results than molluscicides? The necessity of finding an answer to this question led to the St. Lucia project. In 1965, in that small Caribbean island in which *S. mansoni* was endemic, a team led by Peter Jordan and supported financially by the Rockefeller Foundation and by the British Overseas Development Administration, which had replaced the older colonial administrations, set out to test the relative merits of snail control, water supplies, and chemotherapy on the incidence of bilharzia. In a 16-year program, the island became a laboratory in which isolated river valleys were used to test the effectiveness of the various methods. Basically, they discovered what Macdonald had predicted: "Chemotherapy was the cheapest and most rapidly effective method of achieving transmission control."[52] Control became the key word; no longer was the disease and the parasite to be eliminated by entirely removing the snail hosts. Instead the parasite was to be gradually eliminated by breaking its transmission cycle; by reducing the probability that each stage in the life cycle could be successfully completed to such an extent that the parasite would be no longer able to maintain itself. And the key to this break lay in the development of therapeutic drugs with minimal side effects.

Therapeutic drugs

In 1965, when the St. Lucia project began, 6 percent tartar emetic was still the drug of choice in Egypt, despite the fact that a new drug had appeared on the scene during the war when the British Army had overrun the Bayer factory at Elberfeld and had come across the drug lucanthone hydrochloride (Miracil D). In 1927, the Bayer Company had set up a mouse colony infected with the Liberian strain of *Schistosoma mansoni* and, by 1937, had developed the techniques required for screening large numbers of potential drugs; one of them was a new oral drug, Miracil D, which had been synthesized in 1938.[53] But the positive claims for the drug by Bayer scientist, W. Kikuth, had been criticized in another report which claimed that the drug caused serious fatty degeneration of the liver, heart, and kidneys. A free translation of this criticism, prepared for the Colonial Medical Research Committee, commented that Kikuth's more positive report "was written up primarily for the German government with a view to saving some of his laboratory workers from the army; its tone is, therefore, somewhat more optimistic than the results really justify."[54] A series of rather casual laboratory tests by British workers only confused the situation. The Department of Pharmacology at Oxford, for example, seemed to dismiss the negative claims in a rather cavalier manner, even though another paper had disclosed that half the rabbits tested with

Miracil D contained albumin in the urine, a sign of kidney damage. They also seemed to suggest that since the drug's activity varied widely with different animals it was time to test humans.[55]

The Colonial Committee suggested that a team be sent to Egypt, Southern Rhodesia, or Iraq in order to test the efficacy of the drug on humans. With work already underway in Southern Rhodesia, the *fellaheen* were chosen to receive the new drug. In 1947, the physician John Newsome and Dr. S. G. Cowper, who, with a medical degree and a Doctorate in Helminthology, was working on bilharzia in Liverpool, were posted to Cairo to begin trials on Miracil D. The grant of £1100, used to support this work, was the first money spent on bilharzia out of the Colonial Development and Welfare Fund. But they soon discovered that irritation of the gastrointestinal tract "mitigated against the general use of the drug in Egypt."[56]

Better results were obtained in Southern Rhodesia. There a Bilharzia and Malaria Research Unit, set up in 1938, had been busy building latrines, studying molluscs, applying molluscicides, and injecting tartar emetic. After the war, the physician D. M. Blair and the helminthologist William Alves had returned to take up the battle again, and had developed a new method of applying tartar emetic. The speed of injection governed the drug's toxicity, they had concluded, and thus in treating patients "an absolute minimum of five to six minutes was taken to complete the intravenous injection with the piston moving all the time."[57] They also developed what they called a method of "sterilization treatment," in which smaller doses of the drug, given over only one day, were assumed to kill the female worms, and prevent further egg production, yet leave the harmless male worms untouched. Linked to mollusciciding with copper sulfate, mass campaigns were carried out in the 1940s, which aimed at "synchronisation of snail killing with sterilization of the infected."[58]

They were naturally only too pleased to welcome a research team from Britain, which arrived in 1947 to test Miracil D on its native "reservoirs of disease." Taking three groups of African schoolchildren, all apparently healthy and passing schistosome eggs, and exposing them to different dosages, the team described only slight nausea but very little therapeutic action.[59] But a year later, with dosages increased, the Southern Rhodesian authorities claimed to have induced a 90 percent cure rate for *S. haematobium* with some side effects. Mass treatment for Africans now seemed a viable option, they reported.[60] Thus, in 1950, Miracil D hydrochloride (or Nilodin) was introduced as standard treatment for the disease, forming with copper sulfate (and later sodium pentachlorophenate) and DDT the major arsenal in Rhodesian malaria and bilharzia control schemes.[61] By the end of the decade, the Rhodesian authorities claimed that mass treatment with Miracil D, in which 2,230,000 tablets had been distributed by 1960, had led to an "improvement in the weight, health, and efficiency of African farm labourers."[62]

But there were, as always, the side effects. These were, according to Blair, less frequent among Africans than Europeans. They included giddiness, diarrhea, vomiting, anorexia, epigastric pains, rashes, tremors, and sometimes even "neurological manifestations." One such sign, Blair reported, was that "objects, such as doors and trees, seemed to be moving away as they walk toward them, until finally they collide with them." Nevertheless, Blair concluded, "no record can be found of any person having died as a result of the administration of lucanthone hydrochloride."[63] Similar alarming side effects were reported from Egypt, where the U.S. Naval Medical Research Unit No. 3 (NAMRU 3) had been conducting some tests with Miracil D on volunteers from a Cairo reformatory and prison. The drug, they reported, was less effective than tartar emetic and least well tolerated, with "depression and marked anorexia frequently occurring."[64]

But finding better drugs was no easy matter, and testing them on laboratory animals required richly endowed and highly structured laboratory facilities. Such laboratories needed to maintain large snail colonies that would liberate thousands of cercariae each day. They needed mammal colonies, space to house them, and personnel to attend to them, at a level that few institutions could afford. The U.S. Army was one such institution that could set up the required facilities, and as its mollusciciding program began to face problems, the 406th laboratory in Japan began gearing up for an extensive drug testing program using chemicals provided by U.S. drug companies.

This drug testing program began quietly in 1956, after techniques of maintaining colonies of *Oncomelania*, the snail host of *S. japonicum*, had been developed. Therapeutic drugs were not their main concern. With the disease endemic in what the military termed "high-risk areas," such as South America, the Middle East, the Caribbean, and Asia, where U.S. troops could be deployed, they were mainly interested in the discovery of prophylactic drugs that would protect troops from becoming infected.[65] By 1965, the techniques for testing a minimum of 100 such drugs per week had been established by the 406th laboratory. But because *S. mansoni* was far easier to maintain in a laboratory setting, it had replaced *S. japonicum* as the experimental animal.

Establishing these testing techniques was no small feat. It involved what was called a "cabinet draw" method for the mass production of cercariae. A colony of snails with up to 500 of them infected was maintained in a metal drawer arrangement, and from them, three to five million cercariae were released each week.[66] Fast, cheap, and effective methods of assessing the impact of the tested drugs also needed to be developed. Initially, the Pellagrino method, developed in Brazil, was used in the laboratory, but by the end of the decade a cheaper method had been devised. The former method was based on the analysis of the character and number of egg masses found in the gut wall. Under normal circumstances, the egg masses would contain eggs of all ages, but with an effective drug that would prevent egg laying, the "oogram" – or egg picture – would change. Immature eggs would disappear from the oogram, and by the seventh day after testing a successful drug, all viable eggs in the oogram would be mature.[67] But the new method was based on the survival rate of infected mice. Mortality in mice infected with 2,000–2,500 cercariae was predictable and highly reproducible, Radke noted, with 99 percent of the mice dead at the end of the fourth week. Thus, any reduction in the mortality of drug-tested mice would indicate some form of positive drug action. This quick and gruesome method, Radke calculated, could be used to test 100 compounds per week and would require 15 personnel on a five-day work week, whereas the older Pellagrino method could test only 50 compounds and would require 15 personnel on a six-day work week.[68] This prophylactic drug-testing program became operational in 1977 after the Composite Drug Testing Unit had been transferred from the 406th laboratory in Japan to the campus of the University of Brazilica.

But the success of any such laboratory depends on the drugs being provided to it. In this crucial area, they had only one partial success. The drug niridazole, manufactured by the Ciba Company, was subsequently found to be a useful drug against *S. haematobium* in children. But, apart from that, the American drug companies did not produce, and by the time the drug screening unit had been transferred to Brazil, the European companies had already produced a series of drugs such as oxamniquine from Pfizer, Inc., and trichlorfon (also called metrifonate) from Bayer. Also unknown to the U.S. Army as they moved to Brazil, the Bayer Company, using the same old strain of *S. mansoni* and techniques developed in the 1930s, had discovered the new "wonder drug" praziquantel.

In 1972, scientists at the Institut für Chemotherapie at the Bayer laboratory in Wuppertal had demonstrated the potential potency of the pyrazino-isoquinoline ring system. In a joint endeavor with the Merck Company, over 400 related compounds were tested, among which was praziquantel, or, for those who delight in chemical mumbo-jumbo, 2-(cyclohexylcarbonyl)-1,2,3,6,7,11*b*-hexahydro-4*H*-pyrazino [2,1-*a*]isoquinolin 4-one. Its antihelminthic activity and apparent nonpathogenicity were reported in 1977, and, in 1979, the first clinical trials took place. Finally, in 1980, the full significance of this single-dose drug was discussed at a praziquantel symposium held in Nairobi.[69] At this conference it was announced that the drug had been administered to over 3,000 *fellaheen* at the Qaliubiya Bilharziasis Project.

By the 1970s, a new wave of optimism began to be felt. The new drugs, associated sometimes with more powerful molluscicides, and a new theory of breakage transmission seemed to point to a brighter future. As Peter Jordan remarked in 1977, "There is a frontier to cross, but it is at least within sighting distance."[70]

17

Conclusion: The imperial triad

For nearly a century, the Western powers have been engaged in a protracted struggle against tropical diseases. It was an essential part of their attempts to dominate and control countries whose climates were sufficiently hot and humid to house pathogens that threatened to undermine the success of their efforts.

The struggle began in earnest at the very end of the nineteenth century when the major Western powers had already industrialized and were passing through the great "sanitary awakening." Their populations, with the exception of the forgotten victims of industrialization, were becoming relatively affluent and enjoying better health than their predecessors. Medicine, however, had contributed little to these changed circumstances and as yet could bring about few miraculous cures; self-healing, that most maligned of all processes in the modern age, remained medicine's most powerful ally. But the professional middle classes were becoming increasingly powerful, and the medical profession in particular was engaged in a protracted and ultimately successful struggle to gain control over health care. Physicians achieved this as medicine grew more scientific and technical, requiring a highly trained specialist elite corps, practicing curative medicine within increasingly imposing and well-furnished hospitals.

Much of this new scientific rigor rested on the modern germ theory of disease which, by the 1890s, more than a decade after the discoveries of Robert Koch, had become generally accepted. The germ theory fundamentally changed the face of medicine by altering the way we understood the relationships among disease, those who had the disease, and the physical and social environment in which such diseased people lived.

Diseases, before the germ theory, were inseparable from the diseased in that they were indications of physiological imbalance within a diseased person. In cases of "infectious diseases," this imbalance was rooted in environmental causes such as decaying matter, noxious vapors, filth, and lack of sunlight, which created diseases only in persons rendered susceptible by "predisposing causes" – their behavior and the social conditions in which they lived. True, some highly "contagious diseases" such as smallpox were known to involve the passage of "contagions" from one person to another, but even then the disease itself remained part of the human condition, clearly distinct from the contagions. Medical theorists, therefore, were faced with a complex interplay among the disease condition, the diseased person, and the social and physical environment in which they lived (left col., Table 17.1).

Westerners visiting the tropics before the middle of the nineteenth century had been decimated by tropical fevers. Yet, working within these medical theories great strides had been made; by the time of Pasteur and Koch, Westerners in the tropics had learned the necessity of following a strict behavior regimen and, after scrupulous attention to disease topography, had learned where best to live and work. Their increasing ability to survive in the tropics was not, in other words, due entirely to the discovery of cinchona bark and its quinine derivative.

The germ theory, or the idea that specific diseases were caused by specific pathogens, introduced new ways of viewing disease that had a profound influence on tropical medicine. Diseases were now caused by pathogens, and the diseased individual had become merely a person unfortunate enough to have been invaded by them (right col., Table 17.1). The environment, so supremely important before the germ theory, remained only as a possible source of these pathogens. Thus practitioners of tropical medicine working within the parameters of the germ theory of disease focused on the pathogens to the almost total exclusion of all other factors. Indeed, so sharp became this focus, that the pathogens and the diseases caused by them were often viewed as one and the same thing: Malaria is a malarial parasite; tuberculosis is a bacillus; bilharzia is a parasitic worm. As a result Western medicine was transferred to the tropics at a period in its history when the socioeconomic conditions and political circumstances of the population had become largely irrelevant to the practice of medicine.

But the new germ theory did carry with it a message of hope. Before the germ theory, Westerners could only hope to adapt to the disease problems of the tropics and learn to live as best they could. Now, however, they could, in theory, look forward to the complete elimination of these diseases. They could be eliminated, they believed, by destroying the pathogens, a possibility made even more feasible when many of them were found to be transmitted by vectors or to pass part of their life cycles as larval stages within intermediate hosts. Indeed, tropical medicine became almost synonymous with diseases that were caused by such transmitted pathogens (protozoa and helminths), and parasitology and medical zoology became the major components of tropical medicine.

Table 17.1. *Concept of disease according to pre– and post–germ theory*

Pre–germ theory	Post–germ theory
Disease Equals:	
(contagion)	PATHOGEN
+	+
DISEASED	CARRIER OF
	PATHOGEN
+	+
PHYSICAL	SOURCE OF
ENVIRONMENT	PATHOGEN
+	+
SOCIAL	(Social
ENVIRONMENT	environment)

IMPERIAL MEDICINE

Germ theory–based Western medicine began to be imposed on the tropical territories and colonies in the final years of the nineteenth century. And just as an imperial power dominates another society, imposes its own sets of beliefs on that society, and remains impervious to indigenous cultures, so was tropical medicine imperial. It was imperial in that the medical problems of the tropical world and solutions to them were defined and imposed by practitioners of Western-style medicine without involving the indigenous populations in these decisions, and with little reference to the culture and social milieu in which they practiced. *Definition, imposition, and noninvolvement* constitute the triad of beliefs that were established in the earliest years of tropical medicine and remained an essential part of it until the late 1970s; throughout that period, tropical medicine remained an imperial discipline.

This triad of imperial medicine was particularly evident before World War II, when tropical medicine was an important and necessary branch of political imperialism. In those years, the basic problem of survival was defined in terms of disease and their causal parasites. In laying down what I have called the "Rockefeller Creed," Frederick Gates was only taking to the extreme what most then believed. His words are worth repeating again: "Disease is the supreme ill of human life, and it is the main source of almost all other human ills – poverty, crime, ignorance, vice, inefficiency, hereditary traits, and many other evils."

But the human life that was of most concern during the early period of tropical medicine was, quite naturally, their own. Thus, for example, to provide medical care for British officials necessitated a medical service that was as near as possible a copy of what they could expect at home – hospital facilities and physicians capable of diagnosing their problems and treating them when they became ill. The London School of Tropical Medicine was concerned primarily with training such physicians in diagnosing those tropical diseases that had not been addressed during their British medical education and were not to be found in British textbooks. Hence the link that was forged from the start between tropical medicine and the protozoa and helminth parasites.

This concern with their own health became a major factor in defining which diseases were important. Bilharzia provides a particularly fine example of a disease that was initially studied because of its supposed threat to British lives. Normally bilharzia does not present much of a health threat to Westerners (although it may do so for their children), but the strategic importance of Egypt and the Suez Canal, together with Looss's mistaken idea that the bilharzia-causing worm was passed directly from man to man, created the political and scientific conditions that led to Leiper's attachment to the British Army and his important discoveries about the worms and their life cycles in Egypt. But, once the snail hosts were discovered and the impossibility of a camp epidemic of the disease realized, then the British officially lost interest in the disease. The bilharzia problem among the *fellaheen* was left to missionary doctors or to the Egyptians themselves, unless, of course, the International Health Board wished to offer financial help. Similarly in Southern Africa, the threat which bilharzia and those with bilharzia posed to the health and weekend activities of the white community created a fairly substantial interest in the disease, but that interest was never so high as when the disease was found to be endemic among the poor whites of the Transvaal.

American concern with tropical diseases and their definitions of which diseases were important were also generated by the threat posed to their own health. The danger tropical diseases presented to their armies of occupation during and after the Spanish-American War generated the famous tropical disease boards which did so much to uncover the etiology of some of these diseases. But, in contrast to the British, their empire of "tutelage" made it necessary also to address the disease problems of the indigenous populations in order to display the superiority of American medicine and the American way of life. Also, again in contrast to the British, much of the American concern with tropical medicine was home-based. Some tropical diseases were endemic to the U.S. mainland, and some North American cities had been periodically ravished by yellow fever spreading from the West Indies. In addition, there was always the fear that more tropical diseases would be introduced into the country to become endemic in the tropical-like conditions of their own South; and after World War II bilharzia became one of them.

The direct threat tropical diseases posed to the health of Western officials in the tropics was not a factor that drove Gates and the Rockefeller philanthropies into tropical medicine and into defining which diseases were significant.

They believed that diseases were one of the prime causes, if not the prime cause, of Southern backwardness and inefficiency. And if in the South, why not in the world at large? But, of course, some diseases were more significant than others in their capacity to do damage to workers' efficiency and, not surprisingly, they chose to eliminate hookworm first. Hookworm, perhaps more than any other disease at that time, had long been associated with worker inefficiency. But the Rockefeller organizations saw this inefficiency within the broad context of worldwide capitalism; for the capitalistic system to work, efficient work forces were necessary. They were thus prepared to mount health campaigns wherever the conditions met their rather stringent requirements.[1] But the link between tropical diseases and worker efficiency had been made also by General Gorgas during his work in the Panama Canal, and by companies hiring workers from the tropics, such as the Puerto Rican sugar companies, the United Fruit Company, and the Rhodesian and South African mining companies. To this group, the success of their own business ventures, rather than worldwide capitalism, could necessitate building hygienic living and working conditions and providing expert Western curative medicine to their workers. On the other hand, as in the case of Southern Africa with its inexhaustible supply of cheap African labor, maximizing profits could necessitate minimum health care and a workforce that was rapidly circulated through the system and then discharged. It was cheaper to replace the dead, injured, and sick rather than spending money to prevent illnesses and accidents and to nurse the sick back to health.

Thus the priority diseases were defined on Western terms – by their impact on Westerners' own health or their profits (in a very broad or very narrow sense). But, of course, one can take this analysis too far. The etiology and epidemiology of many tropical diseases were investigated simply because they were unknown; scientific curiosity was always a major factor in generating research and interest in a disease. But the lack of scientific curiosity can be equally powerful in causing a decline in interest. Hookworm, for example, initially one of the most important and studied of tropical diseases, rapidly lost that position, but not because it was eliminated. On the contrary, even today perhaps four times as many people are infected with hookworm than the schistosomes. The problem with hookworm, as was told to me on more than one occasion, is that, compared with bilharzia, it generates little scientific interest. There are no subtle relationships with numerous varieties of intermediate hosts to uncover, but simply a nematode worm that passes directly from person to person and needs for its prevention only latrines and shoes.

In the long run, the general impact of these decisions on what constituted the primary concerns of tropical medicine has been that the discipline failed to address some of the most important diseases of the colonial countries; thus the great killers of children remained, for example, outside the scope of tropical medicine. Or, to express this rather differently, one can conclude that before

World War II tropical medicine defined health in terms that were often irrelevant to the real public health needs of the people in these countries.

Imperial medicine defined not only the problems but also the solutions to these problems. Basically, following the dictates of the germ theory, each tropical disease was to be sequentially eliminated by destroying each specific disease-causing pathogen. And, because many of these pathogens were carried in vector or intermediate hosts, the destruction of these hosts often became the chosen method. But, as the bilharzia case repeatedly showed, what began as a simple enough procedure quickly ran into difficulties; destroying mosquitoes, tsetse flies, black flies, and snails was no easy task. Insecticides and molluscicides that killed needed to be produced, and an ever increasing amount of scientific information about the parasites and their hosts were required in order that these chemicals could be effectively applied. Indeed, the technical difficulties became so acute that a series of expert-led pilot projects and campaigns were put into operation specifically to kill snails and mosquitoes, whose success was often measured by the number of kills, not by its impact on disease prevalence.[2] At other times, the desire to destroy the pathogens took on the character of a vicious military campaign. In the Philippines, for example, the medical campaigns against cholera and other diseases were barely distinguishable from the military campaigns against the *insurrectos*.

The imperial nature of tropical medicine was most cogently displayed during the imposition of the desired solutions – the third feature of the imperial triad. All experts were Westerners or were Westernized, and their solutions were imposed without any participation by the communities involved and without reference to the social and economic conditions in which people lived. Indeed, snail and mosquito killing was viewed as the most satisfactory control method precisely because it could be done without upsetting the political and social status quo and without the participation of the indigenous populations. This was as true in the early years of copper sulfate as it was during the first campaigns of the WHO. Thus, as the bilharzia story repeatedly shows, whatever schemes were devised collapsed as soon as the experts left.

In British Africa these experts were by necessity British; in the old Empire, the educational system was not designed to produce African research scientists or fully qualified physicians, and those who slipped through the system via the missionary schools and British universities were placed in a subservient position when they returned home. In turn, these British-trained experts rejected as inherently racist the system of subordinate medical assistants which the British first tried to set up and which paradoxically could have provided the nucleus of an adequate rural health system. The Americans, in contrast, were not averse to training fully qualified Puerto Rican and Filipino scientists and physicians as they were not averse to medical schools for blacks in the United States; it was an important part of their tutelage approach to empire to train

Americanized leaders in universities modeled after those at home. In 1907, they opened the Philippine Medical School which, in 1910, became part of the University of the Philippines, and in the 1920s Columbia University provided funds to open the School of Tropical Medicine at San Juan, Puerto Rico.[3] The result has been that Puerto Ricans and Filipinos have contributed to the literature on bilharzia, whereas Africans have not.

These leaders, however, were trained to be part of a thoroughly Western-ized medical system largely unsuitable for the conditions operating in Third World countries. Nowhere was this made more clear than in the Rockefeller's intent to spread scientific medicine by building replicas of the Johns Hopkins University Medical School. The minuscule number of highly trained physi-cians produced by the Peking Union Medical College was inappropriate to the needs of China, as John Grant and other members of the Rockefeller organiza-tion made clear. Likewise in Thailand, the Johns Hopkins-like medical school was built by the Foundation in the 1920s over the opposition of many Thai officials who argued that such a school was inappropriate for a country needing large numbers of less highly trained medical personnel to deal with the medical problems of a poor, rural, and uneducated population.[4]

Considerable changes took place in tropical medicine after World War II. The British Empire changed direction, as Britain belatedly faced the possibil-ity of their colonies gaining some form of autonomy within the British Empire; the WHO entered the picture, and new academic research-oriented professionals began to exert considerable influence. But although it remains true that the health of indigenous populations became a priority for the first time, the nature of tropical medicine did not change; it remained fundamen-tally imperial in that the "imperial triad" remained in place. Indeed it seems to have returned in considerable force after a brief postwar experiment with social medicine, which appears to have had little long-term effect, and the important Chinese successes following the Chinese Revolution.

The definition of postwar health problems and solutions remained in the hands of Western medicine. The narrowly defined concerns of businessmen, mineowners, and fruit companies over the immediate health needs of their employees were considerably expanded, however, under the menaces of international communism and of peasant and working-class movements that threatened to undermine stability and the status quo. Only people who were sick and impoverished, the American Government believed, would heed communist propaganda, and thus, to the satisfaction of professionals in tropical medicine, their discipline was galvanized to fight the totalitarian enemy. "Through health," the Dean of Public Health of Harvard University noted in 1950, "we can prove to ourselves and to the world, the wholesomeness and rightness of democracy. Through health we can defeat the evil threat of communism."[5] But communism or not, the solutions to their health problems remained as before – technically driven without their participation.

But the Western powers were not merely actors in an already existing disease scenario; they also generated diseases in their colonies and territories. Many of these diseases became real public health problems and, in these cases, were recognized to be so. Bilharzia represents one of the most notorious of such man-made diseases. Ernest Faust's survey of bilharzia in Puerto Rico in the 1930s, for example, had shown that the disease had increased dramatically because of its association with the irrigated sugar plantations in the southeast part of the island, and in Brazil the combination of susceptible snail hosts and the growth of the sugar industry provided the conditions for the parasite to become established in the Northeast region from where it spread to become a serious health problem.[6] Most notorious of all, the production of cotton in Egypt to meet foreign debt and to feed the mills of Lancashire was a major factor in changing the agricultural landscape of the country. The parasites had always existed in Egypt, but the change from annual to perennial irrigation dramatically increased the prevalence and the morbidity of bilharzia to such an extent that, by the early years of the twentieth century, it had become the number one health problem in the country. Cotton first tied bilharzia and Egypt together in a knot that has yet to be untangled.

The prevalence of man-made tropical diseases increased dramatically after World War II. In particular, political stability seemed threatened by overpopulation and famine, in response to which the Western powers imposed agricultural policies that increased the prevalence of malaria, bilharzia, and other water-related diseases. This increased prevalence is understood by most people to be an unfortunate but inevitable result of irrigation schemes that are essential to combat food shortages in countries subject to recurrent famines and droughts. But today there are revisionists among agriculturalists who wonder aloud whether indeed these irrigation projects – and in 1975 there were reported to be 10,000–11,000 dams in the tropics over 15 meters in height – do indeed contribute toward a solution.[7]

If these agriculturalists are to be believed, then there is a disturbing parallel between bilharzia and drought: Both owe as much to man's own activity as to natural events. Just as Western experts have increased the prevalence of bilharzia by irrigation schemes, so have their agricultural practices, these agriculturalists argue, made drought a more serious problem by encouraging the process of "desertification." Desertification is a process brought about by overcultivation, overgrazing, and deforestation, by which the productivity of soil is decreased. In the tropics, this process exposes a nonglaciated, highly weathered, humus-poor soil to leaching and erosion. Thus, what little rain that does fall cannot be retained and immediately runs off, causing further erosion and desertification. Thus famine in such countries is not simply a result of low rainfall; it is a consequence also of desertified soils that are incapable of holding moisture and that have, therefore, become highly susceptible to drought.

Thus, they argue, the problems of drought and famine are a result of an imposed imperial-styled agricultural policy, which has in turn led to imposed Western solutions: food aid, the construction of irrigation dams, and the planting of high-yield varieties of food crops. But such irrigation schemes are usually foreign to African cultures and, like the medical schemes, disintegrate when the Western-trained experts leave. Also, their very presence encourages overcultivation and overgrazing, which leads in turn to increased desertification.

Further problems, these agriculturalists point out, arise from the production of cash crops. These crops, sold abroad to gain foreign currency, are usually grown on the best and often irrigated soils, forcing African farmers to grow their subsistence crops on the poorest soils. Thus, when no rain falls, the Africans' food crops fail first, and starvation appears because they can no longer afford to pay the inflated prices required by the traders who corner the food market.[8]

Bilharzia is also linked to the construction of large hydroelectric dams, none more famous than the Aswan High Dam. It was designed to supply energy for industrialization and to expand the area of cultivated land in order to feed the ever-growing population and to provide foreign exchange through the export of cash crops. But, without the annual deposition of the rich Nile silt, there has been an estimated 10 percent annual loss of production because of a decline in soil fertility. There has been also soil erosion, increased salinity, pesticide pollution of the soil, a rise in the water table, an increased encroachment of the desert, and, I have been told, the collapse of a rich fishing industry along the Mediterranean where the Nile outflow no longer contributes sufficient nutrients to supply the fish feeding grounds.[9] In addition, not only has the prevalence of bilharzia along the Nile Valley increased dramatically as a result of the switch to perennial irrigation, but also the disease pattern has changed. In the Nile Delta, in contrast to the days of Scott and Barlow, *S. mansoni* has today replaced the less pathogenic *S. haematobium* as the commonest species and has also spread south along the Nile Valley where it was previously absent. This change is probably linked to a change in the water flow induced by the Aswan Dam which has altered the relative abundance of the two host snail species.[10] As far as the Egyptian *fellaheen* are concerned, neither the economic benefits nor the medical and human costs of the Aswan Dam seem to have justified its construction.

Many of those who have worked on bilharzia in Egypt insist, however, that although the prevalence of the disease has increased, there has been a reduction in its morbidity. They assume also that the treatment annexes and the almost endless series of pilot projects have contributed to this decreased morbidity. The evidence for reduced morbidity seems to be based on early texts which described more severe pathologies in hospitalized victims than are seen today. This may be true, but without comparative epidemiological studies to measure the morbidity at the community level, there seems no way of their supporting or rejecting either of these claims.

But after World War II, at least, the increased prevalence of malaria and other fly-transmitted diseases induced by irrigation schemes seemed controllable. DDT seemed to be such a successful mosquito-killer that in 1955 the WHO predicted the eradication of malaria in the foreseeable future and Russell published his *Man's Mastery of Malaria*. But no such optimism gripped the imaginations of those engaged in the postwar fight against bilharzia. Here the success stories were limited to areas on the fringes of the parasite's range. In modern Japan, for example, only the Kofu Basin remains a breeding site for the susceptible snails. But there is little evidence that this virtual elimination of the disease was brought about by the elaborate schemes carried out by the Japanese and the U.S. military. The modernization of Japanese agriculture probably had a much greater effect.[11] It led to a decrease in the proportion of the population engaged in agriculture, a decrease in the area taken up by paddy fields, changes in agricultural customs in the paddy fields and a shortening of working hours, a decreased use of draft animals, improved hygiene, and higher living standards. Similarly, in Puerto Rico, the improvement has been dramatic, but again seems to have had little to do with any specific bilharzia campaigns. The decrease in prevalence was paralleled by a marked shift in the pattern of infection, indicating that economic factors played a major role. The 1976 survey showed that whereas the disease had declined in the old sugar areas, it had actually increased in the northeast adjacent to San Juan; bilharzia had changed from a plantation disease to a recreational disease. Puerto Rican officials now claim that most cases result from random, sporadic exposures; the disease is no longer a public health problem. In this new scenario, eradication of the disease from the island through use of the new drugs has become a very distinct possibility.[12] But, as the Chinese experiences seem to indicate, without such socioeconomic changes and a health-care delivery system that involves the diseased population, the antibilharzia schemes in the rest of the world consistently failed, and in the 1960s malaria, too, began its dramatic resurgence.

Professionals in biological research have played a more dominant role in postwar tropical medicine, whether members of the American Society of Tropical Medicine, the South African Council of Scientific and Industrial Research, or the British Colonial Research Service. In many ways, such a complex and fascinating puzzle as bilharzia answers their professional needs and can attract research funding into their laboratories and field stations. In 1976, to give the most obvious example, the Edna McConnell Clark Foundation began to fund a research program geared to the long-range goal of developing practical vaccines against the schistosome parasites.[13] The result has been a research explosion on bilharzia. Between 1950 and 1975, for example, only about 5–10 percent of the papers published in the *American*

Journal of Tropical Medicine and Hygiene dealt with bilharzia. But thereafter, the numbers climbed to between 20 and 30 percent. I think one can say with some degree of certainty that during the early 1980s about one-fifth to one-quarter of the research effort in tropical medicine was devoted to bilharzia. Yet, even *The Strategic Plan* of the McConnell Clark Foundation admits that bilharzia is "not usually fatal or even serious," and Ken Warren, one person who has pushed long and hard in favor of bilharzia research, wrote in 1973 that "studies on morbidity have found remarkably little evidence of overt disease in most endemic areas." Warren justifies the research activity directed toward bilharzia by making the peculiar argument that although only a small proportion in any area become sick, this small proportion, taken in total across the world, grows into a very large number of individuals, and thus bilharzia becomes a "medical problem of the foremost magnitude."[14] But, the question must be put, Who has benefited most from this activity, the *fellaheen* in Egypt, or the academics in the United States where most of the research takes place? Of the $3 million dollars that the Edna McConnell Clark Foundation spent on bilharzia research prior to September 1980, 73 percent went to support programs in American universities and only 3.2 percent was spent in the Third World – the University of Puerto Rico and two universities in Cairo.[15] And have those who are forced to live in the homelands of South Africa benefited from the research activities of South African scientists?

As those in the business admit privately to themselves, this academic research on the schistosome worms has created a great deal more information about the nature of parasitism and the nature of immunity than about the solutions to the problems of bilharzia. "Dazzling advances in biomedical science," John Bryant noted, "are scarcely felt in areas where need is greatest."[16] Even P. Williams, while decrying the failure of WHO to maintain the postwar research impetus, noted nevertheless that research in the area was concentrating more and more in temperate climates where "they made fundamental scientific advances, but, because they were not in the tropics, their work was not orientated to practical problems."[17]

But while this scientific activity was being nourished, awareness grew that tropical diseases were not simply diseases of the tropics, diseases of place, but also diseases of poverty and underdevelopment. By the 1960s, texts had appeared that differed fundamentally from the standard textbooks which restricted themselves almost exclusively to a discussion of protozoan, metazoan, viral, and bacterial diseases. Instead, we read that problems are determined mainly by poverty and that Western models for health care and education are irrelevant for the tropical world. Poverty, we read, creates conditions in which the traditional climatic tropical diseases can flourish, as it also reduces the availability of the equipment and skills needed to combat these diseases. We learn that upgrading the quality of medical care has taken precedence over extending the range of medical coverage. We learn of medical standards being too high; of health professionals taking "lavish provision for the few rather than provision for the many"; and of failing to resist the cliché that "our people deserve nothing but the best."[18] Others have stressed that many tropical diseases, of which bilharzia is certainly a prime example, are actually diseases that arose as a consequence of development, and very few now subscribe to the view that heavy disease concentration is natural in the tropics and that Western medicine has gradually overcome it.[19]

The late Brian Maegraith, Dean of Tropical Medicine at the Liverpool School, was adamant that tropical medicine should not simply be ordinary Western medicine transferred to the tropics. It was a "dangerous" notion, he wrote, inhibiting progress in medical education and in the development of an efficient health care system. What is more, he added, it leads to the production of physicians in the Third World who only mirror those in the West and who think therefore that "what is good for the West must be equally good for everybody else." Tropical medicine is multidisciplinary, he urged, taking place in "areas where communal poverty and low standards of life are basic facts of life." For the past 70 years, he concluded, there has been too much emphasis on certain diseases so that community medicine and the delivery of medical care have been relegated to the periphery. Among those diseases which he thought overemphasized, he named bilharzia.[20]

These criticisms are, in many ways, a reaction to what Andrew Learmouth has called the "overdominance of the germ theory" and the "single-variable explanation," in which the socioeconomic component of disease was almost completely ignored.[21]

HEALTH FOR ALL

By the 1980s, these challenges to the underlying assumptions and beliefs of what I have called "imperial medicine" found expression in the changed medical policies of the WHO. According to David Bradley, these changes were precipitated by events surrounding their antimalarial campaigns, where success seemed to demand good management, good organization, extensive health-care coverage, and low-cost health centers.[22]

In 1979, the 32nd Assembly of the WHO launched what was rather grandly called a "global strategy for health for all by the year 2000," and in doing so endorsed the report of an international conference held the previous year in Alma Ata in the USSR. "Today," that report noted,

health resources are allocated mainly to sophisticated medical institutions in urban areas. Quite apart from the dubious social premise on which this is based, the concentration of complex and costly technology on limited segments of the population does not even have the advantage of improving health. Indeed, the improvement of health is being equated with the provision of medical care dispensed by growing numbers of specialists, using narrow medical technologies for the benefit of the privileged few. . . . Contact has been lost between those providing medical care and those receiving it.[23]

The report urged that primary health care must replace what I have called the imposed imperial-style medicine of the past. Not only must the entire population be reached, but, in contrast to what had occurred previously, "the people have the right and duty to participate individually and collectively in the planning and implementation of their health care." The implementation of the new policies, the report went on, requires teams of health workers including medical auxiliaries, midwives, and community workers. Western medicine, in other words, should no longer provide the model for the developing countries; no longer was health to be achieved by the step-by-step elimination of every disease by such technological processes as snail elimination or specific drug therapies. Such "multiple, integrated, intervention techniques," the WHO Expert Committee on Bilharzia noted in 1984, were beyond the human and financial resources of most countries.[24]

The antibilharzia program responded quickly to this new approach. It came also at an opportune time; attempts to break the transmission cycle of the parasites had not worked, partly because the measurement of "incidence," by which the success of transmission breakage was measured, had proven too difficult to calculate. Not only was it next to impossible to keep track of uninfected people from one year to the next, but, most significantly, the test demanded a foolproof diagnostic technique. But failure to locate schistosome eggs in the urine or feces was never a reliable enough indication that the individual was indeed negative for the parasite, and without that reliability the validity of the statistic of "incidence" itself became problematical. So, if the total elimination of the parasite was impossible and transmission breakage impracticable, what was the future to bring?

The answer was to phase out independent, technologically sophisticated antischistosome campaigns, and to replace them by programs in which "community participation must be considered as a fundamental aspect of schistosomiasis control," and in which control was aimed, not at the parasite, but at the disease. At last came the realization that the parasites were not necessarily a public health problem; any problems that arose were due to the morbidity induced by them. "Public health administrators must realise," Peter Jordan wrote in 1985, "that while high prevalence rates and intensities of infection can usually be easily reduced to low levels, it is more difficult to reduce them further and it is probably uneconomical and unnecessary to do so."[25] Thus the goal of modern programs was not to eliminate snails or the parasite but to reduce the morbidity or illness induced by the worms. The control of morbidity, the emphasis on disease rather than on the parasite, and on man rather than on the snail, was, Kenneth Mott noted in a paper prepared for the crucial Expert Committee meeting of 1984, feasible, attainable, and afford-able.[26]

The success of such programs required an accurate, easily measured assessment of morbidity. This was attained by a new quantitative filtration technique which gave a reliable measure of the number of eggs in the urine or feces, which in turn was linked to the number of worms in the body and thus to the severity of the disease. In very practical terms, the goal of the new program was to reduce the number of eggs of *S. haematobium* to less than 50 eggs per 10 milliliters of urine, and of *S. japonicum* and *S. masoni* to less than 100 eggs in 1 gram of feces.[27]

In addition, because the new antibilharzia campaigns now had to be integrated into each country's primary health care program, the public health importance of the disease had to be assessed, particularly because as a chronic disease it lacked the obvious impact of those with high mortalities and high morbidities. For the first time, assessment of the pathological morbidity and socioeconomic impact of the disease became an essential prerequisite to any bilharzia program; the mere presence of the parasite in the community was no longer sufficient justification for mounting a campaign against it.[28]

By 1985, primary health care programs with a bilharzia component to them had commenced in some countries. In Gambia, for example, two minimally trained part-time health workers had been appointed in some villages, one concerned with curative work and health promotion, and the other a midwife.[29] The former, not Western-trained physicians, delivered the major weapon against bilharzia – praziquantel – but only as one aspect of a total health program that provided pure water, sanitation, environmental management, and, to a lesser degree, focal mollusciciding. Perhaps Mott is correct when he wrote, in 1983, that "never before in the history of schistosomiasis have the prospects for its control been more optimistic."[30]

But as one who has studied the history of bilharzia, I will be forgiven if I remain somewhat skeptical; such positive pronouncements have been made many times before. In 1988, UNICEF was reported by the *Toronto Globe and Mail* to have blamed the debt crisis for the death of a half-million children in 1987. Societies faced with such economic problems cut back disproportionally on services directed to the poor – health, education, and social welfare. But the same article, by pointing out that immunization programs have saved 15 million lives every year, implied that were it not for the medical programs, even more children would have died.[31] Perhaps the article should have stated instead that whereas before, these children would have died of smallpox, they now join those who die of malnutrition and poverty. For, as noted by the WHO in 1952, if those who suffer from tropical diseases continue to live in a state of poverty and semistarvation, "we cannot speak of 'progress.'"[32]

The year 2000 will have passed long before there will be health for all.

NOTES

CHAPTER 1 *Introduction*

1 This point has been made by David Bradley, "Tropical medicine," in J. Walton et al. (eds.), *Oxford Companion to Medicine* (Oxford: Oxford University Press, 1986).

2 Today the word "colonialism" is often used in place of "imperialism," partly, I suspect , because of the evil connotations that have become associated with imperialism. I do not subscribe to this use. Colonialism originally referred specifically to the establishment of overseas colonies, mirrored after the home country, and should be used only in that sense. For a fruitful introduction to these issues, see D. K. Fieldhouse, *Colonialism 1870–1945: An Introduction* (London: St Martin's Press, 1981).

3 H. Harold Scott, *A History of Tropical Medicine* (London: Edward Arnold, 1939). W. D. Foster's *A History of Parasitology* (London: Livingstone, 1965) is another excellent study in this vein.

4 To list a few of these writings: P. C. C. Garnham, "Britain's contribution to tropical medicine," *The Practitioner* 201 (1968): 153–61; J. S. Boyd, "Fifty years of tropical medicine," *British Medical Journal* 1 (1950): 37–43; M. Gelfand, *Tropical Victory: An Account of the Influence of Medicine on the History of Southern Rhodesia, 1890–1923* (Cape Town: Juto, 1953); G. S. Nelson, "Medical aspects – Commented discussion," *Symposium of the British Society of Parasitology* 16 (1978): 15–23, which is, as the author even admits, a rather embarrassing "jingoistic discourse." Every one of these authors practiced tropical medicine or parasitology in the field. The Americans, too, have produced work of a similar nature: M. Yoeli, "The evolution of tropical medicine: A historical perspective," *Bulletin of the New York Academy of Medicine* 48 (1972): 1231–46. In 1976, at a joint meeting of the American Society of Tropical Medicine and the Royal Society of London, a conference was held entitled "Milestones in the history of tropical medicine and hygiene," which has been published in *American Journal of Tropical Medicine and Hygiene* 26, No. 5 (1977): 1053–104. There are also similar works dealing with victories over specific diseases, of which P. Russell's *Man's Mastery of Malaria* (London: Oxford University Press, 1955) and L. J. Bruce-Chwatt and J. de Zulueta's *The Rise and Fall of Malaria in Europe* (Oxford: Oxford University Press, 1980) are probably the best known.

5 Lewis Gann and P. Duignan, *Burden of Empire: An Appraisal of Western Colonialism in Africa South of the Sahara* (New York: Praeger, 1967).

6 Two books dealing with imperial medicine appeared in 1988: R. MacLeod and M. Lewis (eds.), *Disease, Medicine and Empire* (London: Routledge, 1988) and David Arnold (ed.), *Imperial Medicine and Indigenous Societies* (Manchester: Manchester University Press, 1988). MacLeod's introductory chapter to the former book provides a good introduction to the historiography of writing in the general area of imperial

306   *Notes to pp. 2–5*

medicine. These more recent studies often focus on a single disease, often within a short time period and in a single location. They include the chapters in the above books, Gordon Harrison's delightful *Mosquitoes, Malaria and Man: A Story of Hostilities Since 1880* (New York: Dutton, 1978); J. McKelvey, *Man Against Tsetse: Struggle for Africa* (Ithaca, Cornell University Press, 1973); R. E. Dumett, "The campaign against malaria and the expansion of scientific medical and sanitary services in British West Africa, 1898–1910," *African Historical Studies* 1 (1968): 153–97, and many others. A few have dealt with the history of bilharzia. They include G. Hartwig and K. Patterson, *Schistosomiasis in Twentieth-Century Africa: Historical Studies on West Africa and Sudan* (Los Angeles: Crossroads Press, 1984); F. R. Sandbach, "The history of schistosomiasis research and policy for its control," *Medical History* 20 (1976): 259–75 and "Farewell to the God of Plague – The control of schistosomiasis in China," *Social Science and Medicine* 14 (1977): 27–33. Current interest in the field of international development has generated many extremely critical studies of modern policies. Many of these studies have appeared in the *International Journal of Health Services*, and in Vicente Navarro (ed.), *Imperialism, Health and Medicine* (Farmingdale, N.Y.: Baywood Publ., 1981).

7 G. W. Hartwig and K. Patterson (eds.), *Disease in African History* (Durham, N.C.: Duke University Press, 1978), pp. 4, 11. J. Goodyear, "The sugar connection: A new perspective on the history of yellow fever," *Bulletin of the History of Medicine* 52 (1978): 5–21.

8 R. MacLeod, Introduction to *Disease, Medicine and Empire.*

9 Philip Curtin, *The Image of Africa: British Ideas and Actions, 1780–1850* (Madison: University of Wisconsin Press, 1964). There are two pieces by Michael Worboys which are really much too brief to address the issue of medicine and empire: "The emergence of tropical medicine," In G. Lemaine et al. (eds.), *Perspectives on the Emergence of Scientific Disciplines* (London: Mouton, 1976) and "The emergence and early development of parasitology," in K. S. Warren and J. Z. Bowers (eds.), *Parasitology: A Global Perspective* (New York: Springer-Verlag, 1983). In my opinion, David Bradley, Director of the Ross Institute in the London School of Hygiene and Tropical Medicine, has presented the best succinct account of the relationships in his "Tropical Medicine."

10 G. Webbe, "Six diseases of the W.H.O.," *British Medical Journal* 283 (1981): 1104–6. The other five are malaria, filariasis, trypanosomiasis, leishmaniasis, and leprosy.

11 For a bibliography on the disease, see K. S. Warren and V. A. Newill, *Schistosomiasis: A Bibliography of the World's Literature from 1852 to 1962* (Cleveland: The Press of Western Reserve University, 1967), 2 vols. For the past few years a bibliography of current literature is published quarterly in *Schisto Update* (New York: Edna McConnell Clark Foundation). Abstracts of some of the major articles on bilharzia have also been published in K. S. Warren, *Schistosomiasis: The Evolution of a Medical Literature, Selected Abstracts and Citations, 1852–1972* (Cambridge, Mass.: M.I.T. Press, 1973); K. S. Warren and D. B. Hoffman, *Schistosomiasis III: Abstracts of the Complete Literature, 1963–1974*; and D. B. Hoffmann and K. S. Warren, *Schistosomiasis IV: Condensation of the Selected Literature, 1963–75* (Washington, D.C.: Hemisphere Publ., 1978). For general accounts of bilharzia there are Peter Jordan and Gerald Webbe, *Schistosomiasis: Epidemiology, Treatment and Control* (London: William Heinemann, 1982); M. F. Abdel-Wahab, *Schistosomiasis in Egypt* (Boca Baton, Fla.: CRC Press, 1982); J. F. Maldonado, *Schistosomiasis in America* (Barcelona: Editorial Cientifico-Medica, 1967); and D. Rollinson and A. Simpson, *The Biology of Schistosomes: From Genes to Latrines* (London: Academic Press, 1987). For a shorter presentation, see E. Michelson, "Snail intermediate hosts," and A. Mahmoud, "Schisto-

somiasis," in K. S. Warren and A. Mahmoud, *Tropical and Geographical Medicine* (New York: McGraw-Hill, 1986). The WHO has produced many reports about the disease, including *International Work in Bilharziasis, 1948–1958* (Geneva: WHO, 1959).

12 The most recent review of the subject is D. S. Brown, *Fresh Water Snails of Africa and Their Medical Importance* (London: Taylor and Francis, 1980); also F. Frandsen et al., "A practical guide to the identification of African fresh water snails," *Malacological Review* 13 (1980): 95–119.

CHAPTER 2 *1898: A declaration of war*

1 F. A. Lyon, "The imperial functions of the hospital for tropical diseases, London: An appeal to India," *The Indian Medical Gazette* 62 (1927): 277.

2 Figures from P. Burroughs, "The human cost of imperial defence in the early Victorian age," *Victorian Studies* 24 (1980): 1–32. More detailed figures can be found in Philip Curtin, *The Image of Africa: British Ideas and Actions, 1780–1850* (Madison: University of Wisconsin Press, 1964).

3 John Farley, "Parasites and the germ theory of disease," *Milbank Quarterly* 67, Suppl. 1 (1989): 50–68.

4 "Europeans in the tropics," *British Medical Journal*, January 9, 1897, p. 94.

5 For the history of African diseases and attempts to avoid them during the nineteenth century, see P. Curtin, *The Image of Africa*; "The white man's grave: Image and reality, 1780–1850," *Journal of British Studies* 1 (1961): 94–110; "Epidemiology and the slave trade," *Political Science Quarterly* 83 (1968): 190–216; Daniel Headrick, *The Tools of Empire: Technology and European Imperialism in the 19th Century* (Oxford: Oxford University Press, 1981); Dennis Carlson, *African Fever: A Study of British Science, Technology, and Politics in West Africa, 1787–1864* (Canton, Mass.: Science History Publ., 1984).

6 Patrick Manson, *Tropical Diseases: A Manual of the Diseases of Warm Climates* (London: Cassell, 1898), Introduction.

7 Luigi Sambon, "Remarks on the acclimatisation in tropical regions," *British Medical Journal*, January 9, 1897, p. 63.

8 A. Davidson, *Hygiene and Diseases of Warm Climates* (Edinburgh: Pentland, 1893), p. 5.

9 J. R. Seeley, *The Expansion of England* (London: 1883), reprinted by The Chicago University Press, 1971, p. 126.

10 Chairman's remarks before Patrick Manson's address, "A school of tropical medicine," to the Royal Colonial Institute, March 1900, *London School of Tropical Medicine and Hospital for Tropical Diseases: Miscellanea, 1899–1927*, Library archives, London School of Hygiene and Tropical Medicine. [Hereafter, referred to as *London School Miscellanea*.]

11 Address to the opening of third session of the London School of Tropical Medicine, October 16, 1901, *London School Miscellanea*.

12 Patrick Manson, Introductory address at the opening of the London School of Tropical Medicine, October 2, 1899, *London School Miscellanea*.

13 The Church Missionary Society recruited only 12 physicians between 1817 and 1893, but 62 over the next 25 years. In 1891, they formed a Medical Missionary Auxiliary to raise funds specifically for medical work. W. D. Foster, *The Church Missionary Society and Modern Medicine in Uganda: The Life of Sir Albert Cook, 1870–1951* (privately printed, 1973).

14 M. W. Swanson, "The sanitation syndrome: The bubonic plague and urban native

policy in the Cape Colony, 1900–1909," *Journal of African History* 18 (1977): 387–410. This issue has also been discussed by L. Spicer, "The mosquito and segregation in Sierra Leone," *Canadian Journal of African Studies* 2 (1968): 49–61; P. Curtin, "Medical knowledge and urban planning in tropical Africa," *American Historical Review* 90 (1985): 594–613.

15 This transition from "conversion" to trusteeship is succinctly discussed in Philip Curtin, *Imperialism* (New York: Walker, 1971).

16 Quoted in Henry Winkler, *The League of Nations Movement in Great Britain, 1914–1919* (New Brunswick, N.J.: Rutgers University Press, 1952), p. 204.

17 Frederick Lugard, *The Dual Mandate in British Tropical Africa* (London: Blackwell, 1922), p. 615.

18 D. K. Fieldhouse, *The Colonial Empires* (London: Weidenfeld and Nicolson, 1966). I have taken this brief discussion of the British Empire also from Fieldhouse, *Colonialism, 1870–1945* (New York: St. Martin's Press, 1981); and Penelope Hetherington, *British Paternalism and Africa, 1920–1940* (London: Frank Cass, 1978).

19 Gage Brown to the Colonial Office, October 4, 1897, *Miscellaneous Papers Printed for the Use of the Colonial Office*, Public Records Office [hereafter referred to as *Miscellaneous Papers*], CO 885/7/119.

20 Patrick Manson, "Necessity for special education in tropical medicine," Address to St. George's Hospital, October 1, 1897, *Miscellaneous Papers*, CO 885/7/119.

21 Colonial Office memo to General Medical Council and 26 British medical schools, March 11, 1898, *Miscellaneous Papers*, CO 885/7/119.

22 CO 885/7/119 contains all of these replies.

23 N. Cantlie, *A History of the Army Medical Department* (London: Churchill Livingston, 1973). D. G. Crawford, *A History of the Indian Medical Service, 1600–1913* (London: Thacker, 1914). The Netley Hospital, somewhat reminiscent of the Bombay Railway Station, occupied a "grand range of buildings," with a frontage of 480 yards overlooking Southampton Water. But, as even the enthusiastic writer in *The Navy and Army Illustrated* (March 19, 1897) was forced to admit, there was insufficient shelter and the patients found the place rather "exposed." I have been given two reasons for this chilly business. The architect who was asked to design a hospital for the British Army naturally assumed it would be built in India and designed it accordingly. He was wrong. A far better story has it that two plans were submitted – one for India and one for Southampton – but somehow the plans were switched. Is there, therefore, somewhere in India, a small, airless hospital in which the patients slowly roast to death?

24 A. G. McBride, *The History of the Dreadnought Seamen's Hospital at Greenwich* (Greenwich: Seamen's Hospital Management Committee, 1970).

25 Seamen's Hospital Society to Colonial Office, April 16, 1898, *Miscellaneous Papers*, CO 885/7/119.

26 Colonial Office to Treasury, June 14, 1898, *Miscellaneous Papers*, CO 885/7/119.

27 B. G. Maegraith, "History of the Liverpool School of Tropical Medicine," *Medical History* 16 (1972): 354–68. For further details, see *Liverpool School of Tropical Medicine: Historical Record 1898–1920* (Liverpool: Liverpool University Press, 1920). For the life of Alfred Jones, see P. N. Davies, *Sir Alfred Jones: Shipping Entrepreneur Par Excellence* (London: Europa Publ., 1978) and *The Trade Makers: Elder Dempster in West Africa, 1852–1972* (London: George Allen, 1973).

28 The London School of Tropical Medicine, *Report for the Year 1899–1900*, Library archives, London School of Hygiene and Tropical Medicine.

29 Good stories are always worth telling, even in footnotes! The Liverpool School began to offer a Diploma of Tropical Hygiene (DTH) in 1921 to those with

the Diploma in Tropical Medicine (DTM). Naturally, few took the extra classes, and so a questionnaire of 1934 asked these graduates if there were problems with the course. The replies suggested the need for more practical work. So in 1935, the School rented 9.5 acres of land at Melling on the Leeds–Liverpool Canal and built there a model African village complete with corrugated iron walls, reed roofs, and borehole latrines. By 1939, the School reported "numerous thefts of apparatus and willful destruction of demonstration material," so that by 1940 the whole bizarre operation was terminated. In 1946, the DTM and DTH were amalgamated to form the Diploma in Hygiene and Tropical Medicine.

30 The beginnings of tropical medicine and parasitology are discussed by Michael Worboys in two brief articles: "The emergence of tropical medicine," in G. Lemaine et al. (eds.), *Perspectives on the Emergence of Scientific Disciplines* (London: Mouton, 1976); and "The emergence and early development of parasitology," in K. S. Warren and I. Z. Bowers (eds.), *Parasitology: A Global Perspective* (New York: Springer-Verlag, 1983).

31 John Farley, "Parasites and the germ theory of disease."

32 For the life of Manson, see Philip Manson-Bahr and A. Alcock, *The Life and Work of Sir Patrick Manson* (London: Cassell, 1927), and the shorter Philip Manson-Bahr, *Patrick Manson: The Father of Tropical Medicine* (London: Thomas Nelson, 1962). See also Patrick Manson, *Tropical Diseases: A Manual of the Diseases of Warm Climates* (London: Cassell, 1898).

33 Manson-Bahr, *Life and Work of Manson*, p. 89.

34 King's College to Colonial Office, November 22, 1898, *Miscellaneous Papers*, CO 885/7/119. The medical schools had been informed of the Greenwich site for a new institution on November 9. Their claim to have instructed colonial medical officers in the past was a little strained. Of 85 graduates listed as serving overseas and in the colonies, 5 were in Africa, 16 in India, 24 in the United States, 19 in Australasia, and 12 in the tropical expanses of Canada.

35 Ibid., December 5, 1898

36 Wright moved to St. Mary's Hospital in 1902 where, four years later, he was joined by a junior assistant, Alexander Fleming.

37 Manson to Colonial Office, December 26, 1898, *Miscellaneous Papers*, CO 885/7/119.

38 Worboys, "The emergence of parasitology," p. 8.

39 Victoria Harden, "Rocky Mountain spotted fever research and the development of the insect vector theory, 1900–1930," *Bulletin of the History of Medicine* 59 (1985): 449–66. Farley, "Parasites and the germ theory."

40 Patrick Manson's Introductory address, October 2, 1899, *London School Miscellanea*.

41 "Investigation and control of tropical disease." Memorandum to Colonial Office, April 13, 1910, *Miscellaneous Papers*, CO 885/21.

42 A brief story will illustrate that this view is still prevalent. A few years ago, I happened to meet a group of American Peace Corps volunteers on their way to Africa. They were taking a class on tropical diseases at the London School and were, on that particular day, filled with information on bilharzia. They were somewhat confused by my statement that hepatitis, which I contracted in Boston, would be a more serious problem for them in terms of both morbidity and avoidance.

CHAPTER 3 *1898: Another war, another continent*

1 For a comparison of the two empires, see D. K. Fieldhouse, *The Colonial Empires* (London: Weidenfeld and Nicolson, 1966); and Robin Weeks, "American and Euro-

pean imperialism compared," in Richard Miller (ed.), *American Imperialism in 1898* (New York: Wiley, 1970). Quotation from Fieldhouse, p. 343.

2 Elihu Root, "The principles of colonial policy," in *The Military and Colonial Policy of the United States* (Cambridge, Mass.: Harvard University Press, 1916), p. 165.

3 Quotation from T. R. Clark, *Puerto Rico and the United States, 1917–33* (Pittsburgh: University of Pittsburgh Press, 1975).

4 A. Lawrence Lowell, "The colonial expansion of the United States," *Atlantic Monthly* 83 (1899): 145–54; C. Lasch, "The anti-imperialists, the Philippines, and the inequality of man," *Journal of Southern History* 24 (1958): 319–31.

5 E. B. Tompkins, *Anti-imperialism in the United States: The Great Debate, 1890–1920* (Philadelphia: University of Pennsylvania Press, 1970), p. 245.

6 Manuel Quezon, quoted in P. W. Stanley, *A Nation in the Making: The Philippines and the United States, 1899–1921* (Cambridge, Mass.: Harvard University Press, 1974), p. 85.

7 President Taft, quoted in Stanley, *A Nation in the Making*, p. 111.

8 C. Wellman, "The New Orleans School of Tropical Medicine and Hygiene," *New Orleans Medical and Surgical Journal* 64 (1912): 893–915.

9 John Warner, "A Southern medical reform: The meaning of the antebellum argument for Southern medical education," *Bulletin of the History of Medicine* 57 (1983): 364–81. Also Todd Savitt and J. Harvey Young (eds.), *Disease and Distinctiveness in the American South* (Knoxville: The University of Tennessee Press, 1988).

10 Kenneth Ludmerer, *Learning To Heal: The Development of American Medical Education* (New York: Basic Books, 1985), p. 21.

11 "Dr. Edouard Michel Dupaquier, 1858–1928," *New Orleans Medical and Surgical Journal* 80 (1927): 772–4.

12 Quotation taken from Gaines Foster, *The Demands of Humanity: Army Medical Disaster Relief* (Washington, D.C.: Center of Military History, 1983), p. 26.

13 Charles Craig, "The army medical service," *Yale Medical Journal* 16 (1910): 415–27.

14 Faculty minutes of the Army Medical School. Medical History Department, Uniformed Services University of the Health Sciences, Bethesda, Maryland. For other accounts of the school, see G. Lull, "The days gone by: A brief history of the Army Medical School, 1893–1933," *The Military Surgeon* 74 (1934): 78–86; R. S. Henry, *The Armed Forces Institute of Pathology, 1862–1962* (Washington, D.C.: Office of the Surgeon General, 1964); H. Nichols, "Notes on the history of the laboratories of the Army Medical School," *Military Surgeon* 60 (1927): 52–8.

15 M. Warner, "Hunting the yellow fever germ: The principle and practice of etiological proof in late 19th century America," *Bulletin of the History of Medicine* 59 (1985): 361–82.

16 John Gibson, *Soldier in White: The Life of General George Miller Sternberg* (Durham, N.C.: Duke University Press, 1958).

17 J. Hamilton-Stone, "Our troops in the tropics," *Journal of the Military Service Institute of the United States* 26 (1900): 358–69.

18 The quotations are taken from Graham Cosmas, *An Army for Empire* (University of Missouri Press, 1971), Chapter 8. Casualty figures and other information are taken from R. F. Weigley, *History of the United States Army* (Bloomington: Indiana University Press, 1984); and M. A. Kreidberg and M. Henry, *History of Military Mobilization in the U.S. Army, 1775–1945* (Washington, D.C.: Department of the Army, 1955).

19 C. Greenleaf, "A brief statement on the sanitary work so far accomplished in the Philippine Islands," *Reports and Papers of the American Public Health Association* 27 (1901): 157–65.

20 Quotation from P. W. Stanley, *A Nation in the Making*, p. 109.

21 J. Gates, *Schoolbooks and Krags: The U.S. Army in the Philippines, 1898–1902* (Westport, Conn.: Greenwood Press, 1973), p. 136.

22 R. Ileto, "Cholera and the origins of the American sanitary order in the Philippines," in D. Arnold (ed.), *Imperial Medicine and Indigenous Societies* (Manchester: Manchester University Press, 1988); R. Sullivan, "Cholera and colonialism in the Philippines, 1899–1903," in R. MacLeod and M. Lewis (eds.), *Disease, Medicine and Empire* (London: Routledge, 1988).

23 Greenleaf, "Brief statement on sanitary work," p. 162. A similar picture is painted by James Roy, "The Philippine health problem," *The Outlook* 71 (1902): 777–82.

24 Marie Gorgas and B. J. Hendrick, *William Crawford Gorgas: His Life and Work* (Philadelphia: Lea & Febiger, 1924), p. 73.

25 Ibid., p. 85.

26 For details see Clark, *Puerto Rico*; A. M. Carrion, *Puerto Rico: A Political and Cultural History* (New York: Norton, 1983); E. J. Berbusse, *The United States in Puerto Rico, 1898–1900* (Chapel Hill: University of North Carolina Press, 1966).

27 Henry Carroll, *Report on the Island of Porto Rico* (Washington, D.C.: U.S. Government Printing Office, 1899), p. 211.

28 Ashford tells his story in his autobiography, *A Soldier in Science* (New York: William Morrow, 1934). A brief biography is given by G. W. Bachman, "Dr. Bailey K. Ashford (1873–1934), as I knew him," *Boletin – Asociacion Medica de Puerto Rico* 55 (1963): 83–9.

29 B. Ashford and P. G. Igaravidez, "Summary of a ten year's campaign against hookworm in Porto Rico," *Journal of the American Medical Association* 54 (1910): 1757–61.

30 B. Ashford and W. W. King, "A study of uncinariasis in Puerto Rico," *American Medicine* 6 (1903): 391–6, 431–8; "Uncinariasis, an economic question for Porto Rico" [Editorial of September 12, 1903], *American Medicine* 6 (1903): 422.

31 A full report of the campaign is given in B. Ashford and P. G. Igaravidez, *Uncinariasis in Porto Rico: A Medical and Economic Problem* (Washington, D.C.: U.S. Government Printing Office, 1911).

32 Ashford, "Ankylostomiasis in Puerto Rico," *New York Medical Journal* 71 (1900): 553–6.

33 Gorgas and Hendrick, *William Gorgas*, p. 88.

34 A. Agramonte, "The inside story of a great medical discovery," *The Scientific Monthly* (1915): 209–37; William Bean, *Walter Reed: A Biography* (Charlottesville: University Press of Virginia, 1982).

35 Testimony of Dr. Simon Flexner and Dr. L. F. Barker, July 3, 1899, *Report of the Philippine Commission to the President* (Washington, D.C.: U.S. Government Printing Office, 1900), Vol. 2, pp. 231–42.

36 J. J. Curry, "U.S. pathological laboratories in the Philippine Islands," *Boston Medical and Surgical Journal* 144 (1901): 175–7. The history of these boards is being detailed by Mary Gillett's forthcoming study, *The Army Medical Department*, Vol. 1: *1775–1818*; Vol. 2: *1818–1856*; Vol. 3: *1865–1917*; Vol. 4: *1917–1941* (Washington, D.C.: Center of Military History, U.S. Army).

37 Hospital admissions for each disease were given in the Annual Reports of the Surgeon General, U.S. Army. For 1905, for example, among American troops there was a combined admission rate of 236.99 (per 1000 men) for diarrhea and dysentery, whereas among Filipino scouts rates of 94.36 and 74.62 for diarrhea and beriberi, respectively, were reported.

38 Council minutes, March 20, 1903, Archives of the American Society of Tropical Medicine, Countway Library, Harvard Medical School. A brief account of the early

years of the Society is given by E. C. Faust, "The American Society of Tropical Medicine: A brief biographical sketch," *American Journal of Tropical Medicine* 24 (1944): 63–9.

39 Resolution submitted by Isaac Brewer at the Sixth Annual General Meeting in the U.S. Naval Medical School, "Whereas the best interests of the American people who serve their country in the tropics demands that all physicians who practice in the American tropical possessions should be thoroughly instructed in tropical medicine and hygiene before their departure for the tropics, and Whereas there is no place in the United States where such instruction is offered . . . Be it resolved that the American Society of Tropical Medicine endorses the movement to establish in this country an institution for the investigation and teaching of tropical medicine and hygiene, and commends this matter to the consideration of the American Capitalists. . . ." A committee of five (Gorgas, Welch, Matas, Fenton, and Lambert), set up to investigate the matter, never seems to have reported back to the Society.

40 Quoted in Foster, *Demands of Humanity*, p. 26.

41 Nancy Stepan, "The interplay between socio–economic factors and medical science: Yellow fever research, Cuba and the United States," *Social Studies of Science* 8 (1978): 397–423.

42 For details of this discovery, see Ernest Faust, "Studies on schistosomiasis mansoni in Puerto Rico. 1. The history of schistosomiasis in Puerto Rico," *Puerto Rico Journal of Public Health and Tropical Medicine* 9 (1933): 154–68.

43 *Report of the Surgeon-General of the Army for 1908*, p. 98; Capt. B. Ashburn, *The Board for the Study of Tropical Diseases as They Occur in the Philippine Islands*, Fifth Quarterly Report, 1906. Also H. J. Nichols and J. Phalen, "The work of the board for the study of tropical diseases in the Philippine Islands," *Military Surgery* 23 (1908): 361–70, 462–8.

CHAPTER 4 *Bilharzia (1850–1918): The Looss controversies*

1 Figures from M. F. Abdel-Wahab, *Schistosomiasis in Egypt* (Boca Raton, Fla.: CRC Press, 1982), p. 76.

2 W. Ayer, "Napoleon Buonaparte and schistosomiasis or bilharziasis," *New York State Journal of Medicine* 66 (1966): 2295–301.

3 C. C. Scott-Moncrieff, "Irrigation in Egypt," *The Nineteenth Century* 17 (1885): 342–7. Details of Muhammad Ali's irrigation schemes are taken from H. Rivlin, *The Agricultural Policy of Muhammad Ali in Egypt* (Cambridge, Mass.: Harvard University Press, 1961), Chapter 12.

4 M. Khalil and M. Azim, "Further observations on the schistosomiasis infection through irrigation schemes in Aswan Province, Egypt," *Journal of the Egyptian Medical Association* 21 (1938): 95. The lower figure is indicated in J. A. Scott, "The incidence and distribution of the human schistosomes in Egypt," *American Journal of Hygiene* 25 (1937): 566–614.

5 J. Heyworth-Dunne, *An Introduction to the History of Education in Modern Egypt* (London: F. Cass, 1939), p. 127.

6 G. Knabe, *Im Kampf gegen die 11. Plage: Das Leben des Theodor Bilharz* (Nettetal: Steyler-Verlag, 1970). Karl Enigk, *Geschichte der Helminthologie im deutschsprachigen Raum* (Stuttgart: Fischer, 1986).

7 "Ein Beitrag zur Helminthographia humana, aus brieflichen Mitteilungen des Dr. Bilharz in Cairo, *Zeitschrift für wissenschaftliche Zoologie* 4 (1853): 59–62. English translation in B. H. Kean, K. E. Mott, and A. J. Russell (eds.), *Tropical Medicine and Parasitology* (Ithaca: Cornell University Press, 1978), Vol. 2, p. 475. Almost all other

trematode worms are hermaphroditic, with male and female sex organs being carried on the same individual.

8 "Fernere Beobachtungen über das die Pfortader des Menschen bewehnende *Distomum haematobium,*" *Zeitschrift für wissenschaftliche Zoologie* 4 (1853): 72–6. English translation in Kean et al., *Tropical Medicine and Parasitology,* p. 478.

9 J. Heyworth-Dunne, *History of Education,* pp. 303–7.

10 P. Sonzino, "La *Bilharzia haematobia* et son role pathologique en Egypt," *Archives générales de médecine* 1 (1876): 657.

11 R. L. Tignor, *Modernization and British Colonial Rule in Egypt, 1882–1914* (Princeton: Princeton University Press, 1966), p. 48.

12 Ibid., p. 84.

13 E. Hart, "Letters from the East," *British Medical Journal,* April 18, 1885, p. 810. In reading the criticism of the Egyptian school, one should remember that equally harsh things could be said about North American schools and were said 25 years later.

14 Egypt. Ministry of the Interior, Department of Public Health. *Annual Report,* 1909.

15 First meeting of Advisory Board, Tropical Disease Research Fund, November 1, 1904, *Miscellaneous Papers,* CO 885/9/170. The advisory board had been established following a memo from Chamberlain to all colonies, May 28, 1903. *Miscellaneous Papers,* CO 885/9/170. The British Treasury and the India Office both promised to grant £500 per year for five years, while the colonies, depending on their wealth, gave either £100 or £200. The Tropical Disease Fund Advisory Board, made up of unpaid voluntary experts, provided one of the earliest models of Boards that were used by the British Colonial Office until the collapse of the Empire in the early 1960s.

16 Sheila Willmott, "Biographical Note: Robert Thomson Leiper, 1881–1969," *International Journal for Parasitology* 11 (1981): 423–4.

17 In 1864, a schistosome parasite was first discovered in South Africa and given the name *S. capense.* J. Harley, "On the endemic haematuria of the Cape of Good Hope," *Medico-chirurgical Transactions* 47 (1864): 55–72. The South African form was soon recognized to be a variety of *S. haematobium* and not a separate species.

18 August Hirsch, "Trematodes" in *Handbook of Geographical and Historical Pathology,* Vol. 2, pp. 295–9; English translation by C. Creighton (London: The Sydenham Society, 1885).

19 Patrick Manson, *Tropical Diseases: A Manual of the Diseases of Warm Climates,* rev. ed. (New York: William Wood, 1905), pp. 605–16.

20 This controversy has recently been discussed by Eli Chernin, "The curious case of the lateral-spined egg: *Schistosoma mansoni,*" *Transactions of the Royal Society of Tropical Medicine and Hygiene* 77 (1983): 847–50.

21 L. Sambon, "New or little known African Entozoa," *Journal of Tropical Medicine and Hygiene* 10 (1907): 117.

22 P. Manson, "Report of a case of bilharzia from the West Indies," *British Medical Journal* 2 (1902): 1894–5.

23 W. Griesinger, "Klinische und anatomische beobachtungen über die Krankheiten von Egypten," *Archiv für Physiologie Heilkunde* 13 (1854): 561–75; English translation in Kean (ed.), *Tropical Medicine,* Vol. 2, pp. 481–7.

24 J. Harley, "On the endemic haematuria of the Cape of Good Hope," *Medico-chirurgical Transactions* 47 (1864): 55–72.

25 L. Sambon, "The part played by metazoan parasites in tropical pathology," *Journal of Tropical Medicine and Hygiene* 11 (1908): 29–36.

26 Discussion of paper. *Journal of Tropical Medicine and Hygiene* 11 (1908): 44.

27 A. Looss, "What is *Schistosoma mansoni* Sambon 1907?" *Annals of Tropical Medicine and Parasitology* 2 (1908): 153–91.

28 Ibid., p. 154.
29 Ibid., pp. 156–9.
30 The egg cells and yolk-containing cells are passed into the so-called ootype before entering the "uterus." In the ootype they receive secretions that eventually lead to the production and hardening of the egg shell.
31 *Annals of Tropical Medicine and Parasitology* 2 (1908): 166.
32 Ibid., p. 191.
33 L. Sambon, "What is *Schistosoma mansoni* Sambon 1907?" *Journal of Tropical Medicine and Hygiene* 12 (1909): 1–11.
34 Ibid., quotes from pp. 4, 5, and 8.
35 Piraja da Silva, "Contributions to the study of schistosomiasis in Bahia, Brazil," English translation of original paper in *Journal of Tropical Medicine and Hygiene* 12 (1909): 159–64; "La schistosomose à Bahia," *Archives de Parasitologie* 13 (1908): 231–302.
36 Manson to da Silva, June 25, 1909. Reprinted in E. de Cerqueira Falcao, *Novas Achegas as Estudo da Determinacao da Especifidade do S. mansoni* (Rio de Janeiro, 1953). Da Silva was, according to Falcao, "the first researcher in the world really to discover and recognize *S. mansoni*." Unfortunately this argument is somewhat invalidated by da Silva's belief that his worm was neither *mansoni* nor *haematobium*, but a new species. I would like to thank Dr. E. Michelson for drawing Falcao's book to my attention.
37 A. Looss, "Some notes on the Egyptian *Schistosoma haematobium* and related forms," *Journal of Tropical Medicine and Hygiene* 14 (1911): 180.
38 Leiper to da Silva, July 2, 1909. Reprinted in Falcao, *Novas Achegas*.
39 Ibid.
40 R. Leiper, "Stale-mate in the bilharzia controversy: A new theory." *Journal of the London School of Tropical Medicine* 1 (1911): 20.
41 Looss, "Some notes," p. 181.
42 For details, see Edward Reinhard, "Landmarks in Parasitology I. The discovery of the life-cycle of the liver fluke." *Experimental Parasitology* 6 (1957): 208–32.
43 P. Manson, *Tropical Diseases: A Manual of the Diseases of Warm Climates*, 2nd ed. (London: Cassell, 1905), p. 608.
44 A. Looss, "Bemerkungen zur Lebensgeschichte der *Bilharzia haematobia* in Anschlusse an G. Sandison's Brock's Arbeit über denselben Gegendstand," *Zentralblatt für Bakteriologie und Parasitologie* 16 (1894): 342–3.
45 Looss, "What is *S. mansoni?*" 178.
46 Ibid., p 177.
47 An English translation of some of Looss's hookworm papers is given in Kean et al., *Tropical Medicine and Parasitology*, pp. 301–14.
48 Ibid., pp. 309–10.
49 F. Sandwich, *The Medical Diseases of Egypt* (London: H. Kimpton, 1905), pp. 211–40; F. C. Madden, *Bilharziosis* (London: Cassell, 1907), p. 15.
50 B. S. Elgood, "Bilharziasis among women and girls in Egypt," *British Medical Journal* 2 (October 31, 1908): 1356; Looss, "Bilharziasis of women and girls in Egypt in light of the 'skin infection theory,'" *British Medical Journal* 1 (March 27, 1909): 773–7.
51 J. Cattoi, "*Schistosoma cattoi*, a new blood fluke of man," *British Medical Journal* 1 (1905): 11–13.
52 An English summary of this very important Japanese work can be found in M. Sasa, "A historical review of the early Japanese contributions to the knowledge of schistosomiasis japonica," in M. Yokagawa (ed.), *Research in Filariasis and Schistosomiasis*, Vol. 2 (Baltimore: University Park Press, 1972). English translations of some of

these Japanese papers appear also in Kean et al. *Tropical Medicine*, Vol. 2, pp. 513–45. My summary of the events is taken from these translations.

53 A. Looss, "The life-cycle of the bilharzia worm," *Cairo Journal of Science* 4 (1910): 134–9.

54 Advisory Committee of the Tropical Disease Research Fund. *Report for the Year 1910*.

55 *Miscellaneous Papers*, CO 885/22/274. For details, see *Liverpool School of Tropical Medicine: Historical Record, 1898–1920* (Liverpool: Liverpool University Press, 1920).

56 R. J. Cottell, "Notes on cases of *Bilharzia haematobia* collected at the Royal Hospital, Chelsea," *Journal of the Royal Army Medical Corps* 18 (1912): 434–8.

57 At the first meeting of the Advisory Board of the Tropical Disease Research Fund, the London School was granted £1000 per year for five years, whereas the Liverpool School received only £500 for the same period, *Miscellaneous Papers*, CO 885/9/173, November 1, 1904.

58 Ibid., CO 885/18/202, February 1907.

59 Ross Archives, Box 33, London School of Hygiene and Tropical Medicine. This strange episode is described by E. Chernin, "Sir Ronald Ross vs. Sir Patrick Manson: A matter of libel," *Journal of the History of Medicine* 43 (1988): 262–74.

60 Meeting of the Advisory Committee, Tropical Disease Research Fund, October 24, 1913, *Miscellaneous Papers*, CO 885/22/274.

61 Parasitology provides a curious link between the frigid poles and the steamy tropics. The race for the poles took place during the same period as the race for Africa. In 1899, the Norwegian Carsten Borchgrevink opened the race for the South Pole by wintering at Cape Adare and sledging farthest south to 78° 58′. The British became involved with the 1902 National Antarctic Expedition on *The Discovery* with Robert Scott and Ernest Shackleton and the Scottish National Antarctic Expedition of the same year. Leiper worked with the Scottish expedition's parasite collection, and Atkinson was well known to the British public as the chief medical officer on Scott's 1911–12 expedition to the South Pole. He was the one who had actually found the bodies of Scott, Wilson, and Bowers. Atkinson, on his return from Antarctica in 1912, spent time at the London School working on the helminths collected by him during the Scott expedition. More detail of Atkinson and his involvement with Leiper is found in G. S. Nelson, "A milestone on the road to the discovery of the life-cycles of the human schistosomes," *American Journal of Tropical Medicine and Hygiene* 26 (1977): 1093–1100.

62 Leiper to his wife, June 7, 1914. Archives of the London School of Hygiene and Tropical Medicine.

63 K. Miyairi and M. Suzuki, "The intermediate host of *Schistosoma japonicum*." English translation in B. H. Kean and K. Mott, *Tropical Medicine and Parasitology: Classical Investigations* (Ithaca: Cornell University Press, 1978), Vol. 2, 544.

64 The Advisory Committee for the Tropical Disease Research Fund. *Report*, 1914.

65 Kitchener's reply in Foreign Office to Colonial Office, January 7, 1914, *Miscellaneous Papers*, CO 885/23/301.

66 V. Heiser, "Notes on 1915 trip," July 17, Rockefeller Foundation Archives.

67 Leiper's report to the Tropical Disease Research Fund, October 21, 1915, *Miscellaneous Papers*, CO 885/23/301.

68 *Planorbis* is one of the names by which the genus *Biomphalaria* was previously known. As I shall explain later on, there has been much time and effort wasted on classifying schistosome-carrying snails. I have decided to ignore this aspect of the bilharzia story and will try to avoid confusing the reader not familiar with snails by either using the modern names or denoting the modern name as follows: *Planorbis* [Biomphalaria]

boissyi. Of course the species names also have changed, but that I shall ignore entirely.

69 R. T. Leiper, "Report on the results of the bilharzia mission in Egypt, 1915, Part I. Transmission," *Journal of the Royal Army Medical Corps* 25 (1915): 1–55.

70 Ibid., pp. 47–8.

71 Leiper, "Report on the bilharzia mission, Part IV. Egyptian mollusca," *Journal of the Royal Army Medical Corps* 27 (1916): 175, 177.

72 Leiper, "Report on the bilharzia mission, Part V. Adults and ova," *Journal of the Royal Army Medical Corps* 30 (1918): 241.

73 Ibid., p. 243.

74 Leiper, "Report on the bilharzia mission, Part II. Prevention and eradication." *Journal of the Royal Army Medical Corps* 26 (1915): 147–92.

75 Leiper, "Report on the bilharzia mission, Part I," pp. 47–8.

76 Leiper, "Report on the bilharzia mission, Part V," pp. 248.

77 A. R. Ferguson, "Some notes on bilharziasis," *Journal of the Royal Army Medical Corps* 29 (1917): 57–65.

78 Colonial Office to Treasury, December 28, 1916, *Miscellaneous Papers*, CO 885/25/321.

CHAPTER 5 *The International Health Board*

1 At its founding, this organization was called the International Health Commission. In 1916, however, after the formation of the Rockefeller Foundation, it was renamed the International Health Board. This name was retained until 1927, when the International Health Division was formed.

2 This 1901 quotation of the Surgeon-General's report was included in a hookworm report from British Guiana, May 24, 1909, *Miscellaneous Papers*, CO 885/20/238.

3 The complex story of the hookworm in the South, including the stormy relationship between Stiles and Ashford, is best told in John Ettling, *The Germ of Laziness: Rockefeller Philanthropy and Public Health in the New South* (Cambridge, Mass.: Harvard University Press, 1981). The quotation of Stiles is taken from p. 35.

4 G. B. Wood and F. Bache, *The Dispensatory of the United States of America*, 17th ed. (Philadelphia: J. B. Lippincott, 1896).

5 *Squire's Companion to the British Pharmacopoeia* (London: Churchill, 1916).

6 This is discussed further in Ettling, *Germ of Laziness*, pp. 169–71.

7 R. Fosdick, *The Story of the Rockefeller Foundation* (New York: Harper, 1952), p. 15.

8 The Rockefeller Foundation, *Annual Report*, 1913–14, p. 11.

9 Quotation from Fosdick, *The Rockefeller Foundation*, p. 23.

10 Gates and Rose, *Founding Document of the International Health Commission*, presented to the Rockefeller Foundation on June 27, 1913. Rockefeller Foundation Archives, RG 3, Series 908, Box 11, Folder 123.

11 John Ferrell to Looss, November 14, 1913, Rockefeller Foundation Archives, RG 5, Series 1.2, Box 15, Folder 213.

12 "Correspondence relating to ancylostomiasis," *Miscellaneous Papers*, CO 885/23/297.

13 "Prevalence of ankylostomiasis in the British Empire," August 7, 1913, *Miscellaneous Papers*, CO 885/23/297.

14 Colonial Office to Colonies, etc., August 26 and October 13, 1913, *Miscellaneous Papers* CO 885/23/297.

15 "Note on ankylostomiasis in Egypt," March 1914. *Miscellaneous Papers*, CO 885/23/304.

16 Victor Heiser, "Notes on 1915 trip," p. 274, Rockefeller Foundation Archives.

17 A. F. MacCallan, "Preliminary note on the ankylostomiasis campaign in Egypt, 1914," *Foreign Office Papers*, FO 141/466/1492.

18 MacCallan to Rose, June 2, 1914, Rockefeller Foundation Archives, RG 5, Series 1.2, Box 15, Folder 214.

19 A. F. MacCallan, "Note on the ankylostomiasis campaign in Egypt, 1913–14," Rockefeller Foundation Archives, RG 5, Series 2 (812 Egypt), Special Reports, Box 61.

20 Ibid.

21 Rose to Ferrell, April 3, 1914, Rockefeller Foundation Archives, RG 5 Series 1.2, Box 15, Folder 213.

22 Rose to Foreign Office, September 6, 1915; Cairo to Foreign Office, October 25, 1915, *Foreign Office Papers*, FO 141/466/1492.

23 Cairo to Foreign Office, January 2, 1916, *Foreign Office Papers*, FO 141/466/1492.

24 H. L. Finley to Rose, July 31, 1913; Rose to Ferrell, April 3, 1914, Rockefeller Foundation Archives, RG 5, Series 1.2, Box 15, Folder 213.

25 George Cox, "Economic value of the treatment of hookworm infection in Costa Rica," Report dated November 27, 1918, Rockefeller Foundation Archives, RG 5, Series 3, Box 138, Folder 176.

26 That the activities of American foundations, such as the Rockefeller, represent a blatant form of economic and cultural imperialism has been argued many times. See, in particular, Robert Arnove (ed.), *Philanthropy and Cultural Imperialism: The Foundations At Home and Abroad* (Boston: G. K. Hall, 1980); E. Richard Brown, "Public health in imperialism: Early Rockefeller programs at home and abroad," *American Journal of Public Health* 66 (1976): 897–903; and *Rockefeller Medicine Men: Capitalism and Medical Care in America.* (Berkeley: University of California Press, 1979). I believe their analyses to be far too simplistic.

27 Elizabeth Fee, "Competition for the first school of hygiene and public health," *Bulletin of the History of Medicine* 57 (1983): 339–63. For another account of this competition from the point of view of the "loser," see Greer Williams, "Schools of public health – Their doing and undoing," *Milbank Memorial Fund Quarterly* 54 (1976): 489–527. Elizabeth Fee has now extended her study, *Disease and Discovery: A History of the Johns Hopkins School of Hygiene and Public Health, 1916–1939* (Baltimore: Johns Hopkins University Press, 1987).

28 Quoted in Fee, "Competition for the first school of hygiene," p. 351.

29 "Copy of a memorandum prepared by Dr. William H. Welch and Dr. Wickliffe Rose, outlining the need for and general plan of an Institute of Hygiene," p. 9. Chesney Medical Archives, Johns Hopkins University.

30 This report and its implications are discussed at far greater length in Fee's article, pp. 351–4, and in her book.

31 "Memorandum" from Frederick Gates to J. D. Rockefeller, forwarded to Rockefeller Snr. by his son, August 2, 1911. Copy in Chesney Medical Archives, Johns Hopkins University, Box 49.

32 *New York Tribune*, October 23, 1913; *Baltimore Evening Sun*, October 25, 1913.

33 Visit to Johns Hopkins, January 18, 1916, Rockefeller Foundation Archives, RG 1.1, Series 200, Box 184.

34 "Institute of Public Health. Final Report of the General Education Board," January 26, 1916. Copy in Welch Papers, Box 70. Chesney Medical Archives, Johns Hopkins University.

35 The Johns Hopkins University School of Hygiene and Public Health. *Preliminary Announcement*, January 1918, p. 6.

36 William Welch, Report to the Rockefeller Foundation, December 1919, Chesney Medical Archives, Johns Hopkins University.

37 The University of Illinois began, in 1868, as the Illinois Industrial University, with funds generated out of the Morrill Land Grant Act of 1862. In 1885, in keeping with a desire to broaden the base of its curriculum, the University took on its modern name, and, under the leadership of Stephen Forbes, the Zoology and Entomology Department moved to develop such fields as economic entomology, and freshwater ecology. Ward, who succeeded Forbes, brought to the campus the new field of parasitology, which fitted into both the medical and agricultural interests of the University. Details are from H. B. Ward Papers, Archives of the University of Illinois in Champaign. Among his most famous graduates were William Cort, Ernest Faust, George LaRue, Harold Manter, Justus Mueller, Thomas Magrath, Horace Stunkard, and H. van Cleave. The history of the Illinois Department is told in Harley van Cleave, "A history of the Department of Zoology in the University of Illinois," *Bios* 18 (1947): 75–97. The early history of parasitology in the United States is discussed by Calvin Schwabe, "A brief history of American parasitology: The veterinary connection between medicine and zoology," in K. S. Warren and E. Purcell (eds.), *The Current Status and Future of Parasitology* (New York: Joseph Macy, 1981); also by John Farley, "Parasites and the germ theory of disease," *Milbank Quarterly* 67 (Suppl. 1, 1989): 50–68.

38 "The reminiscences of William Walter Cort." Oral History Collection, Columbia University, 1966. A copy is also available in the archives of the American Society of Parasitology, Harold Manter Laboratory, University of Nebraska.

39 Minutes of the International Health Board, May 20, 1919, Rockefeller Foundation Archives, RG 1.1, Series 401, Box 1, Folder 8.

40 Ibid., October 25, 1921.

41 Post-Graduate Medical Committee, *Report*, London, May 1921.

42 "Proposed School of Hygiene," Ministry of Health to Trustees of the Rockefeller Foundation, August 1921, Rockefeller Foundation Archives, RG 1.1, Series 401, Box 2, Folder 10.

43 Leiper to George Vincent, January 9, 1921, Rockefeller Foundation Archives, RG 1.1, Series 401, Box 2, Folder 10.

44 For details of these events, see Donald Fisher, "Rockefeller philanthropy and the British Empire: The creation of the London School of Hygiene and Tropical Medicine," *History of Education* 7 (1978): 129–43.

45 Four major diplomas were offered by the London School, including the Diploma in Statistical Methods, the Diploma of Bacteriology, the Diploma in Public Health, and the Diploma in Tropical Medicine and Hygiene (formerly the Diploma in Tropical Medicine). By 1932, over 1,000 medical graduates and senior medical students had been granted the Diploma in Tropical Medicine and Hygiene, whereas only 127 had received the public health qualification, indicating the continued and unchanged emphasis of the London School. At the same time, Johns Hopkins had awarded 185 medical students the Certificate in Public Health (changed to the Master's of Public Health in 1931); 124 medical graduates and students the Doctor of Public Health degree; and 118 medical and science graduates the D.Sc. degree. Figures are from the London School of Hygiene and Tropical Medicine, *Annual Reports*, and "Report of Dr. Howell to the President of Johns Hopkins," 1931, Chesney Archives, Johns Hopkins Medical School.

46 Warren I. Cohen, *America's Response to China* (New York: Wiley, 1977), p. 25. Much of the background information on China is drawn from this book and from John

Fairbank, *The United States and China*, 4th ed. (Cambridge, Mass.: Harvard University Press, 1983).

47 This account of the Rockefeller work in China leading to the formation of the Peking Union Medical College is drawn from Mary Ferguson, *China Medical Board and Peking Union Medical College* (New York: China Medical Board, 1970); John Bowers, *Western Medicine in a Chinese Palace: Peking Union Medical College, 1917–51* (New York: John Macy Foundation, 1972); and Mary Bullock, *An American Transplant: The Rockefeller Foundation and Peking Union Medical College* (Berkeley: University of California Press, 1980).

48 Ferguson, *China Medical Board*, p. 17.

49 For the best account of this early period, see Bowers, *Western Medicine*.

50 "Peking Union Medical College," *China Medical Journal* 31 (1917): 568–71.

51 Editorial, *China Medical Journal* 33 (1919): 457–63.

52 An account of these week-long activities is presented in *China Medical Journal* 36 (1922): 9–43, and published separately in *Dedication Ceremonies and Medical Conference: Peking Union Medical College, September 15–22, 1921* (Peking: 1922).

53 The complete song is given in Bullock, *An American Transplant*. The British also taught the "colonials" to play British games, but were far more successful at it than the Americans. The West Indies regularly crush the English and the Australians at cricket, whereas the Americans will not even allow their "colonials" to play baseball in what they arrogantly call a "World Series!"

54 These issues have been discussed by C. C. Chen, *Medicine in Rural China* (Berkeley: University of California Press, 1989).

55 Bowers, *Western Medicine*.

56 This information is given in *China Medical Journal* 40 (1926): 699–820, a volume given over to a consideration of education.

57 I found the best account of Faust's early life in a student essay from the University of Nebraska based on an oral interview. John Bergner, "Dr. E. C. Faust," Paper for Zoology 207, March 20, 1965. A biographical record of American parasitologists is maintained with the archives of the American Society of Parasitology, housed in the Harold Manter Laboratory at the University of Nebraska in Lincoln.

58 H. B. Ward to F. C. McLean (China Medical Board), April 8, 1919, H. B. Ward Papers, University of Illinois Archives.

59 Reminiscences of Dr. John B. Grant. Transcript of interviews conducted by Saul Benison. Oral History Research Office, Columbia University. Copy in Rockefeller Foundation Archives, S. 900 Hist. Gra., Vol. 1.

60 Ernest Faust, "The present state of the schistosome problem," *China Medical Journal* 35 (1921): 405–10.

61 Henry Meleney to Faust, August 12, 1922, Faust Papers, National Library of Medicine, Bethesda, Maryland. For the British reader: "I'm from Missouri" is a strange American expression meaning "I am very skeptical," or "I have to be convinced." As a result, car license plates from Missouri carry the message "Show me!"

62 H. Meleney and E. Faust, "The intermediate host of *Schistosoma japonicum* in China. I. Its discovery in the Soochow Region," *China Medical Journal* 37 (1923): 541–5; and "II. Its distribution in China," ibid., 545–54; Faust and Meleney, "The life history of *Schistosoma japonicum*," ibid., 726–34.

63 E. C. Faust and H. E. Meleney, *Studies on Schistosomiasis Japonica, American Journal of Hygiene Monograph Series*, No. 3 (1924), pp. 171–2.

64 Ibid., pp. 254–60.

65 Meleney to Faust, July 3, 1923, Faust Papers.

66 New sites for the disease were reported in *China Medical Journal* 38 (1924): 270–6; 47 (1933): 837; 50 (1936, Suppl.): 449–56; 52 (1937): 650; 54 (1938): 159–62. Treatment campaigns were reported in ibid., 38 (1924): 276–8; 47 (1933): 1411–20. In 1925, the *China Medical Journal* became the official journal of the China Medical Association, rather than of the China Medical Missionary Association which had founded and run the journal up until that time. In 1932, the China Medical Association and the National Medical Association merged, and the journal became the *Chinese Medical Journal*.

CHAPTER 6 *Bilharzia: Optimism in Egypt (1918–1939)*

1 F. O. Lasbrey & R. B. Coleman, "One thousand cases of bilharziasis treated by antimony tartrate," *British Medical Journal* 1 (1921): 299–301. Their optimism is in contrast to Patrick Manson, *Tropical Diseases: A Manual of the Diseases of Warm Climates* (London: Cassell, 1898), p. 615.

2 J. B. Christopherson, "The successful use of antimony in bilharziosis," *Lancet* 2 (September 7, 1918): 325–7; "Intravenous injections of antimonium tartrate in bilharziosis," *British Medical Journal* 2 (December 1918): 652–3.

3 *The Dispensatory of the U.S.A.*, 18th ed. (Philadelphia: Lippincott, 1899), p. 180. A grain, based on the average weight of a grain of wheat, is equivalent to approximately 0.06 gram.

4 *Squire's Companion to the British Pharmacopoeia*, 19th ed. (London: Churchill, 1916), p. 211.

5 Lasbrey and Coleman, "One thousand cases."

6 M. Khalil, "The history and progress of anti-ankylostomiasis and anti-bilharziasis work in Egypt, Part III. Resumption of the campaign in 1919," in *Ankylostomiasis and Bilharziasis in Egypt: Reports and Notes of the Public Health Laboratories, Cairo* (Cairo: Government Press, 1924).

7 Because of Egypt's great strategic importance, the British refused to grant it total independence. But, unfortunately for Egypt, although the British were able to play off the Egyptian King, the liberals, and the nationalistic Wafd Party against one another, they were unable to negotiate a treaty that satisfied any of the parties, all of whom wanted not only to oust the British but also to control the Sudan. Finally, in 1922, the frustrated British unilaterally declared Egypt to be an independent sovereign state while at the same time retaining for themselves responsibility for the Sudan, the protection of foreign interests, and the defense of the country, including, of course, the Suez Canal. And, although the new constitution stated that all public officials were to be Egyptian, the British remained in control of the Egyptian army, and European officials were allowed to remain in service for some years. Thus, when responsibility for bilharzia and hookworm was passed to the Endemic Disease Section of the Public Health Department, in 1928, both this section and the Public Health laboratories remained under the direction of Englishmen – Dr. J. Tomb and Lt.-Col. Perry, respectively. Perry resigned in 1930, to be replaced by Dr. Ali Tewfik Shousha Bey, and, a year later, the parasite work was passed to the jurisdiction of the newly opened Research Institute and Endemic Disease Hospital headed by Leiper's protégé, Dr. Mohammed Khalil. The 1936 treaty took this so-called independence one step further by confining British troops to the Suez Canal zone, but gave them the right to reenter the country in time of war.

8 M. Khalil, "Parasitic diseases at Saft el Enab village," in *Ankylostomiasis and Bilharziasis*, pp. 159–71.

9 Khalil, "The control of bilharziasis in Egypt," in *Ankylostomiasis and Bilharziasis*, p. 96.
10 Khalil, "The history and progress," Part III, pp. 30, 32.
11 Ibid., Appendix II, p. 47.
12 M. Khalil and M. H. Betache, "The treatment of bilharziasis with a new compound 'Fouadin,'" *Lancet* (February 1, 1930): 234–5. Whatever the figures mean, they claimed a 68.6 percent cure rate with the new drug compared to 43.2 percent with tartar emetic. By 1932, Fouadin had replaced tartar emetic for use on a regular basis in the Egyptian annexes, with a claimed cure rate of 86 percent.
13 A. C. Chandler, "Control of the fluke diseases by destruction of the intermediate host," *Journal of Agricultural Research* 20 (1920): 193–208.
14 M. Khalil, "The eradication of bilharziasis," *Lancet* 2 (December 10, 1927): 1235.
15 Egypt. Ministry of the Interior, Department of Public Health, Research Institute and Endemic Disease Hospital. *Annual Reports.* Helminthological Section. *Annual Reports*, 1931 and 1936. Also M. Khalil and Abdel Azim, "On the history of the anti-bilharzial campaign in the Dakhla Oasis," *Journal of the Egyptian Medical Association* 21 (1938): 102–5.
16 R. T. Leiper, Report to the Undersecretary of Public Health on the problem of bilharzia control in Egypt, 1928 [typed manuscript], Rockefeller Foundation Archives, Barlow Papers, Series 4, Box 7, Folder 93, pp. 12–13.
17 Ibid., p. 7.
18 Heiser to Wilbur Sawyer, November 21, 1927, Rockefeller Foundation Archives, RG 1.1, Series 485H, Box 2, Folder 11.
19 Scientific Director's Meeting, International Health Division, February 4, and June 29, 1929, Rockefeller Foundation Archives, RG 1.1, Series 485H, Box 1, Folder 5.
20 Barlow to J. D. Rockefeller, Jr., October 13, 1922. Included in Welch Papers, Chesney Medical Archives, Johns Hopkins University, Baltimore.
21 J. D. Rockefeller, Jr., to Barlow, November 22, 1922, Rockefeller Foundation Archives, Barlow Papers, Series 1, Box 1, Folder 1.
22 Newspaper cutting, fall 1925, Rockefeller Foundation Archives, Barlow Papers, Series 1, Box 1, Folder 2.
23 Cort to Frederick Russell, February 13, 1929. Rockefeller Foundation Archives, RG 1.1, Series 485H, Box 1, Folder 5.
24 Russell to Barlow, May 16, 1929. Rockefeller Foundation Archives, Barlow Papers, Series 1, Box 1, Folder 2.
25 Barlow to J. Franklin (Foreign Secretary to American Baptist Mission Society), May 10, 1929, Rockefeller Foundation Archives, Barlow Papers, Series 1, Box 1, Folder 2.
26 W. W. Cort, "Schistosome dermatitis in the United States," *Journal of the American Medical Association* 90 (1928): 1027–9. Cort, years later, wrote an excellent review: "Studies on schistosome dermatitis. XI. Status of knowledge after more than twenty years," *American Journal of Hygiene* 52 (1950): 251–307. Swimmer's itch has a worldwide distribution, but is a particular nuisance where migratory bird flyways coincide with lakes frequented by North American families who build "cottages" on their banks to escape the heat of some of their cities.
27 Barlow to Victor Heiser, August 17, 1929. Encloses the report: "A suggested program for research work in Egypt resulting from a series of conferences held at Douglas Lake, Michigan. August – 1929," Rockefeller Foundation Archives, RG 1.1, Series 485H, Box 1, Folder 5.
28 Barlow to American Baptist Foreign Mission Society, November 29, 1930, Rockefeller Foundation Archives, Barlow Papers, Series 1, Box 1, Folder 3.
29 Barlow, Egyptian-Hookworm Studies, *Annual Report*, 1930. Rockefeller Foundation Archives, Barlow Papers, Series 4, Box 6, Folder 82.

30 Barlow, *Annual Report*, 1931. Rockefeller Foundation Archives, Barlow Papers, Series 4, Box 6, Folder 82.

31 Scientific Director's Meeting, International Health Division. October 29, 1932; November 1, 1935; October 29, 1936, Rockefeller Foundation Archives, RG 1.1, Series 485H, Box 1, Folder 5.

32 J. A. Scott, "Infestation rates of *S. haematobium, S. mansoni*, hookworms, and *Ascaris* in Egyptian villages following sanitation." *Preliminary Report,* October 1935, Rockefeller Foundation Archives, RG 1.1, Series 485H, Box 1, Folder 5.

33 Scott and Barlow, "Limitations to the control of helminth parasites in Egypt by means of treatment and sanitation." *American Journal of Hygiene* 27 (1938): 619–48.

34 Barlow, *First Quarterly Report*, August 28, 1930, Rockefeller Foundation Archives, Barlow Papers, Series 1, Box 1, Folder 3.

35 L. W. Hackett, *Malaria in Europe: An Ecological Study* (London: Oxford University Press, 1937). The campaign is discussed in Gordon Harrison, *Mosquitoes, Malaria and Man: A History of the Hostilities Since 1880* (New York: Dutton, 1978). Barlow received a copy of Hackett's report in July 1930.

36 Russell to Barlow, June 4, 1930, Rockefeller Foundation Archives, Barlow Papers, Series 1, Box 1, Folder 3.

37 An account of this visit is given in Barlow, *First Quarterly Report*, August 28, 1930, Rockefeller Foundation Archives, Barlow Papers, Series 1, Box 1, Folder 3.

38 Barlow, *Annual Report*, 1932, Rockefeller Foundation Archives, Barlow Papers, Series 4, Box 6, Folder 83.

39 Barlow, "The effect of the 'winter rotation' of water upon snails involved in the spread of schistosomiasis in Egypt, 1930–31 and 1931–32," *American Journal of Hygiene* 17 (1933): 724–42.

40 Barlow to Heiser, March 1, 1931, Rockefeller Foundation Archives, Barlow Papers, Series 1, Box 1, Folder 4.

41 Barlow, "The effect upon snails of clearing canals of vegetation and snails." Included in *Annual Report*, 1931, Rockefeller Foundation Archives, Barlow Papers, Series 4, Box 6, Folder 84.

42 Barlow, "The value of canal clearance in the control of schistosomiasis in Egypt," *American Journal of Hygiene* 25 (1937): 327–48.

43 Scientific Director's Meeting, November 1, 1935, Rockefeller Foundation Archives, RG 1.1, Series 485H, Box 1, Folder 5.

44 Barlow to Cort, May 22, 1932, Rockefeller Foundation Archives, Barlow Papers, Series 1, Box 1, Folder 5.

45 Cort interview with Russell, July 6, 1934. Also a series of letters passed between Cort and Russell in August 1934 (Rockefeller Foundation Archives, RG 1.1, Series 485H, Box 1, Folder 7). Cort was "astonished" by the discovery that infected snails have a very spotty distribution and that the prevalence of snail infection is so extraordinarily low in a country where so many humans carry the worm. These findings explain the difficulty experienced by earlier workers in finding the snail host, as they also raise questions about Leiper's ease in discovering infected snails in 1915.

46 Memo from George Strode, September 15, 1936. Discussed also in Scientific Director's Meeting, October 29, 1936, Rockefeller Foundation Archives, RG 1.1, Series 485H, Box 1, Folder 8.

47 Barlow, *Annual Report*, 1938. Rockefeller Foundation Archives, Barlow Papers, Series 4, Box 6, Folder 86.

48 Scientific Director's Meeting, November 6, 1939, Rockefeller Foundation Archives, RG 1.1, Series 485H, Box 1, Folder 5.

49 W. A. Sawyer to A. J. Warren, April 17, 1939, Rockefeller Foundation Archives, RG 1.1, Series 485H, Box 1, Folder 8.
50 J. A. Scott, "The incidence and distribution of the human schistosomes in Egypt," *American Journal of Hygiene* 25 (1937): 566–614.
51 "Consultation of experts on bilharziasis," Geneva, December 1938. League of Nations Health Organization, CH 1395. The Rockefeller Foundation was opposed to forming a commission, because of what they deemed to be the limited distribution and seriousness of the disease. As a result, Barlow was advised not to attend the meeting to which he had been invited.

CHAPTER 7 *Into the 1930s: Economics of disease*

1 These words are taken in part from Charles Wilson, *Ambassadors in White: The Story of American Tropical Medicine* (New York: Holt, 1942), p. 23. He wrote, "Behind every bunch of bananas stands a man, and that man cannot be a sick man." For some strange reason this book was reissued in 1972, by arrangement with the Kennikat Press, Port Washington, N.Y.
2 Gregory Mason, "The humanity of the dollar: How American business lifts backward peoples to health and happiness." *The World's Work* 54 (1927): 294–302.
3 "The native workers on the Witwatersrand gold mines," *The Mining Survey* 1 (1947): 12.
4 Mason, "The humanity of the dollar," p. 300.
5 Wilson, *Ambassadors in White*, p. 277.
6 Mason, "The humanity of the dollar," p. 302.
7 G. Mason, "Has the dollar a heart?" *The World's Work* 54 (1927): 197–207.
8 Frederick Adams, *Conquest of the Tropics* (New York: Doubleday, 1914). This book was part of a series entitled "Romance of Big Business."
9 For details see Gordon Lewis, *Puerto Rico: Freedom and Power in the Caribbean* (New York: MR Press, 1963).
10 Bailey Diffie and J. W. Diffie, *Porto Rico: A Broken Pledge* (New York: Vanguard Press, 1931).
11 John C. McClintock (1954) quoted in Robert Arnove, *Philanthropy and Cultural Imperialism: The Foundations At Home and Abroad* (Boston: G. K. Hall, 1980), p. 126.
12 A. P. Cartwright, *Doctors of the Mines* (Cape Town: Purnell, 1971), p. 2.
13 G. D. Maynard, "An enquiry into the etiology, manifestations and prevention of pneumonia amongst natives on the rand recruited from tropical areas," *Memoir No. 1, South African Institute of Medical Research* (Johannesburg, 1913).
14 Details in Marie Gorgas and Burton Hendrick, *William Crawford Gorgas: His Life and Work* (Philadelphia: Lea & Febiger, 1924).
15 Charles van Onselen, *Chibaro, African Mine Labour in Southern Rhodesia, 1900–1933* (London: Pluto Press, 1976), p. 33.
16 Quotation from ibid., p. 73.
17 "The native workers on the Witwatersrand gold mines," *The Mining Survey* 1 (1947): 3.
18 Cartwright, *Doctors of the Mines*, p. 80.
19 D. J. Bradley, "The health implications of irrigation schemes in man-made lakes in tropical environments," in R. Feachem et al. (eds.), *Water, Wastes, and Health in Hot Climates* (London: Wiley, 1977).
20 I. Gonzalez-Martinez, "Investigations on the prevalence and clinical features of intestinal bilharziasis (schistosomiasis mansoni) in Porto Rico," *New Orleans Medical Surgical Journal* 69 (1916): 352–94.

21 William Hoffman, "Studies on schistosomiasis (*S. mansoni*) in Porto Rico. I. Preliminary report on the distribution of *S. mansoni*," *Porto Rico Review of Public Health and Tropical Medicine* 3 (1927): 231–4.

22 The east–west ridge of high ground, running down the backbone of Puerto Rico, causes the prevailing northeasterly winds to drop up to 200 inches of rain on the northern slope of these hills. But south of the hills, conditions are dry, and any large-scale sugar production demands irrigation.

23 W. Hoffman and E. C. Faust, "The epidemiology and geographical distribution of schistosomiasis mansoni in Puerto Rico. 1. Epidemiology of the infection on the island," *Puerto Rico Journal of Public Health and Tropical Medicine* 9 (1933): 154–68. Nothing was done to address the problem. Instead Faust and Hoffman carried out a standard academic study of the parasite and its snail host. They described, for example, the sizes and shapes of the schistosome eggs, the structure and behavior of the released miracidia, their penetration into the snail, and the stages in the snail. Finally, using experimental rats, rabbits, and monkeys, they described the stage-by-stage migration of the young stages through the tissues into the liver and gut blood vessels.

24 This is discussed further by William Jobin, "Sugar and snails: The ecology of bilharziasis related to agriculture in Puerto Rico," *American Journal of Tropical Medicine* 29 (1980): 86–94.

25 The story of the Gezira scheme is told in Arthur Gaitskell, *Gezira: A Story of Development in the Sudan* (London: Faber and Faber, 1959); and in the much more critical Tony Barnett, *The Gezira Scheme: An Illusion of Development* (London: Frank Cass, 1977). Surprisingly, neither of these authors mentioned the bilharzia problem generated by the irrigation works.

26 I have chosen not to discuss bilharzia and the Gezira project any further than this brief introduction to it. The problem is discussed at length by Gerald Hartwig, "Schistosomiasis in the Sudan," in G. Hartwig and K. D. Patterson (ed.), *Twentieth-Century Africa: Historical Studies on West Africa and Sudan* (Los Angeles: Crossroads Press, 1984). In 1985, by which time the scheme covered over two million acres or 8,000 square kilometers, the bilharzia problem still remained. As a report noted: "For many years it has been the objective of programmes aimed at the control of schistosomiasis by means of molluscicides, but evaluation of these in terms of human infection had shown little effect." "The Blue Nile Health Project," Special edition of the *Journal of Tropical Medicine and Hygiene* 88, No. 2 (1985).

27 A. Rupert Hall and B. A. Bembridge, *Physic and Philanthropy: A History of the Wellcome Trust 1936–1986* (Cambridge: Cambridge University Press, 1986).

28 C. C. Chesterman, "The training and employment of African natives as medical assistants," *Proceedings of the Royal Society of Medicine* 25 (1932): 1068.

29 J. F. Murray, "History of the South African Institute of Medical Research," *South African Medical Journal* 37 (1963): 389–95.

30 A. H. Watt et al., *Silicosis (Miners' Phthisis) on the Witwatersrand* (Pretoria: Government Printing Office, 1913); W. Watkins-Pitchford, "The industrial diseases of South Africa," *South African Medical Record* 12 (1914): 33–50. Of the white miners, 26.1 percent also had silicosis, with an annual death rate of 13.8 per thousand.

31 Isaac Brewer, "An American school of tropical medicine: Shall there be one? Where shall it be located? What shall be its organization?" *New Orleans Medical and Surgical Journal* 60 (1907): 763–9.

32 *The Picayune*, July 2, 1911.

33 *The Times-Democrat*, July 2, 1911.

34 John Dyer, *Tulane: The Biography of a University, 1824–1965* (New York: Harper &

Row, 1966); and Tulane University of Louisiana, Medical Department, *Bulletin*, 1901–12.

35 "Dr. Wellmann quits Tulane Medical," *The Picayune*, January 14, 1914.

36 Faculty Minutes, Medical Department, Tulane University, February 10, 1914.

37 C. Kay-Scott (F. Creighton Wellman), *Life Is Too Short*, (Philadelphia: J. B. Lippincott, 1943). Wellman had one son, Creighton, by Elsie Dunn, who stayed with his father through his life. He married Pabla Pearson from Taos, New Mexico, and fathered five children, one of whom, Frederick, is the entomologist at the Nova Scotia Museum in my home town, Halifax. In 1974, Fred applied through CUSO (almost the Canadian equivalent of the VSO and Peace Corps) for a two-year position in Papua New Guinea. I chaired the interview that CUSO gives to all potential volunteers. We naturally asked him why he wanted to go to the tropics. "Well," I can still remember him saying "I really have to go because of my grandfather." And so he told us this fascinating story.

38 The story of these commissions has been told by J. Davies, "The cause of sleeping sickness? Entebbe 1902–03," *East African Medical Journal* 39 (1962): 81–99, 145–60.

39 The history of tropical medicine at Harvard is told in George C. Shattuck, *Tropical Medicine at Harvard, 1909–1954* (Boston: Harvard School of Public Health, 1955).

40 "The necessity of a department of tropical medicine at Harvard," Archives, Harvard Medical School. A general publicity and fund-raising letter which was presented to Mr. Preston of the United Fruit Company in February 1914.

41 Edward Tobey, "Tropical medicine," *The Harvard Graduates Magazine* 16 (1908): 793–5.

42 Strong to Preston, July 30, 1914. Strong Papers, Archives, Harvard Medical School.

43 "The necessity of a department at Harvard."

44 F. R. Hart to S. Schermerhorn, April 8, 1916, Strong Papers.

45 Dean Bradfield to President Lowell, March 4, 1915, Archives, Harvard Medical School.

46 List of gifts to tropical medicine and financial balance of the Department, Archives, Harvard Medical School.

47 Application for aid from Rockefeller Foundation for School of Tropical Medicine, Harvard University, March 27, 1915, Archives, Harvard Medical School.

48 R. Strong, "An institution devoted to the medical and economic interests of tropical and exotic countries," January 21, 1915, Archives, Harvard Medical School.

49 For details, see Jean Curran, *Founders of the Harvard School of Public Health, 1909–1946* (New York: Josiah Macy, Jr. Foundation, 1970); and Shattuck, *Tropical Medicine at Harvard*.

50 For a brief account of the modern period, see Eli Chernin, *Tropical Medicine at Harvard: The Weller Years, 1954–1981* (Boston: Harvard School of Public Health, 1985).

51 The George Williams Hooper Foundation. The Pacific Institute of Tropical Medicine [typewritten budget proposal for 1935, including outline of purpose, etc.]. Also A. Reed, "The first five years" [typed memo], April 20, 1934, Archives, University of California at San Francisco.

52 Alfred Reed, "Organized tropical medicine in the Western United States," *California and Western Medicine* 35 (1931): 185–9.

53 Annie Porter, "A survey of the intestinal entozoa both protozoal and helminthic, observed among natives in Johannesburg," South African Institute for Medical Research Memoir No. 11 (Johannesburg, 1918).

54 Southern Rhodesia. *Reports on Public Health for the Year 1931*.

55 *Report of the Committee Appointed To Inquire into the Training of Natives in Medicine and Public Health* (Pretoria: Government Printing Office, 1928), p. 4.

56 Ibid., p. 7.

57 The Molema episode is discussed in B. K. Murray, *WITS-The Early Years* (Johannesburg: Witwatesrand University Press, 1982).

58 For details on C. T. Loram, see R. H. Davis, "Charles C. Loram and an American model for African education in South Africa," *African Studies Review* 19 (1976): 87–99; reprinted in P. Kallaway (ed.), *Apartheid and Education* (Johannesburg: Raven Press, 1984). Loram was also a key figure on the Phelps–Stokes African Education Commissions of the early 1920s, where he was regarded as the African representative. For details of the relationship between education in the American South and in black Africa, see the essay by Edward Berman, "Educational colonialism in Africa: The role of American foundations, 1910–1945," in Robert Arnove (ed.), *Philanthropy and Cultural Imperialism* (Boston, Mass.: G. K. Hall, 1980).

59 Murray, *WITS: The Early Years.*

60 E. N. Thornton, "A medical and nursing service for natives in South Africa," *Journal of the Medical Association of South Africa* 4 (1930): 507–11.

61 C. C. Chesterman, "The training and employment of African natives as medical assistants," *Proceedings of the Royal Society of Medicine* 25 (1932): 1067–76. Chesterman was the director of a missionary hospital in the Belgian Congo who argued that although the African was intellectually capable of becoming a British-type physician, the rural problems would not be solved by such a group. They would never be content, he argued, to spend their lives in rural dispensaries. But he was more concerned about what allowing such intellectually equal Africans into the medical service would do to the prestige of the profession.

62 Annual Meeting of the Medical Association of South Africa, Durban, *Journal of the Medical Association of South Africa* 4 (1930): 505–22.

63 Memorandum of the Federal Council, Medical Association of South Africa, October 1931, *Journal of the Medical Association of South Africa* 5 (1931): 683–4.

64 W. S. Carter, "Medical education in South Africa" [typed report], Rockefeller Foundation Archives, RG 1.1, Series 487, Box 2, Folder 6.

65 R. Pearce, Internal memo, June 1, 1926, Rockefeller Foundation Archives, RG 1.1, Series 487, Box 1, Folder 3.

66 Rockefeller Foundation to C. Loram, November 13, 1929, Rockefeller Foundation Archives, RG 1.1, Series 487, Box 1, Folder 3.

67 House of Assembly, May 15, 1930, Rockefeller Foundation Archives, RG 1.1, Series 487, Box 1, Folder 4.

68 Loram to Carter, May 27, 1930, Rockefeller Foundation Archives, RG 1.1, Series 487, Box 1, Folder 4.

69 Ibid., March 1, 1932. The Rockefeller Foundation continued to be ignored by the South African Government, and their offer of £70,000 remained unacknowledged. They finally decided to withdraw their offer in 1932, but, in obvious embarrassment, were not sure to whom the letter of withdrawal should be sent!

70 "Hofmeyer details new native welfare plans: Courses for 'medical aids' at Fort Hare," *Rand Daily Mail*, April 18, 1934.

71 Quoted in A. Kerr, *Fort Hare, 1915–48* (London: C. Hurst, 1968).

72 These issues are discussed in the health reports of Southern Rhodesia, 1928–31.

73 Southern Rhodesia, *Medical Report*, 1936, pp. 10–13.

74 These figures are derived from Southern Rhodesia, *Reports on Public Health*, 1921–7.

75 William Blackie, *A Helminthological Survey of Southern Rhodesia*. London School of Hygiene and Tropical Medicine Memoir Series No. 5, 1932.

76 *Schistosoma matthei*, first described in 1929, is found mainly in domestic and wild animals in the southern part of Africa, replacing *S. bovis* which occupies the same

niche in the northern part of the continent. Humans, however, are more susceptible to the former species.

77 G. A. Turner, *Report on the Principal Diseases Existing in the Kraals of the Natives in Portuguese East Africa Territory, South of Latitude 22* (Johannesburg, 1907); "An account of some of the helminthes occurring among the South African natives," *Journal of Tropical Medicine and Hygiene* 13 (1910): 33–40, 50–9.

78 A. Porter, *The Larval Trematoda Found in Certain South African Mollusca with Special Reference to Schistosomiasis (Bilharziasis)* (Johannesburg: The South African Institute for Medical Research, 1938).

79 Details of these surveys are given in the South African Institute for Medical Research, *Annual Reports*, 1932–50.

80 Pamphlet No. 339, *Bilharzia (Human Redwater) Disease*, prepared by the Union Department of Public Health.

81 Not surprisingly, hookworm was initially blamed for poor whitism, but a survey revealed the prevalence of the worm to be low. However, the same set of surveys revealed that the disease was a problem in the mines, not only for the "East Coast Boys," nearly 50 percent of whom were infected, but more ominously for white miners who were picking up the larvae in the less than hygienic conditions in the mines. Naturally, since the whites were infected, preventive measures were immediately taken, including mass treatment of the African workers. E. Cluver, "Ancylostomiasis: Occurrence and possibility of spread in the Union of South Africa," *Journal of the Medical Association of South Africa* 2 (1928): 319–23.

82 Reports of these campaigns were given in Union of South Africa. Department of Public Health. *Annual Report*, for the years after 1927.

83 The report was issued in five volumes: Vol. 1: J. F. W. Grosskopf, *Economic Report: Rural Impoverishment and Rural Exodus*; Vol. 2: R. W. Wilcocks, *Psychological Report: The Poor White*; Vol. 3: E. G. Malherbe, *Educational Report: Education and the Poor White*; Vol. 4: W. A. Murray, *Health Report: Health Factors in the Poor White Problem*; Vol. 5: J. Albertyne and M. E. Rothmann, *Sociological Report: The Poor White Society and the Mother and Daughter in the Poor Family*. Each of these volumes is self-contained in that the joint findings and recommendations of the entire program are included.

84 Murray, *Health Report*, pp. 117–19.

85 "Joint findings and recommendations," pp. xiv and xx of each report.

86 These measures are discussed very briefly in T. H. R. Davenport, *South Africa: A Modern History* (Toronto: University of Toronto Press, 1977); and W. Vatcher, *White Laager: The Rise of Afrikaner Nationalism* (London: Pall Mall Press, 1965).

CHAPTER 8 *The 1930s: Empires in transition*

1 These records are derived from *Southern Nigeria, Annual Reports Medical Department*, 1905–14; *Northern Nigeria, Annual Reports Medical Department*, 1907–14; *Nigeria, Annual Medical and Sanitary Reports*; *Uganda Protectorate, Annual Medical and Sanitary Reports*. The latter report of 1922 includes Appendix 6, "A report on helminthiasis in the West Nile District," by R. E. McConnell.

2 These figures are derived from *Nyasaland Protectorate, Annual Medical Reports*, 1911–32.

3 W. Dye, "Schistosomiasis in the North Nyasa District with special reference to intestinal schistosomiasis," *Nyasaland Medical Report*, 1922.

4 W. Gopsill, "Some notes upon schistosomiasis in the Lower Shire district of Nyasaland," *Nyasaland Medical Report*, 1929 and 1931. There are other genera of trema-

todes that produce forked-tailed cercariae, and an inexperienced observer could easily assume them to be schistosomes.

5 E. Eldred, "Ankylostomiasis in North Nyasa District," *Nyasaland Medical Report*, 1913.

6 Quotations from Stephen Constantine, *The Making of British Colonial Development Policy, 1914–1940* (London: Frank Cass, 1984). Much of my discussion of the Empire during this period is taken from this work.

7 *House of Lords Debates*, 5th Series, Vol. 75, col. 173. This argument is made by George Abbott, "A reexamination of the 1929 Colonial Development Act," *Economic History Review* 24 (1971): 68–81. For the opposite conclusion, see E. R. Wicker, "Colonial development and welfare, 1929–1957: The evolution of a policy," *Social and Economic Studies* 7 (1958): 170–92.

8 These figures are taken from Constantine, *British Colonial Development Policy*, p. 205.

9 Advisory Committee on Colonial Development, First meeting, August 1, 1929, *Miscellaneous Papers*, CO 970/1.

10 *Nyasaland Medical Reports*, 1930, 1931, and 1932.

11 These figures are one-tenth of the present level of about 0.5 percent of the GNP, which most developed countries spend on foreign aid. Today, however, this aid is even more tightly tied to the purchase of donor goods and services than was the case with the British act.

12 Advisory Committee, 117th meeting, April 25, 1939, *Miscellaneous Papers*, CO 970/3.

13 Constantine, *British Colonial Development Policy*, p. 220.

14 Figures from E. C. Faust, "The American Society of Tropical Medicine: A brief biographical sketch," *American Journal of Tropical Medicine* 24 (1944): 69–76.

15 Articles of Incorporation, Archives American Society of Tropical Medicine, Countway Library, Harvard University Medical School.

16 Perry Burgess to the Council of American Academy of Tropical Medicine, July 17, 1934. Archives, American Society of Tropical Medicine.

17 Earl McKinley, "The development of tropical medicine in the United States," Archives, American Society of Tropical Medicine.

18 Pierce, "A carefully worked out case for tropical medicine," Director's meeting, American Foundation of Tropical Medicine, April 22, 1936, Archives, American Society of Tropical Medicine.

19 Progress report to Board members of the American Foundation and Council members of American Academy, November 11, 1937, Archives, American Society of Tropical Medicine.

20 Quotation from Fieldhouse, *Colonialism* (New York: St. Martins, 1981), p. 44.

21 These critics included Dr. Norman Leys, who practiced in Kenya and Nyasaland before his retirement in 1918. His critical writings included *Kenya* (London, 1924); and *Last Chance in Kenya* (London, 1931). For details of these critics and events of the 1930s see Constantine, *British Colonial Development Policy*; P. Hetherington, *British Paternalism and Africa, 1920–1940* (London: Frank Cass, 1978); John Flint, "MacMillan as a critic of empire: The impact of an historian on social policy," in H. MacMillan and S. Marks (eds.), *Africa and Empire: W. M. MacMillan, Historian and Social Critic* (London: Gower, 1989).

22 Constantine, *British Colonial Development Policy*, p. 259.

23 The place of Coupland is discussed by R. Robinson, "Oxford in imperial historiography," in F. Madden and D. K. Fieldhouse (eds.), *Oxford and the Idea of Commonwealth* (London: Croom Helm, 1982).

24 E. Barton Worthington, *The Ecological Century: A Personal Appraisal* (Oxford: Clarendon Press, 1983).

25 William MacMillan, *Africa Emergent* (London: Penguin, 1947), p. 34.

26 "Draft statement of policy on Colonial development and welfare," presented to Cabinet, February 15, 1940, *Colonial Office Papers*, CO 859/40/12901/Part B.

27 Colonial Office to all Colonies, February 16, 1940, *Colonial Office Papers*, CO 859/40/12901/Part I.

28 *Parliamentary Debates* (Commons), May 21, 1940, 5th Series, Vol. 361, pp. 42–5. By this time, Malcolm MacDonald had moved from the Colonial Office to become the Minister of Health in Churchill's coalition cabinet established only a week before. The bill was seen as his "swan song."

29 For details of the debate, see ibid., pp. 41–126, 1204–11; and Fifth Series, Vol. 363, p. 161. For details of the House of Lords debate, see *Parliamentary Papers* (Lords), 5th Series, Vol. 116, p. 724.

30 *Colonial Office Papers*, CO 859/40/12901, includes a set of press clippings prepared for the Colonial Secretary, Lord Lloyd.

31 *Parliamentary Debates* (Lords), April 10, 1945, Vol. 135, line 946.

32 Secretary Ickes (1935), quoted in Gordon Lewis, *Puerto Rico: Freedom and Power in the Caribbean* (New York: MR Press, 1963), p. 92.

33 Luis Marin, "The sad case of Puerto Rico," in K. Wagenheim (ed.) *The Puerto Ricans: A Documentary History* (New York: Praeger, 1973). Luis Marin, born in 1898 and brought up in the United States, eventually became the island's first elected governor.

34 J. C. Rosario, "The Porto Rico peasant," in V. Clark (ed.) *Porto Rico and Its Problems* (Washington, D.C.: The Brookings Institute, 1930), Appendix A.

35 Ibid.

36 Quoted in Bailey Diffie and J. W. Diffie, *Porto Rico: A Broken Pledge* (New York: Vanguard Press, 1931), p. 45.

37 Quoted in Clark, *Porto Rico*, p. 69.

38 Bryce Wood, *The Making of the Good Neighbor Policy* (New York: Columbia University Press, 1961), p. 4.

39 From 1936 Buenos Aires Protocol Article 1, in *Making of the Good Neighbor Policy*, p. 120.

40 Secretary's report to the Sixth Annual Meeting of the American Academy of Tropical Medicine, Archives, American Society of Tropical Medicine.

41 Secretary of American Society of Tropical Medicine to the Secretary of the American Academy of Tropical Medicine, January 31, 1940, Archives, American Society of Tropical Medicine.

42 These Latin-American scholarships were discussed at the Seventh Annual Meeting of the Academy in Louisville, 1940; the Eighth Meeting in St. Louis and Ninth Annual Meeting in Richmond. The American Foundation agreed, in its 1941 meeting, that business would be more likely to support these scholarships if North Americans were eligible. This seems to have had the desired result: In 1943, 23 Latin Americans and two North Americans held scholarships at Tulane.

43 *History of the Office of the Coordinator of Inter-American Affairs* (Washington, D.C.: U.S. Government Printing Office, 1947).

44 George Dunham, "Role of tropical medicine in international relations," *Science* 102 (1945): 105–7.

45 Charles Wilson, *Ambassadors in White: The Story of American Tropical Medicine* (New York: Holt & Co., 1942), p. 8.

46 Ibid., p. 23.

47 Ibid., p. 9.

48 Sam Zmuri gave millions of dollars to good causes. He founded the Doris Zemurray Stone Chair of English Literature at Radcliffe College in Cambridge, Massachusetts,

and gave over $1 million to Tulane University, whose President today lives in a fine old house that once belonged to Zmuri. For an inside look by an ex-public relations director of the company, see Thomas McCann, *An American Company* (New York: Crown, 1976).

CHAPTER 9 *Bilharzia: World War II*

1 Thomas Mackie, Presidential Address to Annual Meeting of the American Society of Tropical Medicine, April 1941. Archives, American Society of Tropical Medicine, Countway Library, Harvard University Medical School.
2 The Society always met with the Southern Medical Association at sites determined by that body. As a result, although interested in the tropical world, it hypocritically maintained a color bar. The subject was first broached publicly in 1944, when the Secretary of the American Society of Tropical Medicine wrote to a Captain Hakanssen, pointing out that it was a very touchy subject, that the constitution of the society did not exclude blacks, but that they were forced to meet with the Southerners because of their size and meager finances. "As long as we meet with the Southern Medical Association," he concluded, "we cannot have negros to meetings." Six years later, however, despite their larger size, they still met with the Southern Medical Association. A letter to the Secretary of the Society in 1950, reminded him that the hotel in Savannah, where the annual meeting was to be held that year, did not admit blacks. The author of the letter argued that the hotel should be told of foreign scientists attending the meeting, "such as Hindus, who might be mistaken for Negroes, although they do not have any black blood."
3 Announcement of funding presented at the General Meeting, American Society of Tropical Medicine, St. Louis, November 1944. Archives, American Society of Tropical Medicine.
4 Report of the Committee on War and Postwar Problems, July 7, 1944, Archives, American Society of Tropical Medicine; C. Stiles, "A new species of parasite in man," Third A. G. M. American Society of Tropical Medicine, 1906; Gonzalez Martinez, "Investigations on the prevalence and clinical features of bilharziasis in Puerto Rico," 13th A. G. M., 1916; Discussion, "Is the importance of intestinal parasites in tropical pathology exaggerated," *American Journal of Tropical Diseases and Preventive Medicine* 1 (1913): 169–72; A. Reed, "Schistosomiasis japonica," *American Journal of Tropical Diseases and Preventive Medicine* 3 (1915): 250–73.
5 J. S. K. Boyd, "Advances in Tropical Medicine," in V. Zachery Cope (ed.), *History of the Second World War: Medicine and Pathology*, (London: H. M. Stationery Office, 1952), Chapter 7.
6 Allan Walker, "Schistosomiasis," in *Australia in the War of 1939–45* (Canberra, 1952), Series 5: *Medical*, Vol. 1: *Clinical Problems of the War*, Chapter 13.
7 "Schistosomiasis," in *Official History of the Indian Armed Forces in the Second World War: Medical Services*, Vol. 4: *Preventive Medicine*, Chapter 29.
8 M. S. Ferguson and F. B. Bang, "Schistosomiasis," in *Medical Department of the U.S. Army: Preventive Medicine in World War II*, Vol. 5: *Communicable Diseases*, Chapter 6. This is the most detailed account of bilharzia in the war.
9 War Department Technical Bulletins dealing with schistosomiasis: *TB MED* 30 [Formosa], April 1944; ibid. 67 [Celebes], July 1944; ibid. 68 [Philippines], July 1944; ibid. 171 [Southeast China], June 1945; ibid. 179 [Mozambique], July 1945; ibid. 160 [Japan], May 1945; ibid. 214 [Egypt], February 1946; ibid. 220 [Northeast China], April 1946.

10 P. M. Mendoza-Guazon, "Schistosomiasis in the Philippines," *Philippine Journal of Science* 21 (1922): 535–67; M. A. Tubangui, "The molluscan intermediate host in the Philippines of the Oriental blood fluke, *Schistosoma japonicum*," ibid. 49 (1932): 295–304; M. A. Tubangui and A. M. Pasco, "Studies on the geographical distribution, incidence, and control of schistosomiasis japonica in the Philippines," ibid. 74 (1941): 301–27.

11 S. E. Morison. *History of the United States Naval Operations in World War II*, Vol. 12: *Leyte, June 1944–January 1945* (Boston: Little, Brown, 1958).

12 Ibid., p. 394.

13 The 118th Field Hospital Figures are taken from W. L. Winkenwerder et al., "Studies on Schistosomiasis japonica. 2. Analysis of 364 cases of acute schistosomiasis with report of results of treatment with Fuadin in 184 cases," *Bulletin of Johns Hopkins Hospital* 79 (1946): 406–35. The number of cases admitted was, in November, 4; December, 80; January, 155; February, 74; March, 24; April, 8; May, 3.

14 Ferguson and Bang, "Schistosomiasis," p. 63.

15 This account of the outbreak is derived mainly from Ferguson and Bang, "Schistosomiasis."

16 Adjutant's Report, Johns Hopkins Hospital No. 118 in Philippines and Australia, Chesney Archives, Johns Hopkins Medical School.

17 For details and examples, see Ferguson and Bang, "Schistosomiasis."

18 R. Sullivan and M. S. Ferguson, "Studies on schistosomiasis japonica III. An epidemiological study of schistosomiasis japonica," *American Journal of Hygiene* 44 (1946): 324–47.

19 T. B. Magath and D. R. Mathieson, "Important factors in the epidemiology of schistosomiasis in Leyte," *American Journal of Hygiene* 43 (1946): 152–63.

20 D. B. McMullen, "The control of schistosomiasis japonica. I. Observations on the habits, ecology, and life-cycle of *Oncomelania quadrasi*, the molluscan intermediate host of *Schistosoma japonicum* in the Philippine Islands," *American Journal of Hygiene* 45 (1947): 259–73.

21 D. B. McMullen and O. H. Graham, "The control of schistosomiasis japonica. II. Studies on the control of *Oncomelania quadrasi*, the molluscan intermediate host of *Schistosoma japonicum* in the Philippine Islands," *American Journal of Hygiene* 45 (1947): 274–93.

22 M. S. Ferguson et al., "Studies on schistosomiasis japonica V. Protection experiments against schistosomiasis japonica," *American Journal of Hygiene* 44 (1946): 367–78.

23 W. H. Wright et al., "The control of schistosomiasis japonica. VI. Studies on the chemical impregnation of uniform cloth as a protection against *Schistosoma japonica*," *American Journal of Hygiene* 47 (1948): 33–43; and "VII. Studies on the value of repellents and repellent ointments as a protection against *Schistosoma japonicum*," ibid., 44–52.

24 D. Carroll and A. V. Hunninen, "Studies on schistosomiasis japonica in the Philippine Islands. 3. A clinical study of 72 cases treated with tartar emetic," *Bulletin of Johns Hopkins Hospital* 82 (1948): 366–72. Also see Winkenwerder, "Analysis of 364 cases."

25 F. B. Bang and N. G. Hairston, "Studies on schistosomiasis japonica IV. Chemotherapy of experimental schistosomiasis japonica," *American Journal of Hygiene* 44 (1946): 348–66.

26 E. C. Faust et al., "The diagnosis of schistosomiasis japonica I. The symptoms, signs, and physical findings," *American Journal of Tropical Medicine* 26 (1946): 87–112, quotation on p. 92.

27 W. H. Wright et al., "The diagnosis of schistosomiasis japonica V. The diagnosis of

schistosomiasis japonica by means of intradermal and seriological tests," *American Journal of Hygiene* 45 (1947): 150–63.

28 These techniques dominated the reports in the *Bulletin of the U.S. Army Medical Department*: "Laboratory diagnosis of infection with *S. japonicum*," 89 (1945): 73–5; "Schistosomiasis japonica – Laboratory diagnosis," 5 (1946): 673–80.

29 G. W. Hunter et al., "Studies on schistosomiasis japonica II. Summary of further studies on methods of recovering eggs of *S. japonicum* from stools," *Bulletin of the U.S. Army Medical Department* 8 (1948): 128–31.

30 Articles on schistosomiasis japonica appeared in the *Bulletin of the U.S. Army Medical Department* 86 (1945): 23–4; 89 (1945): 73–5; 4 (1945): 57–61; 178–80; 197–202; 273–6; 5 (1946): 673–80; 8 (1948): 128–31.

31 Allan Walker, "Schistosomiasis," in *Australia in the War*.

32 Ibid., p. 219.

33 Winkenwerder, "Analysis of 364 cases."

34 J. D. Frank, "Emotional reactions of American soldiers to an unfamiliar disease," included in records of 118th General Hospital, Chesney Archives, Johns Hopkins Medical School.

35 Ferguson and Bang, "Schistosomiasis," p. 81.

CHAPTER 10 *New ideas*

1 The best general account of this movement is George Rosen, "What is social medicine? A genetic analysis of the concept," *Bulletin of the History of Medicine* 21 (1947): 674–733. Also by the same author, "What is social medicine?" in *From Medical Police to Social Medicine* (New York: Science History Publications, 1974).

2 *Malaria Commission: Report on Its Tour of Investigation in Certain European Countries in 1924* (Geneva: League of Nations Health Organization, 1925), Document C.H. 273, pp. 19, 25, 27. This confrontation has been discussed more fully in G. Harrison, *Mosquitoes, Malaria and Man: A History of the Hostilities Since 1880* (New York: Dutton, 1978); and H. Evans, "European malaria policy in the 1920s and 1930s," *Isis* 80 (1989): 40–59.

3 N. Swellengrebel, "Some aspects of the malarial problem in Italy," Annex II, in *Malaria Commission Report*, pp. 168–71.

4 *Principles and Methods of Antimalarial Measures in Europe: Second General Report of the Malaria Commission* (Geneva: League of Nations Health Organization, 1927), Document C.H./Malaria/73, p. 13.

5 For details, see Jane Lewis, *What Price Community Medicine?* (Brighton: Wheatsheaf Books, 1986).

6 J. Lewis and Barbara Brookes, "The Peckham Health Centre, "PEP," and the concept of general practice during the 1930s and 1940s," *Medical History* 27 (1983): 151–61.

7 John Ryle, "Health of the people," Radio broadcast S.A.B.C., January 21, 1948 [typed ms], Ryle Papers, File 301/2, Wellcome Institute for the History of Medicine, Oxford University.

8 John Ryle, "Social medicine: Its meaning and scope," *British Medical Journal* 2 (1943): 633–36.

9 Elizabeth Fee, "Henry E. Sigerist: From the social production of disease to medical management and scientific socialism," *Milbank Quarterly* 67 (Suppl. 1, 1989): 127–50.

10 Lord Hailey, *An African Survey: A Study of Problems Arising in Africa South of the Sahara* (London: Oxford University Press, 1938), p. 1114.

11 Ibid., p. 1122.

12 The issue is discussed in Michael Worboys, "The discovery of colonial malnutrition between the wars," in D. Arnold (ed.), *Imperial Medicine and Indigenous Societies* (Manchester: Manchester University Press, 1988), pp. 208–31. My short account of this issue is drawn from this paper.

13 John Boyd Orr and J. L. Gilks, *Studies in Nutrition: The Physique and Health of Two African Tribes* (London: H.M.S.O., 1931).

14 "Colonial Medical Policy," Conference of African Governors, 1947, Memo C.A.M.C. 6/47 Revised, *Miscellaneous Papers*, CO 994/3.

15 Quoted in Worboys, "Colonial nutrition."

16 Alan Gregg, "Statement on social medicine," June 7, 1943, Rockefeller Foundation Archives, RG 3, Series 900, Box 25, File 196.

17 G. K. Strode, "The International Health Division in the world of tomorrow," March 7, 1944; "I.H.D. excerpt from plans for the future work of the Rockefeller Foundation," November 1944, Rockefeller Foundation Archives, RG 3. Series 908, Box 13, File 135.

18 Meeting of Scientific Directors, I.H.D., October 1944, Rockefeller Foundation Archives, RG 3, Series 908, Box 16, File 194a.

19 Grant wrote an account of his and his family's early life in an untitled typed MS., housed in the Acadia University Archives, Wolfville, Nova Scotia. In addition to other material in the Acadia archives, there is "Reminiscences of Dr. John B. Grant," a transcript of interviews conducted by Saul Benison, Oral History Research Office, Columbia University. The draft I consulted is housed in the Rockefeller Archives, Series 900, History Grant. My account is taken from these sources and from Mary Bullock, *An American Transplant: The Rockefeller Foundation and Peking Union Medical College* (Berkeley: University of California Press, 1980). See also John Farley, "John Black Grant (B.A. 1912): The Rockefeller Bolshevik," *Acadia University Alumni Bulletin*, Vol. 74, 1990.

20 Selskar Gunn, "China and the Rockefeller Foundation," January 23, 1934, Rockefeller Foundation Archives, RG 3, Series 900, Box 22, File 169. This aspect of the Rockefeller's work in China is explored more fully in Mary Bullock, *An American Transplant*.

21 John Grant, "Medical care," Memo for Scientific Directors' meeting, September 1946, Rockefeller Foundation Archives, RG 3, Series 900, Box 25, File 197.

22 Grant, "Reminiscences," Vol. 6. The report, "International Trends in Health Care" in which he failed to mention his visit to South Africa, was presented to the Scientific Directors in their December 1947 meeting, Rockefeller Foundation Archives, RG 3, Series 900, Box 25, File 198. It was eventually published in *American Journal of Public Health* 38 (1948): 381–97.

23 Henry Gluckmann, Speech to South African Parliament, February 17, 1942. Details in Henry Gluckmann, *Abiding Values* (Johannesburg: Caxton Press, 1970), pp. 411–27.

24 "Draft of Medical Association of South Africa to National Health Commission," *South African Medical Journal* 17 (1943): 199–206. This draft was approved by the membership, 789 votes to 72.

25 *The Health of the Nation: A Summary of the Report of the National Health Service Commission*, New Africa Pamphlet No. 6 (Johannesburg: South Africa Institute of Race Relations, 1946), Part 1, Chapter 3.

26 Ibid., Part 2, p. 7.

27 Ibid., Part 2, p. 9.

28 Ibid., Part 1, Chapter 3.

29 Editorial, "The Health Commission's Report," *South African Medical Journal* 19 (1945): 17.

30 Meeting of Federal Council, February 3, 1945, *South African Medical Journal* 19 (1945): 65–7.

31 Government Statement of Policy, October 9, 1944, *South African Medical Journal* 20 (1946): 538.

32 Union of South Africa, Department of Public Health, *Annual Report for 1947* (Pretoria: 1947).

33 J. B. Grant, "International trends in health care," p. 2. Also "Trends of health care in social welfare," *The Almoner* 2 (1949): 1–7.

34 R. F. Chester Barnard, "Memo to Commission on Review," March 7 and April 13, 1950, Rockefeller Foundation Archives, RG 3, Series 908, Box 13, File 140. Similar ideas are to be found in Files 142 and 143.

35 "Report of the Rockefeller Foundation Commission on Review of the International Health Division," November 1951, Rockefeller Foundation Archives, RG 3, Series 908, Box 14, File 147.

36 These figures were presented in the 1951 report. Other expenses of the Foundation included $36.6 million on the natural sciences, $53.9 million on the social sciences, and $22.9 million on the humanities.

37 Brock Chisholm, "The W.H.O.," *British Medical Journal* 1 (May 6, 1950): 1021–7.

38 Grant, "International trends," p. 19.

CHAPTER 11 *Bilharzia: Pessimism in Egypt (1940–1955)*

1 A. Hallawani, "Obituary to Mohammed Khalil Abdel Khalik Bey," *Journal of the Egyptian Medical Association* 33 (1950): 864–8.

2 Barlow to Minister of Public Health, September 8, 1939, Rockefeller Foundation Archives, Barlow Papers, Series 1, Box 1, Folder 8.

3 Khalil's version of the affair is to be found in M. Khalil, "The national campaign for the treatment and control of bilharziasis from the scientific and economic aspects," *Journal of the Royal Egyptian Medical Association* 32 (1949): 817–56.

4 Barlow to Dr. A. Warren, October 10, 1939, Rockefeller Foundation Archives, Barlow Papers, Series 1, Box 1, Folder 8.

5 Barlow to his wife, October 24, 1939, Rockefeller Foundation Archives, Barlow Papers, Series 1, Box 1, Folder 8.

6 Barlow's story of the affair is told in "The status of Dr. Barlow's contract with the Egyptian Government," memo to the American Ambassador to Egypt, April 1941, Rockefeller Foundation Archives, Barlow Papers, Series 1, Box 1, Folder 10.

7 Barlow, "The status of the Bilharzia Snail Destruction Section," copy included in memo to the American Ambassador, Rockefeller Foundation Archives, Barlow Papers, Series 1, Box 1, Folder 10.

8 Khalil, "The credit of Bilharzia Destruction in the Fayum. The requests of Dr. Barlow." English translation in Barlow, memo to the American Ambassador, Rockefeller Foundation Archives, Barlow Papers, Series 1, Box 1, Folder 10.

9 Hussein Sirry to Ahmed Helmy, February 9, 1941. English translation in Barlow, memo to the American Ambassador, Rockefeller Foundation Archives, Barlow Papers, Series 1, Box 1, Folder 10.

10 Barlow to Ali Shousha, March 8, 1941, in memo to the American Ambassador, Rockefeller Foundation Archives, Barlow Papers, Series 1, Box 1, Folder 10.

11 Ali Shousha to Barlow, March 16, 1941, in Barlow, memo to the American Ambassador, Rockefeller Foundation Archives, Barlow Papers, Series 1, Box 1, Folder 10.

12 Barlow, "Myself," undated typed document, Rockefeller Foundation Archives, Barlow Papers, Series 3, Box 5, Folder 71.

13 Barlow, untitled, undated typed document, Rockefeller Foundation, Archives, Barlow Papers, Series 1, Box 1, Folder 8.

14 *First Annual Report of the Bilharzia Snail Destruction Section* (Cairo, 1945).

15 *Seventh Annual Report of the Bilharzia Snail Destruction Section* (1948–9), pp. 4–5.

16 Ali Shousha, "Schistosomiasis (bilharziasis), a world problem," *Bulletin of the WHO* 2 (1949): 19–30. M. Khalil, "The national campaign . . ."

17 Shousha, "Schistosomiasis," p. 26.

18 Ibid, p. 28.

19 Khalil, "The national campaign," p. 843.

20 Ibid., p. 845.

21 Ibid., p. 843.

22 Ibid., p. 849.

23 Barlow, "A reply to Prof. Khalil's article," unpublished memo, Rockefeller Foundation Archives, Barlow Papers, Series 5, Box 8.

24 Barlow, "Bilharzia work in China," Rockefeller Foundation Archives, Barlow Papers, Series 2, Box 2, Folder 18.

25 Khalil, "The national campaign," p. 850.

26 M. F. Abdel-Wahab, *Schistosomiasis in Egypt* (Boca Raton, Fla: CRC Press, 1982).

27 For details of Soper's work, see G. Harrison, *Mosquitoes, Malaria and Man: A History of the Hostilities Since 1880* (New York: E. P. Dutton, 1978).

28 G. Strode to F. Soper, November 12, 1946, Rockefeller Foundation Archives, RG 1.2, Box 1003, unprocessed Series 485J, "Rural Health Service."

29 J. M. Weir, *Report on the Medical Services and Public Health Facilities of Egypt,* 1948, Rockefeller Foundation Archives, RG 1.2, Box 1003, unprocessed Series 485J, "Rural Health Services." In this report he made the important remark that although treatment did little to reduce the prevalence of the disease, it had reduced the complications that arise in nontreated cases.

30 Scientific Directors' Meeting, International Health Division, October 31, 1947, Rockefeller Foundation Archives, bound Minutes Books.

31 Docket Item for Egypt in 1948, Rockefeller Foundation Archives, RG 1.2, Box 1003, unprocessed Series 485J, "Rural Health Service."

32 D. B. Wilson to G. Strode, August 7, 1947, covering letter with docket item for Egypt in 1948, Rockefeller Foundation Archives, RG 1.2, Box 1003, unprocessed Series 485J, "Rural Health Service."

33 J. M. Weir, "Sanitation and health in rural Egypt," Report of interview with J. M. Weir, 1953. Rockefeller Foundation Archives, RG 1.2, Box 1003, unprocessed Series 485J, "Rural Health Service."

34 J. M. Weir, I. M. Wasif, F. R. Hassan, S. Din Moh, and M. Kader, "An evaluation of health and sanitation in Egyptian villages," *Journal of the Egyptian Public Health Association* (1952): 55–114.

35 Diaries of John Weir, Rockefeller Foundation Archives. I had the pleasure of visiting Dr. Weir in 1987, at which time he graciously granted me permission to read his diaries.

36 Ibid., entries for October 27 and December 21, 1949, and March 27, 1950.

37 Weir et al., "An evaluation of health," p. 76.

38 Ibid., p. 109.

39 Ibid., p. 92.

40 *New York Times*, May 1 and 5, 1952. The major story was also published in *The Times* of London and Cairo's *El Ahram*.

41 Hugh Smith, June 3, 1952, Rockefeller Foundation Archives, RG 1.2, Box 1003, unprocessed Series 485J, "Rural Health Service."

42 H. Baity (WHO) to R. Burden, December 16, 1954, Rockefeller Foundation Archives, RG 1.2, Box 1003, unprocessed Series 485J, "Rural Health Service."

43 M. C. Balfour to A. J. Warren, July 15, 1952. Rockefeller Foundation Archives, RG 1.2, Box 1003, unprocessed Series 485J, "Rural Health Service."

44 Minister of Health, Israel, to Rockefeller Foundation, September 10, 1956. Rockefeller Foundation Archives, RG 1.2, Box 1003, unprocessed Series 485J, "Rural Health Service."

45 Weir to Warren, February 2, 1952, Rockefeller Foundation Archives, RG 1.2, Box 1003, unprocessed Series 485J, "Rural Health Service." Unfortunately, I have been unable to locate this film in any of the American archives.

46 Weir, "Sanitation and health in rural Egypt," p. 22.

47 Weir et al., "An evaluation of health," p. 110.

48 Quoted in letter from R. Burden to H. Baity, December 9, 1954, Rockefeller Foundation Archives, RG 1.2, Box 1003, unprocessed Series 485J, "Rural Health Service."

49 Tarraf to Rockefeller Foundation, October 1954, Rockefeller Foundation Archives, RG 1.2, Box 1003, unprocessed Series 485J, "Rural Health Service."

50 J. Grant, "The place of the health centre in providing adequate health care," Memo of April 1949, Rockefeller Foundation Archives, RG 3, Series 900, Box 25, Folder 198.

CHAPTER 12 *Bilharzia: Victory in China?*

1 Tien Hsi-cheng, "Schistosomiasis in mainland China. A review of research and control programs since 1949," *American Journal of Tropical Medicine* 20 (1971): 26–53.

2 F. Kierman, "The blood fluke that saved Formosa," *Harper's Magazine* (April 1959): 45–7. A less polemic account is given by Wu Zhili, "Brief history of medical service in Chinese People's Liberation Army." Typed manuscript. Uniformed Services University of the Health Sciences, Bethesda. I would like to thank Col. Robert Joy for showing this manuscript to me.

3 Editorial, *Chinese Medical Journal* 67 (1949): 397. For general discussion of health care in China, I have used David Lampton, *The Politics of Medicine in China* (Folkestone, J. K.: Dawson, 1977).

4 C. Ling, W. Cheng, and H. Chung, "Clinical and diagnostic features of schistosomiasis japonica," *Chinese Medical Journal* 67 (1949): 347–66.

5 "Our journal" [Editorial], *Chinese Medical Journal* 69 (1951): 1–2.

6 F. Lien-chang, "Summing up report on the activities of the Chinese Medical Association since the Eighth General Conference," Report given to the Ninth General Conference, Peking, August 1952, *Chinese Medical Journal* 71 (1953): 229–40.

7 F. Lien-chang, "Learning from advanced Soviet medicine," *Chinese Medical Journal* 71 (1953): 241–7.

8 Kung Nai-chuan, "New China's achievements in health work," *Chinese Medical Journal* 73 (1955): 87–92.

9 "Some aspects of research in the prevention and treatment of schistosomiasis japonica in New China," *Chinese Medical Journal* 73 (1955): 100–6.

10 *Handbook of the Prevention and Treatment of Schistosomiasis*, English translation, U.S. Department of Health, Education and Welfare (Publication No. NIH 77-1290, 1977).

11 This account of the campaign is taken from Ch'ien Hsin-chung, "Summing up of mass technical experiences with a view to expediting eradication of the five major parasitic diseases," *Chinese Medical Journal* 77 (1958): 521–32. The campaign has been discussed also by F. R. Sandbach, "Farewell to the God of Plague – The control of schistosomiasis in China," *Social Science and Medicine* 14 (1977): 27–33.

12 Hsin-chung, "Summing up," p. 523.

13 News and Notes, *Chinese Medical Journal* 77 (1958): 103.

14 Ibid., p. 513.

15 Wei Wen-po, "The people's boundless energy during the current leap forward. 1. New victories on the anti-schistosomiasis front." *Chinese Medical Journal* 77 (1958): 107–11.

16 Mao Tse-tung, "Farewell to the God of Plague," printed in *Chinese Medical Journal* 1 (1973): 81–2. Quoted by permission of the Chinese Medical Association.

17 "All-China Conference on Parasitic Diseases," *Chinese Medical Journal* 77 (1958): 519–20.

18 "Our leap forward," *Chinese Medical Journal* 77 (1958): 1–2.

19 "Let the technical revolution in medicine, pharmacology and public health blossom and yield fruit," reprinted in *Chinese Medical Journal* 78 (1959): 1–3.

20 Li Teh-chuan, "Ten years of public health in New China," *Chinese Medical Journal* 79 (1959): 483–8.

21 "Battle against schistosomiasis" [reprint of article in *Red Flag*], *Chinese Medical Journal* 80 (1960): 299–305.

22 Hsu Yun-pei, "Advance the great work of protecting the people's health," *Chinese Medical Journal* 80 (1960): 405–14.

23 Lampton, *Politics of Medicine*, p. 118.

24 Ibid., p. 131.

25 *People's Daily*, January 24, 1964. Quoted in Lampton, *Politics of Medicine*, p. 173.

26 Quoted in Lampton, *Politics of Medicine*, pp. 185–6. In fact, rural health teams were sent out for a few months at a time from the urban centres before the speech was delivered. See "Medical service in the countryside" [Editorial], and Huang Chia-su, "Our medical team in the countryside," *Chinese Medical Journal* 84 (1965): 799–803.

27 "Apply Chairman Mao's teaching and do an even better job in the service of the workers, peasants and soldiers" [Editorial], *Chinese Medical Journal* 85 (1966): 73–8. Health care during the Cultural Revolution is discussed in S. M. Hillier and J. Jewell, *Health Care and Traditional Medicine in China, 1800–1982* (London: Routledge, 1983).

28 "Apply Chariman Mao's Teaching" [Editorial]; and "Health work serving the peasants: Chang Kai, Vice-Minister of Health, on why and how medical services are directed to the countryside," *Chinese Medical Journal* 85 (1966): 143–9. Also discussed in Lampton, *Politics of Medicine*.

29 Ruth and Victor Didel, *The Health of China* (London: Zed Press, 1983).

30 Ch'ien Hsin-chung, "Prelude to the great march of orientating health work towards the rural areas. Some questions concerning the work of the rural mobile medical teams," *Chinese Medical Journal* 85 (1966): 209–22.

31 Ts'ao Feng-kang, "The second half of my life shall be dedicated to rural health work," *Chinese Medical Journal* 85 (1966): 532–5.

32 Editorial, "Never forget the class struggle," *Chinese Medical Journal* 85 (1966): 362–7. The same volume of the journal reprinted also editorials from the *Liberation Army Daily* and the *People's Daily* dealing with the same issues: "routing the bourgeois specialists, scholars, authorities, venerable masters," "holding high the great red

banner," and sweeping away "all monsters." These articles included such titles as "Hold high the great red banner of Mao Tse-tung's thought and actively participate in the great socialist Cultural Revolution"; "Sweep away all monsters"; "Long live Mao Tse-tung's thought"; "Long live the great proletarian revolution"; "A new stage of socialist revolution in China."

33 "Profound revolution on the health front," *Chinese Medical Journal* 1 (1975): 311–14. Between 1967 and 1972 the journal ceased publication, and in 1973 and 1974 changed its long-standing language policy by publishing articles only in Chinese, with English text reduced to short abstracts.

34 *Chinese Medical Journal* 2 (1976), September issue.

35 Ibid., p. 347.

36 United Nations Relief Organization, quoted in S. M. Hillier and J. A. Jewell, *Health Care*.

37 Sandbach, "Farewell to the God of Plague," p. 27.

38 Paul Basch, "Schistosomiasis in China: An update," *American Journal of Chinese Medicine* 14 (1986): 17–25.

39 "Report of the American Schistosomiasis Delegation to the People's Republic of China," *American Journal of Tropical Medicine and Hygiene* 26 (1977): 427–57.

40 Hsi-cheng, "Schistosomiasis in mainland China," p. 48.

41 J. S. Horn, *Away with All Pests: An English Surgeon in People's China, 1954–1969* (New York: Monthly Review Press, 1969).

42 James Grant, Foreword to C. C. Chen, *Medicine in Rural China* (Berkeley: University of California Press, 1989), p. xi.

CHAPTER 13 *The new British Empire: Finding the experts*

1 British policy toward higher education for the African is discussed in Eric Ashby's definitive study, *Universities: British, Indian, African – A Study in the Ecology of Higher Education* (Cambridge, Mass.: Harvard University Press, 1966).

2 *Report of the Advisory Committee on Native Education in the British Tropical African Dependencies*, 1925. Parliamentary Papers. Cmd 2374.

3 Personnel reports from Southern Nigeria, *Annual Reports of the Medical Department*, (1905–1914). Also Ralph Schram, *A History of the Nigerian Health Services* (Ibadan, Nigeria: Ibadan University Press, 1971).

4 Uganda Protectorate, *Annual Medical and Sanitary Report for the Year 1923*.

5 Ibid., 1926.

6 H. B. Owen, Report on the Uganda Medical School, Mulago. In Uganda Protectorate. *Annual Medical and Sanitary Report for the Year 1928*, Appendix II.

7 Proposal from the Government of Uganda to Ormsby–Gore Committee, 1924, in Ashby, *Universities*, p. 192.

8 Owen, "Medical education in Uganda," *Tropical Disease Bulletin* 30 (1933): 659–68.

9 N. Fendall, "A history of the Yaba School of Medicine, Nigeria," *West African Medical Journal* 16 (1967): 118–24. Reports on the school also in Nigeria, *Annual Medical and Sanitary Reports*, 1933 and 1934.

10 H. B. Owen, "Medical education."

11 Ashby, *Universities*, p. 234.

12 Obafemi Awolowo, *Awo: The Autobiography of Chief Obafemi Awolowo* (Cambridge: Cambridge University Press, 1960). For details of the political activities of missionary-trained African physicians, see A. Adeloye, "Nigerian pioneer doctors and early West African politics," *Nigeria Magazine* 121 (1976): 2–24; and *African Pioneers of*

Modern Medicine: Nigerian Doctors of the 19th Century (Ibadan, Nigeria: Ibadan University Press, 1985).

13 E. B. Worthington, *Science in Africa: A Review of Scientific Research Relating to Tropical and Southern Africa* (London: Oxford University Press, 1938), pp. 490–8.

14 Ibid., p. 505.

15 Lord Hailey, *An African Survey* (London: Oxford University Press, 1938).

16 Roger Jeffery, "Recognizing India's doctors: The institutionization of medical dependency, 1918–1939," *Modern Asian Studies* 13 (1979): 301–26.

17 The Currie Report, December 1933; reprinted in Ashby, *Universities*, pp. 476–81.

18 *Higher Education in East Africa: Report of the Commission Appointed by the Secretary of State for the Colonies*, September 1937, in Ashby, *Universities*, pp. 197–200.

19 Ashby, *Universities*, p. 203.

20 These issues were reported in Uganda, *Annual Report of the Medical Department*, 1936–40.

21 Nigeria, *Annual Medical and Sanitary Reports*, 1937 and 1938.

22 The four commissions were *Report of the Commission on Higher Education in the Colonies*, 1945 (chair: Mr. Justice Asquith). British Parliamentary Papers, Cmd. 6647; *Report of the Commission on Higher Education in West Africa*, 1943 (chair: W. Elliot), Cmd. 6655; *Report of the West Indies Committee of the Commission on Higher Education in the Colonies* (chair: J. Irvine), Cmd. 6654; *Report of the Commission on University Education in Malaya*, 1948, Col. 229.

23 The Asquith Commission.

24 *Interuniversity Council for Higher Education Overseas*, Report, 1946–54. Parliamentary Papers, Cmd. 9515 (1955). This story is told in M. MacPherson, *They Built for the Future: A Chronicle of Makerere University College, 1922–62* (Cambridge: Cambridge University Press, 1964); K. Mellanby, *The Birth of Nigeria's University* (London: Methuen, 1958); J. T. Saunders, *University College Ibadan* (Cambridge: Cambridge University Press, 1960).

25 Ashby, *Universities*, p. 218.

26 Hailey, *African Survey*, p. 1611.

27 Worthington, *Science in Africa*, p. 23.

28 Hailey, *African Survey*, p. 1662.

29 *Nutrition in the Colonial Empire*, First Report, 1939, Cmd. 6050, p. 133. The report was summarized in *British Medical Journal* 2 (1939): 294–6.

30 Michael Worboys, "The discovery of colonial malnutrition between the wars," in David Arnold (ed.), *Imperial Medicine and Indigenous Societies* (Manchester: Manchester University Press, 1988).

31 Hailey, *African Survey*, p. 1628.

32 Minutes of meeting of East African Medical Research Scientific Advisory Committee, January 12, 1960, *Miscellaneous Papers*, CO 913/11.

33 Memorandum by the Colonial Advisory Medical Committee on Medical Research in the Colonies. Memo C.A.M.C. 22/43. January 7, 1944, *Miscellaneous Papers*, CO 994/3.

34 Colonial Research Committee, *Progress Report*, 1944–45, Cmd. 6663, p. 7.

35 Ibid., p. 10.

36 Third reading of the Colonial Development and Welfare Bill, February 16, 1945, *Parliamentary Debates* (Commons), 5th Series, Vol. 408, line 541. Many members were also conscious of the monetary assistance given by the Rockefeller Foundation to fight disease and were anxious to end that embarrassing dependence.

37 Ibid., Col. Stanley, line 552.

38 *Parliamentary Debates* (Lords), April 10, 1945, 5th Series, Vol. 135, line 936.

39 *Parliamentary Debates* (Commons), February 7, 1945, 5th Series, Vol. 407, line 2121.

40 *Parliamentary Debates*, (Lords), April 10, 1945. 5th Series, Vol. 135, line 932.
41 "Colonial Research Fellowships," Appendix II, *Colonial Research, 1948–49*, Colonial Research Council, Cmd. 7739.
42 Colonial Medical Research Committee, Eighth meeting, June 12, 1946, *Miscellaneous Papers*, CO 913/1.
43 Colonial Medical Research Committee, 13th Meeting, March 24, 1947, *Miscellaneous Papers*, CO 913/2.
44 The Colonial Office's proposal, "Colonial Research Service: Proposals for Terms of Service," was presented to the Committee on May 10, 1947. It was discussed critically at the Committee's May meeting and a memo presented to the Colonial Office (Memo CMR 47/19. June 23, 1947), *Miscellaneous Papers*, CO 913/2.
45 Colonial Office reply (Memo CMR 47/22. June 24, 1947), *Miscellaneous Papers*, CO 913/2.
46 Colonial Medical Research Committee, First Annual Report, 1945–6, *Colonial Office Papers*, Col. No. 208.

CHAPTER 14 *South Africa (1950–1960): Social medicine versus scientific research*

1 For a detailed discussion of the South African National Health Service, see Shula Marks and Neil Anderson, "Industrialization, rural health and the 1944 National Health Services Commission in South Africa," in S. Feierman and J. Janzen (eds.), *Health and Society in Africa* (Berkeley: University of California Press, in press).
2 See, in particular, *South African Medical Journal* 19 (1945): 121, 159, 161, 199–200, 367.
3 D. O'Keeffe, "Medical practitioners in chains," *South African Medical Journal* 19 (1945): 199–200.
4 Dr. A. Sweetapple, Presidential Address. *South African Medical Journal* 21 (1947): 203–6.
5 "Objections to draft ordinances of Transvaal and Cape re public hospitals," *South African Medical Journal* 20 (1946): 537.
6 Dr. Sweetapple, "Civil servants with a bedside manner," *South African Medical Journal* 22 (1948): 235–7.
7 Henry Gluckmann, "National Health Service," *South African Medical Journal* 20 (1946): 655–63.
8 Press statement, December 5, 1946. *South African Medical Journal* 20 (1946): 800.
9 "Statement of policy," *South African Medical Journal* 21 (1947): 62–3.
10 Press statement, *South African Medical Journal* 22 (1948): 237.
11 G. Gale, "Health Centre practice in relation to private practice: A memorandum," *South African Medical Journal* 22 (1948): 370–2.
12 *Summary of the Report of the Commission for the Socio-Economic Development of the Bantu Areas Within the Union of South Africa*, Union Government Report No. 61 (1955).
13 W. E. Barker, "Apartheid – The only solution," *Journal Racial Affairs* 1 (1949): 27. The division of Nationalist opinion was discussed in John Lazer, "The role of the South African Bureau of Racial Affairs in the formulation of apartheid ideology, 1948–61," in a paper to a postgraduate seminar at the Institute of Commonwealth Studies, University of London. I remain extremely grateful to Dr. Shula Marks for her invitation to attend these seminars.
14 Quoted in Lazer, "The role of the South African Bureau of Racial Affairs."
15 For details see David Smith, *UPDATE: Apartheid in South Africa* (Cambridge: Cambridge University Press, 1987).

16 K. Hartshorne, *Native Education in the Union of South Africa: A Summary of the Report of the Commission on Native Education in South Africa.* U.G. 53–1951 (Johannesburg: Institute of Race Relations, 1953).

17 *Report of the Commission on the Separate University Education Bill* (Parow: Cape Times, 1958). This Commission was preceded by the Holloway Commission which was asked to report on separate training facilities for non-Europeans at universities.

18 Minister of Education to Malherbe, February 26, 1957, Rockefeller Foundation Archives, RG 1.2, Series 487, Box 1005, folder unprocessed, "University Natal Family Practice." For further details see E. H. Brookes, *A History of the University of Natal* (Pietermaritzburg, Natal: University of Natal Press, 1966).

19 Rockefeller Foundation Archives, RG 1.2, Series 487A, Box 1005, (unprocessed material, "University of Natal Medical School,") contains all this material. For histories of the Durban Medical School, see I. Gordan, "The Durban Medical School," *South African Medical Journal* 34 (1960): 414–16; B. T. Naidoo, "A history of the Durban Medical School," ibid. 50 (1976): 1625–8.

20 D. F. Malan, quoted in G. C. Oosthuizen, *Challenge to a South African University: The University of Durban-Westville* (London: Oxford University Press, 1981).

21 S. L. Kark, "Family and community practice in the medical curriculum," *Journal of Medical Education* 34 (1959): 905–10.

22 Docket Item, "Durban Medical School, University of Natal, Union of South Africa," June 12, 1954, Rockefeller Foundation Archives, "University of Natal Family Practice."

23 Gale to Warren, June 14, 1954, Rockefeller Foundation Archives, "University of Natal Family Practice."

24 Foundation to Malherbe, September 24, 1954, Rockefeller Foundation Archives, "University of Natal Family Practice."

25 "Grant from the Rockefeller Foundation to the Durban Medical School" [Press release], Rockefeller Foundation Archives, "University of Natal Family Practice."

26 G. Gale to R. Morrison, January 24, 1955, Rockefeller Foundation Archives, "University of Natal Medical School."

27 Kark to Malherbe, April 4, 1957; Malherbe to Rockefeller Foundation, April 24, 1957, Rockefeller Foundation Archives, "University of Natal Family Practice." Kark was also Jewish, well aware of Prime Minister Verwoerd's anti-Semitism and support for the Nazis during World War II.

28 Thereafter the Durban Medical School was left untouched until the decision to phase out African students was finally implemented in 1976. In its place, the government opened the Medical University of Southern Africa (MEDUSA) near Pretoria, which admitted its first African students in 1978.

29 Weir report to the Rockefeller Foundation, April 1960. Rockefeller Foundation Archives, "University of Natal Family Practice."

30 General Circular from the Secretary for Bantu Administration and Development, December 12, 1967. Appendix II in Donald Moerdijk, *Anti-Development: South Africa and Its Bantustans* (UNESCO, 1981).

31 For details of these settlements, see Moerdijk, *Anti-Development,* Appendix II.

32 Many of these health figures are presented in *Apartheid and Health* (Geneva: WHO, 1983).

33 This aspect of South African health policy is discussed in S. Marks and N. Andersson, "Typhus and social control: South Africa, 1917–50," in R. MacLeod (ed.), *Disease, Medicine and Empire* (London: Routledge, 1988).

34 S. Annecke, R. J. Pitchford, and A. Jacobs, "Some further observations on bilharziasis in the Transvaal," *South African Medical Journal* 29 (1955): 314–23.

35 "Resolution of the Urological Section of the Medical Association of South Africa, presented to meeting of Federal Council, October 1947," *South African Medical Journal* 21 (1947): 875.

36 R. J. Pitchford, "Bilharzia and its control in relation to waters of the northern and eastern Transvaal lowvelt," *Public Health [Johannesburg]*, 17 (1953): 339–41, 345.

37 G. C. Thomson, "Cytoscopic examination in the Witwatersrand Native Labour Association Hospital," *Proceedings of the Transvaal Mine Medical Officers Association* 31 (1951): 12–14.

38 B. de Meillon, "Aspects of the natural history of bilharzia in South Africa," *South African Medical Journal* 22 (1948): 253–60.

39 J. A. Keiser, "Schistosomiasis: An educational problem," *South African Medical Journal* 21 (1947): 854.

40 F. G. Loveridge, W. F. Ross, and D. M. Blair, "Schistosomiasis: The effect of the disease on educational attainment," *South African Medical Journal* 22 (1948): 260–2.

41 B. de Meillon and S. Patterson, "Experimental bilharziasis in animals. VI. The effect of bilharziasis on growth, reproduction, and longevity in white mice," *South African Medical Journal* 31 (1957): 281.

42 H. I. Lurie, "Experimental bilharziasis in animals. V. Immunity in mice produced by repeated small infections." *South African Medical Journal* 31 (1957): 68–9.

43 R. J. Pitchford, "Observations on the mass treatment of bilharziasis in South Africa," *Bulletin of the WHO* 18 (1958): 1112–13.

44 B. de Meillon and S. Patterson, "Effect of a low protein diet on bilharziasis in white mice," *South African Medical Journal* 32 (1958): 1086–8.

45 W. B. DeWitt, "Experimental schistosomiasis mansoni in mice maintained on nutritionally deficient diets. I. Effects of a torula yeast ration deficient in factor 3, vitamin E, and cystine." *Journal of Parasitology* 43 (1957): 119–28; and "II. Survival and development of *Schistosoma mansoni* in mice maintained on a torula yeast diet . . . ," ibid., pp. 129–35.

46 Report of Bilharzia Natural History Unit, in *12th Annual Report (1956–57) of the South African Council of Scientific and Industrial Research*.

47 H. Lurie and B. de Meillon, "Early diagnosis of bilharziasis," *South African Medical Journal* 26 (1952): 1005–8; "Correlation of biochemistry and histopathological changes in the liver in early bilharziasis," ibid. 27 (1953): 950–4.

48 B. de Meillon, E. C. England, and G. Laemmler, "Chemoprophylaxis in bilharziasis," *South African Medical Journal* 30 (1956): 611–13.

49 *Apartheid, Poverty and Malnutrition*, FAO Economic and Social Development Paper No. 24 (Rome, 1982).

CHAPTER 15 *Bilharzia: Second to only one*

1 *Official Records of the World Health Organization*, No. 5 (New York: WHO, 1947), p. 139.

2 Aly Shousha, "Schistosomiasis (bilharziasis): A world problem," *Bulletin of the WHO* 2 (1949): 19–30.

3 *Official Records* 7 (1949): 39, 201.

4 Programme Committee of First World Health Assembly, 11th meeting, July 8, 1948, Minutes (Geneva, 1948); reported also in *Offical Records*, 13 (1948): 141.

5 The first 11 were in malaria, TB, VD, maternal and child care, epidemiology and quarantine, health statistics, biological standardization, pharmacopoeias, drugs, insecticides, and nutrition. The six added later included sanitation, mental health, and plague.

6 The recommendation for this study team was adopted at the Second World Assembly of the WHO, 1949. *Official Records* 21 (1949). In 1907, the 12th International Sanitary Conference in Rome agreed to set up the OIHP to be run by a permanent committee of member states with headquarters in Paris. A little of its history is told in *The First Ten Years of the World Health Organization* (Geneva: WHO, 1958), Chapter 1.

7 W. H. Wright, "Medical parasitology in a changing world: What of the future?" Presidential address, published in *Journal of Parasitology* 37 (1951): 1–12; "Work of the W.H.O.," Annual Report of the Director General to the Third World Assembly (Geneva 1950); *Official Records* 30 (1951); Seventh Meeting, Helminth Subcommittee of Colonial Medical Research Advisory Committee, April 18, 1951, *Miscellaneous Papers*, CO 913/13.

8 Norman Stoll, "This wormy world," *Journal of Parasitology* 33 (1947): 1–18.

9 Special business session of the American Society of Tropical Medicine, November 1943. Archives, American Society of Tropical Medicine, Countway Library, Harvard Medical School.

10 Resolution to President Truman, presented at General Meeting, American Society of Tropical Medicine, December 1945. Archives, American Society of Tropical Medicine.

11 "Report of the Society's representative to the NRC Division of Biology and Agriculture," Annual Meeting, American Society of Parasitology, Boston 1946. Minutes, American Society of Parasitology, H. W. Manter Laboratory, University of Nebraska, Lincoln.

12 These 12 societies were the American societies of bacteriology, botany, development and growth, genetics, horticulturalists, limnology, mycology, physiology, plant physiology, poultry science, zoology, and parasitology.

13 Motion to approve the principle of amalgamation of the AATM with the ASTM and Hygiene. Annual General Meeting of the ASTM and Hygiene, Louisville, Kentucky, November 1943. Minutes of the American Academy of Tropical Medicine.

14 Walter Daniels (ed.), *The Four Point Program* (New York: H. W. Wilson, 1951).

15 Annual Meeting, American Society of Tropical Medicine, 1950 in Savannah, Georgia.

16 Ralph Hancock, *Puerto Rico: A Success Story* (New York: Van Nostrand, 1960).

17 A Puerto Rican side to the story is told in K. Wagenheim (ed.), *The Puerto Ricans: A Documentary History* (New York: Praeger, 1973).

18 Details in Samuel Bailey, *The United States and the Development of South America (1945–75)* (New York: New Viewpoints, 1976), Chapter 3.

19 Critics argue that the program took advantage, once again, of cheap Puerto Rican labor, and led to the total integration of the island's economy with that of the United States. This led to an increased maldistribution of wealth similar to the situation in the United States, increased unemployment, and mass migration by the poorer citizens to the slums of New York and other U.S. cities. Also, the money that entered the country favored special interest groups in the United States: Money had to be spent in the United States, and goods had to be transported in U.S. ships. There was, in other words, economic development but no social reform and redistribution of wealth.

20 A fascinating account of these activities is provided in Thomas McCann, *An American Company* (New York: Crown Publ., 1976), and its involvement in Guatemala is told in S. Schlesinger and S. Kinzer, *Bitter Fruit* (New York: Anchor Books, 1983). Sam Zmuri, the colorful old rogue who ran the company during its battles with the Nazis, had died in 1953. Eventually, the United Fruit Company was taken over by the United Brands multinational corporation.

21 E. Whitman, *How an American Company, Through Advertising and Public Relations, Has Combatted Communism in Latin America* (New York: International Advertising Assoc., 1955).

22 B. Belitt (ed. and trans.), *Selected Poems of Pablo Neruda* (New York: Grove Press, 1985). Reproduced by permission of the Grove Press, New York.

23 Stoll, "This wormy world."

24 Ibid., p. 1.

25 Andrew Warren, "Report of the Committee on War and Postwar Problems," Annual Meeting, American Society of Tropical Medicine, 1944.

26 These experiments are described in *Studies on Schistosomiasis*, National Institutes of Health Bulletin No. 189 (Washington, D.C.: U.S. Government Printing Office, 1947).

27 E. B. Cram and V. S. Files, "Laboratory studies on the snail host of *Schistosoma mansoni*," *American Journal of Tropical Medicine* 26 (1946): 715–20; E. B. Cram, V. S. Files, and M. F. Jones, "Experimental molluscan infection with *Schistosoma mansoni* and *Schistosoma haematobium*," in *Studies on Schistosomiasis*, pp. 81–94.

28 Paul Ward, D. Travis, and R. Rue, "Experimental molluscan infection with *S. japonicum*," *Studies on Schistosomiasis*, pp. 95–100.

29 Cram et al., "Experimental infection with *S. mansoni* and *S. haematobium*."

30 H. Stunkard, "Possible snail hosts of human schistosomiasis in the United States," *Journal of Parasitology* 32 (1946): 539–52.

31 W. H. Wright to Barlow, September 11, 1943; November 26, 1943, January 24, 1944. Rockefeller Foundation Archives, Barlow Papers, Series 1, Box 1, Folder 11.

32 Barlow, "Diary of self-affliction of *S. haematobium*." Ibid., Series 3, Box 5, Folder 73. An account of his agonies was eventually published: Barlow and C. H. Meleney, "A voluntary infection with *S. haematobium*," *American Journal of Tropical Medicine* 29 (1949): 79–87.

33 E. C. Andrus to Barlow, March 21, 1945, Rockefeller Foundation Archives, Barlow Papers, Series 1, Box 1, Folder 11.

34 Barlow, "Diary."

35 George Hunter, III, to Barlow, March 2, 1945, Rockefeller Foundation Archives, Barlow Papers, Series 1, Box 1, Folder 11.

36 This model is discussed in W. S. Thompson, "Population growth and the industrial revolution," *Population Problems* (McGraw Hill, 1953), Chapter 5. Edward Deevey has presented a broader view of this model in "The human population," *Scientific American* 203 (September 1960): 195–204.

37 Kingsley Davis, "The population specter: Rapidly declining death rate in densely populated countries. The amazing decline of mortality in underdeveloped areas," *American Economic Review* 46 (1956): 305–18.

38 Dichloro-diphenyl-trichloroethane (DDT) was first synthesized in 1941 by Paul Mueller of the Swiss Company, J. R. Geigy. In 1942 it was marketed as the antilice agent Neocid. The Americans and British began experimenting with it, and, in 1944, it was first tested against *Anopheles* mosquitoes in Italy by members of the Rockefeller Foundation. By the 1950s, the WHO had become advocates of mass DDT-centered malaria campaigns, and the total eradication of malaria became a viable proposition.

39 These and other surveys are discussed in Thomas Poleman, "World food: A perspective," *Science* 188 (May 1975): 510–18.

40 P. Erhlich, *The Population Bomb* (San Francisco: Sierra Club, 1969); W. Paddock, *Famine 1975! America's Decision: Who Will Survive?* (Boston: Little Brown, 1967).

41 U.S. Department of Agriculture, *The World Food Budget, 1962 and 1966* (Foreign Agricultural Economic Report No. 4, 1961).

42 Wright, "Medical parasitology."

43 Susan George, *How the Other Half Dies* (London: Penguin, 1977), represents one of the most articulate and widely respected of these critics. Also S. Weissman, "Why the population bomb is a Rockefeller baby," *Ramparts* 8 (1970): 43–7.

44 John Hunter, L. Rey, and D. Scott, "Man-made lakes and man-made disease: Towards a policy resolution," *Social Science and Medicine* 16 (1982): 1127–43.

45 G. Macdonald, "Medical implications of the Volta River project," *Transactions of the Royal Society of Tropical Medicine and Hygiene* 49 (1955): 13–27.

46 I. Paperna, "Snail vector of human schistosomiasis in the newly formed Volta Lake," in L. E. Obeng (ed.), *Man-Made Lakes: The Accra Symposium* (Accra: Ghana University Press, 1969).

47 I. Paperna, "Study of an outbreak of schistosomiasis in the newly formed Volta Lake in Ghana, *Zeitschrift für Tropenmedizin und Parasitologie* 21 (1970): 411–25.

48 Hunter et al., "Man-made lakes," 1128.

49 Joint OIHP/WHO Study Group on Bilharziasis in Africa, Report on the First Session, *WHO Technical Report Series*, No. 17 (Geneva: WHO, 1949). It was this committee which proposed that the genus of the worm be called "bilharzia," and the disease "bilharziasis." (See my earlier discussion of this problem.)

50 "Work on the WHO," Annual Report of the Director General to the Third World Assembly, Geneva, 1950, *Offical Records* 30 (1951); Resolution adopted by the Fourth World Assembly, May 1951, *ibid.*, 35 (1951): 23.

51 These surveys included J. A. Meira, "Schistosomiasis mansoni: A survey of its distribution in Brazil," *Bulletin of the WHO* 2 (1949): 31–7; W. H. Wright, "Bilharziasis as a public health problem in the Pacific," *ibid.* 2 (1950): 581–95; D. Blair, "Bilharziasis survey in British East and West Africa," *ibid.* 15 (1956): 203–73.

52 Four of the seven members were American: E. Faust, D. B. McMullen, J. Oliver-Gonzales, and W. H. Wright, but only one, D. M. Blair from Southern Rhodesia, represented British interests.

53 Expert Committee on Bilharziasis, First Report, *WHO Technical Report Series*, No. 65 (Geneva: WHO, 1953).

54 E. D. Pridie, "Reflections on recent African tours," Memo to Colonial Medical Research Advisory Committee, 1950, *Miscellaneous Papers*, CO 994/2.

55 *Parliamentary Debates*, House of Commons, May 24, 1946. Fifth Series, Vol. 423, line 784. For any American reader, the term "Poona mentality" used to be a commonly used term expressing total contempt of those British characters who viewed everyone not of British heritage to be totally incapable of behaving correctly or performing efficiently.

56 N. Hamilton Fairley and F. Hawking, "Proposals for Research in Helminthic Diseases with Specific Reference to Schistosomiasis, Filariasis, and Onchoceriasis," Memo CMR 46 (45), *Miscellaneous Papers*, CO 913/1.

57 *Parliamentary Debates* (Commons), May 27, 1949.

58 Seventh Meeting, Helminth Subcommittee, April 18, 1951, *Miscellaneous Papers*, CO 913/13.

CHAPTER 16 *Bilharzia (1950–1970s): A strategic change*

1 Details of the "new outlook" and these demonstration areas were given in 1950 by Brock Chisholm, Director General of the WHO. Chisholm, "The W.H.O.," *British Medical Journal* 2 (May 6, 1950): 1021–27.

2 "The work of the W.H.O., 1954," *Offical Records of the WHO*, No. 59, 1954.

3 John Weir, "Report of visit to Egypt, to review changes that have occurred in Egypt," Rockefeller Foundation Archives, RG 2, Series 485, Box 65, Folder 427.

4 Weir interview with Dr. A. Kamal, December 16, 1955, Weir Diaries, 1955.

5 John Weir, "Report," p. 5.

6 H. van der Schalie, "WHO Project Egypt – 10: A case history of a schistosomiasis control project," in M. T. Farvar and J. Milton (eds.), *The Careless Technology: Ecology and International Development* (Garden City, NJ: Natural History Press, 1972).

7 Expert Committee on Bilharziasis, Second Report, *WHO Technical Report Series*, No. 214 (Geneva: WHO, 1961).

8 Van der Schalie, "Vector snail control in Qalyub, Egypt," *Bulletin of the WHO* 19 (1958): 263–83.

9 E. G. Beery, "Investigation of bilharziasis control through use of molluscicides in the Warraq El-Arab project near Cairo, Egypt, 1953–63" [typed memo], November 1963, in Schisto-Egypt 1958–64 file, Parasitic Diseases Programme, WHO.

10 W. H. Wright, "Observations on bilharziasis research and control programmes in Egypt," November 21–December 4; December 11–20, 1957. Schisto-Egypt 1957 file; D. B. McMullen, "Report on the preliminary survey by the bilharziasis advisory scheme – 1958," 20 Feb. 1959, in Schisto-Egypt 1958–64 file, Parasitic Diseases Programme, WHO.

11 P. L. Le Roux, "Report on the African Conference on Bilharziasis – Brazzeville," November 26–December 3, 1956, Document CMRC (H) 57 (20). 4, in *Miscellaneous Papers*, CO 913/13.

12 African Conference on Bilharziasis. *WHO Technical Report Series*, No. 139. (Geneva: WHO, 1957).

13 U.S. Army 406th Medical General Laboratory. *Annual Historical Report.* Japan, 1950.

14 Ibid., 1951. Also G. Hunter et al., "Studies on schistosomiasis VI. Control of the snail host of schistosomiasis in Japan with sodium pentachlorophenate (Santobrite)," *American Journal of Tropical Medicine and Hygiene* 1 (1952): 831–47.

15 U. S. Army 406th Medical General Laboratory. *Professional Report.* Japan, 1954.

16 Ibid., 1963. Making accurate counts of snails collected from weedy and murky water is a nearly impossible task. Using snails collected per hour probably gives a more reliable figure for comparative purposes than trying to reach absolute numbers.

17 Ibid., 1964.

18 Second African Conference on Bilharzia. *WHO Technical Report Series* No. 204 (Geneva: WHO, 1960), p. 20.

19 My brief account of the groundnut scheme is taken mostly from Alan Wood, *The Groundnut Affair* (London: The Bodley Head, 1950).

20 George Hall to the House of Commons, July 9, 1946. *Parliamentary Debates* (Commons), 5th Series, Vol. 425, col. 253.

21 *Parliamentary Debates* (Commons), 5th Series, Vol. 443, col. 2033 (Nov. 7, 1947).

22 "A plan for the mechanized production of groundnuts in East and Central Africa," February 1947, Cmd. 7030.

23 Colonial Research (1946–7). I. The Colonial Research Committee, Cmd. 7151, p. 16.

24 East Africa Medical Survey and Research Institute. *Annual Report*, 1955–6.

25 Helminth Subcommittee, 15th meeting, February 25, 1955, *Miscellaneous Papers*, CO 913/13.

26 Ibid., 17th meeting, October 21, 1955.

27 G. Covell and G. Macdonald, "Report on tour of East Africa," Document CMR (57) 11, Colonial Medical Research Committee (CMRC), 42nd meeting, November 1957, *Miscellaneous Papers*, CO 913/8.

28 G. Covell and G. Macdonald, "Report on visit to East Africa," Document CMR (58). 6, CMRC, 43rd meeting, May 21, 1958, *Miscellaneous Papers*, CO 913/9.

29 Macdonald was only 64 years old when he died in 1967. Obituaries to him were published in the *Lancet*, December 23, 1967; *British Medical Journal*, December 23, 1967; and *Nature* 217, February 1968.

30 East African Institute for Medical Research, *Annual Report*, 1960–1.

31 D. Forsyth and D. Bradley, "Radiological manifestations of urinary schistosomiasis in apparently normal, healthy, primary schoolchildren," *Transactions of the Royal Society of Tropical Medicine and Hygiene* 58 (1964): 291; "Irreversible damage by *Schistosoma haematobium* in schoolchildren," *Lancet* 2 (1964): 169–71.

32 East African Institute for Medical Research, *Annual Report*, 1961–2.

33 G. Webbe, "Laboratory and field trials of a new molluscicide, Bayer 73, in Tanganyika," *Bulletin of the WHO* 25 (1961): 525–31; "The transmission of *S. haematobium* in an area of Lake Province, Tanganyika," *Bulletin of the WHO* 27 (1962): 59–85; "Control of transmission of *Schistosoma mansoni* in the Mirongo River," *East African Medical Journal* 41 (1964): 508–19.

34 These concerns are discussed in a letter from Dr. Ansari to the Director General, WHO, briefing him for a forthcoming visit to Egypt; October 27, 1964, Schisto-Egypt 1958–64 file, Parasitic Diseases Programme, WHO.

35 For examples of incidence, see J. E. Gordon "The newer epidemiology," in *Tomorrow's Horizon in Public Health*. Transactions of the 1950 Conference of the Public Health Association of New York (New York: Public Health Assoc., 1950). The first use in tropical medicine may have been J. A. Doull et al., "The incidence of leprosy in Cordova and Talisay, Cebu, Philippine Islands," *International Journal of Leprosy* 10 (1942): 107–31. Dr. Jordan and Dr. Shurrock first pointed out this paper to me.

36 D. B. McMullen et al., "WPRO Report on the schistosomiasis team to the Philippines," September 30, 1952, Philippine – 1958 file, Parasitic Diseases Programme, WHO. (Also published in *Journal of the Philippine Medical Association* 30 (1954): 615–27.)

37 T. P. Pesigan et al., "Studies on bilharziasis in the Philippines." Paper prepared for the Brazzaville Conference on Bilharziasis, 1956 (WHO/Bil. Conf./2 August 21, 1956). Details also published in "Studies on *Schistosoma japonicum* infection in the Philippines. I. General considerations and epidemiology," *Bulletin of the WHO* 18 (1958):428–30.

38 M. Farooq and N. G. Hairston, "The epidemiology of *Schistosoma haematobium* and *S. mansoni* infections in the Egypt-49 project area. IV. Measurement of the incidence of bilharziasis," *Bulletin of the WHO* 35 (1966): 331–8.

39 These and other like findings were reported in *Egypt-49 Quarterly Field Reports*. File Egypt-49, Parasitic Diseases Programme, WHO. Most of the conclusions were given in the *Second-Quarter Report* of 1966. The very positive conclusion was given in a 1965 memo entitled "The effect of area-wide snail control on endemicity of bilharziasis in Egypt," a selected and a slightly more restrained version of which appeared in *Bulletin of the WHO* 35 (1966): 369–75; and also in "Progress in bilharziasis control: The situation in Egypt," *WHO Chronicle* 21 (1967): 175–84.

40 Egypt-49. *Fourth Quarter Report*, 1967.

41 D. Forsyth, M. Soussa, and K. Chu, "Final evaluation of Project UAR-0049," *Fourth Quarter Report*, 1968.

42 Egypt-49 Project, *Fourth-Quarter Report*, 1969.

43 H. M. Gillis et al., "Results of a 7 year control project on the endemicity of

Schistosoma haematobium infection in Egypt," *Annals of Tropical Medicine and Parasitology* 67 (1973): 45–65.

44 P. Jordan, "Incidence rates of *Schistosoma haematobium* infection. UAR-0049," *Annals of Tropical Medicine and Parasitology* 68 (1974): 243. Gilles believed that Farooq had "diluted" his data, by using only the 0- to 6-year-olds in his yearly samples. According to Gilles, in the second year of sampling from which the initial incidence measurement was obtained, Farooq had ignored those who had become 7 years of age and counted those born that year, thus replacing a group with a high probability of becoming infected (the 7-year-olds) with a group with a very low probability (the babies). In that way, the second sample would be "diluted" and the number of noninfected individuals and thus the incidence figure would be too low. Jordan explained, however, that Farooq had found 101 preschoolers negative in 1962 and that in 1963, 78 of this same group were still negative, giving an incidence of 22.8 percent. Then, in 1963, he had also found 273 negative preschoolers in a new group of 0- to 6-year-olds, and that in 1964, 253 of them were still negative, giving an incidence of 7.3 percent.

45 L. J. Olivier, "Assessment report, Egypt 2101," May 23, 1973, Egypt-49 file, Parasitic Diseases Programme, WHO.

46 F. S. Barbosa, "Duty travel report on U.A.R., 0049. Schistosomiasis control pilot project," February–March 1971, Egypt-49 file, Parasitic Diseases Programme, WHO.

47 T. H. Weller and G. Dammin, "The incidence and distribution of *S. mansoni* and other helminths in Puerto Rico," *Puerto Rico Journal of Public Health and Tropical Medicine* 21 (1945): 125–47; 56.5 percent were also found to carry hookworm, the forgotten disease.

48 J. R. Palmer et al., "The control of schistosomiasis on Patillas, Puerto Rico," *Public Health Reports* 84 (1969); 1003–7; F. Ferguson et al., "Control of schistosomiasis on Vieques Island, Puerto Rico," *American Journal of Tropical Medicine and Hygiene* 17 (1968): 258–63; W. Jobin et al., "Control of schistosomiasis in Guayama and Arroyo, Puerto Rico," *Bulletin of the WHO* 42 (1970): 151–6.

49 See, for example, I. G. Kagan and J. Pellegrino, "A critical review of immunological methods for the diagnosis of bilharziasis," *Bulletin of the WHO* 25 (1961): 611–74.

50 H. Negron-Aponte, and W. R. Jobin, "Schistosomiasis control in Puerto Rico: 25 years of operational experience," *American Journal of Tropical Medicine and Hygiene* 28 (1979): 515–25.

51 G. Macdonald, "The dynamics of helminth infections, with special reference to schistosomes," *Transactions of the Royal Society of Tropical Medicine and Hygiene* 59 (1965): 489–506, quotation from p. 495. The "contamination factor" was an estimate of the number of schistosome eggs in the water. It depended on mean worm loads in the human population, the daily egg output of each worm pair, and the proportion of eggs that were not trapped in the tissues but passed into the water. The "snail factor" was an estimate of the number of infected snails and their cercarial output. The "exposure factor" estimated the probability of the cercariae finding a human in which to develop; and the "longevity factor" was a measure of the life-span of the parasite in the host.

52 P. Jordan, "Schistosomiasis: Research to control," *American Journal of Tropical Medicine and Hygiene* 26 (1977): 877–86. A full report of the project was published in Peter Jordan, *Schistosomiasis: The St. Lucia Project*, (Cambridge: Cambridge University Press, 1985). The drug of choice, introduced into the project in 1974, was oxamniquine.

53 W. Kikuth, "Maintenance of a strain of *S. mansoni*," translation of a document found

at Elberfeld, Memo CMR 46 (H) 5, *Miscellaneous Papers*, CO 913/13. The drug was subsequently reported by W. Kikuth, R. Goennert, and H. Mauss, "Miracil, ein neues Chemotherapeuticum gegen die Darmbilharziose," *Naturwissenschaften* 33 (1946): 253.

54 Hecht, "Pharmacology of Miracil," free translation of a report of April 14, 1943 found in *CIOS* 25: 54–124, Memo CMR 47(H) 2, *Miscellaneous Papers*, CO 913/13. I have no idea as to the identity of *CIOS*.

55 D. R. Wood, "Further information about Miracil," Memo CMR 47(H) 3; W. F. Ross and F. Hawking, "The toxicity of Miracil," Memo CMR 47 (H) 5, *Miscellaneous Papers*, CO 913/13.

56 Colonial Medical Research Committee, *Fourth Annual Report*, May 23, 1949, *Miscellaneous Papers*, CO 913/3.

57 William Alves, "Intensive treatment of schistosomiasis with antimony," *South African Medical Journal* 19 (1945): 171.

58 Alves, "The 'public health cure' of bilharziasis with one-day course of antimony," *South African Medical Journal* 20 (1946): 146; Alves and D. M. Blair, "Schistosomiasis: A review of work in Southern Rhodesia," ibid. 21 (1947): 352–7; Blair, "Schistosomiasis in Southern Rhodesia: Public health aspects," ibid. 22 (1948): 462–7.

59 F. Hawking and W. F. Ross, "Report on the clinical trial of Miracil D for the treatment of schistosomiasis," Memo CMR 47 (33), *Miscellaneous Papers*, CO 913/2. This trial was paid for by the wealthy Southern Rhodesian Government, enjoying the fruits of a "self-governing colony," not by the Colonial Development and Welfare Fund. Southern Rhodesia, *Report on Public Health for the Year 1947.*

60 Southern Rhodesia, *Report on Public Health for the Year 1948.*

61 D. M. Blair, "Lucanthone hydrochloride: A review," *Bulletin of the WHO* 18 (1958): 989–1010.

62 *Annual Report on the Public Health of the Federation of Rhodesia and Nyasaland*, 1958 and 1960.

63 Blair, "Lucanthone hydrochloride," and J. E. McMahon, "History of chemotherapy of bilharziasis: (1) Development of schistosomicides," *East African Medical Journal* 53 (1976): 296–305.

64 NAMRU 3 was set up in 1946, taking over the site of the American Typhus Commission which had been disbanded a year before. Bilharzia was never a major component of their work, although Lt. R. Kuntz did some important work searching for reservoir hosts of the disease in Egypt.

65 The discovery of prophylactic rather than therapeutic drugs has always been a major concern of the U.S. military. Very recently they have discovered that a well-known therapeutic drug, niclosamide, also acts to prevent cercariae from entering the skin. J. Cherfas, "New weapon in the war against schistosomiasis," *Science* 246 (1989): 1242–3.

66 D. G. Sandt, J. Bruce, and M. G. Radke, "A system for mass producing the snail *Australorbis glabratus* and cercariae of *Schistosoma mansoni*," *Journal of Parasitology* 51 (1965): 1012–13.

67 J. Pellagrino et al., "New approach to the screening of drugs in experimental schistosomiasis mansoni in mice," *American Journal of Tropical Medicine and Hygiene* 11 (1962): 201–15.

68 M. G. Radke, "*Schistosoma mansoni* mouse mortality test system for mass screening for prophylactic drugs," *Experimental Parasitology* 30 (1971): 1–10.

69 J. Seubert et al., "Synthesis and properties of praziquantel, a novel broad spectrum antihelminthic with excellent activity against schistosomes and cestodes," *Experimentia* 33 (1977): 1036–7. G. Leopold et al., "Clinical pharmacology in normal

volunteers of praziquantel, a new drug against schistosomes and cestodes," *European Journal of Clinical Pharmacology* 14 (1978): 281–91. Its effectiveness against infected laboratory animals was reported in the 1977 issue of *Zeitschrift für Parasitenkunde*, Vol. 52. This volume includes articles by G. Webbe, who had moved to the Bayer Laboratory from Mwanza, and by R. Goennert, who had been, many years before, the codiscoverer of Miracil D. The Nairobi conference proceedings were published in *Arzneimittelforschung* 3a (1981): 535–618.

70 P. Jordan, "Schistosomiasis: Research to control," *American Journal of Tropical Medicine and Hygiene* 26 (1977): 877–86.

CHAPTER 17 *Conclusion: The imperial triad*

1 Franco-Agudelo takes a narrower perspective than I do in arguing that the Rockefellers' health campaigns were set up to increase the profit margin of the Rockefeller empire, and thus that they behaved in much the same way as the United Fruit Company. "The Rockefeller Foundation's antimalarial program in Latin America: Donating or dominating?" *International Journal of Health Services* 13 (1983): 51–67. This argument becomes difficult to rebut when he claims, from what sources I do not know, that the Rockefeller network garners one-third of the sum total of profits reaped by U.S. companies in the world. But in my reading of their archival sources, I saw no indication that a program was actually set up with such self-centered motives in mind – and it certainly didn't apply to their campaigns in the Nile Delta.

2 This has been discussed also by F. R. Sandbach, "The history of schistosomiasis research and policy for its control," *Medical History* 20 (1976): 259–75.

3 For details of the Philippine school see Dean C. Worcester, *The Philippines: Past and Present* (New York: Macmillan, 1930). Details of the Puerto Rican school can be found in the Columbiana Collection, Columbia University.

4 Peter Donaldson, "Foreign intervention in medical education: A case study of the Rockefeller Foundation's involvement in a Thai medical school," in V. Navarro (ed.), *Imperialism, Health, and Medicine* (Farmingdale, N.Y.: Baywood Publ., 1981).

5 J. Simmons, address given at Conference on Health Problems of Industries Operating in Tropical Countries, Harvard School of Public Health, 1950. This quotation was taken from H. Cleaver, "Malaria and the political economy of public health," *International Journal of Health Services* 7 (1977): 557–79.

6 K. Kvale, "Schistosomiasis in Brazil: Preliminary results from a case study of a new focus," *Social Science and Medicine* 15D (1981): 489–500. The issue is discussed further in W. Jobin, "Sugar and snails: The ecology of bilharziasis related to agriculture in Puerto Rico," *American Journal of Tropical Medicine and Hygiene* 29 (1980): 86–94; and K. Haddock, "Control of schistosomiasis: The Puerto Rican experience," *Social Science and Medicine* 15 (1981): 501–14.

7 Figures quoted in John Hunter, L. Rey, and D. Scott, "Man-made lakes and man-made disease," *Social Science and Medicine* 16 (1982): 1127–45.

8 These issues are discussed in D. Owen, "Drought and desertification in Africa: Lessons from the Nairobi conference," *Oikos* 33 (1979): 139–51; Janet Raloff, "Africa's famine: The human dimension," *Science News* 127 (May 11, 1985): 299–301; G. Obasi, "Understanding the drought," *Bulletin of Atomic Scientists* 41, No. 8 (1985): 43–5; Lloyd Timberlake, *Only One Earth* (London: B.B.C. Books, 1987).

9 M. Kishk, "Land degradation in the Nile Valley," *Ambio* 15 (1986): 226–30.

10 M. F. Abdel-Wahab et al., "Changing patterns of schistosomiasis in Egypt, 1935–

1979," *Lancet* 2 (1979): 242. Abdel-Wahab, *Schistosomiasis in Egypt* (Boca Raton, Fla.: CRC Press, 1982), pp. 78–81.

11 N. Nihei, S. Asami, and H. Tanaka, "Geographical factors influencing the population numbers and distribution of *Oncomelania nosophora* and the subsequent effect on the control of schistosomiasis japonica in Japan," *Social Science and Medicine* 115D (1981): 149–57.

12 The changing economic situation in Puerto Rico was accompanied also by mass migrations to U.S. cities. Many of these migrants were infected with *S. mansoni*, and so, in 1959, the Walter Reed Army Institute of Research began testing wild mammals in the Washington area for susceptibility to *S. mansoni*. Woodchucks, field mice, and squirrels were, they concluded, "potential reservoirs of infection."

13 These plans are outlined in the various editions of *Schistosomiasis Research: The Strategic Plan* (New York: The Edna McConnell Clark Foundation.) Four times each year the Foundation also publishes *Schisto Update*, which contains a list of articles concerned with bilharzia.

14 K. S. Warren, "Regulation of the prevalence and intensity of schistosomiasis in man: Immunology and ecology," *Journal of Infectious Diseases* 127 (1973): 595–609.

15 The Edna McDonnell Clark Foundation. *Annual Report*, 1981.

16 John Bryant, *Health in the Developing World* (Ithaca: Cornell University Press, 1969).

17 P. O. Williams, "The scientific neglect of tropical medicine," in Clive Wood (ed.), *Tropical Medicine: From Romance to Reality* (New York: Academic Press, 1978).

18 Maurice King (ed.), *Medical Care in Developing Countries: A Primer on the Medicine of Poverty* (Nairobi: Oxford University Press, 1966). Also Bryant, *Health in the Developing World*.

19 C. Hughes and J. Hunter, "Disease and 'development' in Africa," *Social Science and Medicine* 3 (1970): 443–93; M. Turshen, *The Political Ecology of Disease in Tanzania* (New Brunswick, N.J.: Rutgers University Press, 1984).

20 Brian Maegraith, "Tropical medicine: What it is not, what it is," *Bulletin of the New York Academy of Medicine* 48 (1972): 1210–30. These issues were also discussed in his *One World* (London: Athlone Press, 1973).

21 A. Learmouth, *Disease Ecology* (London: Blackwell, 1988).

22 Bradley, "Tropical medicine." in J. Walton et al. (eds.), *Oxford Companion to Medicine*, (Oxford: Oxford University Press, 1986), Vol. 2, 1393–9.

23 *Primary Health Care*, Report of the International Conference on Primary Health Care, Alma Ata, USSR, September 1978 (Geneva: WHO, 1978). The endorsement by the WHO was published as *Global Strategy for Health for All by the Year 2000* (Geneva: WHO, 1981).

24 *The Control of Schistosomiasis*, Report of a WHO expert committee, *WHO Technical Report Series* No. 728 (Geneva: WHO, 1985).

25 "Management and organization of schistosomiasis control in primary health care," Proceedings from the GTZ/WHO/AFRO Seminar, Nairobi, December 1985, *Tropical Medicine and Parasitology* 37 (1986): 233.

26 K. Mott, The strategy of morbidity reduction in schistosomiasis, report prepared for the Expert Committee on the Control of Schistosomiasis, WHO/SCHISTO/83.68; and "Schistosomiasis control," in D. Rollinson and A. Simpson (eds.), *The Biology of Schistosomes: From Genes to Latrines* (London: Academic Press, 1987).

27 The reason for these numbers is discussed in *The Control of Schistosomiasis*.

28 In 1965, the question of public health importance had been addressed for the first time by the WHO, *Measurement of the Public Health Importance of Bilharziasis*, Report of a WHO scientific group, *Technical Report Series* 349 (Geneva: WHO, 1967). Also,

the new interest in morbidity is indicated by two recent review articles by M. G. Chen and K. Mott: "Progress in assessment of morbidity in *S. haematobium* infection," *Tropical Disease Bulletin* 86 (1989): R1–R36; "Progress in assessment of morbidity in *S. mansoni* infection," *Tropical Disease Bulletin* 85 (1988): R1–R56.

29 Details are given in the Proceedings from the GTZ/WHO/AFRO Seminar, 1985.

30 Mott, "Strategy of morbidity reduction."

31 "UNICEF blames Third World debt for half-million children's deaths," *Toronto Globe and Mail*, December 20, 1988.

32 *Official Records, WHO* No. 39 (1952), p. 2. See also Vicento Navarro, "The nature of imperialism and its implications in health and medicine," in Navarro (ed.), *Imperialism, Health and Medicine.*

INDEX

Abbas I, 48

Africa. *See individual countries*

Africans. *See* British Empire; South Africa; Southern Rhodesia

African Survey (Hailey), 148, 176, 222–24, 227–28, 229

Agramonte, Aristides, 41, 43

Ali, Muhammad, 46–47, 48

Alves, William, 287

American Academy of Tropical Medicine, 146, 153, 251, 252

American empire: administration of, 31; difference from British Empire, 31–33, 294, 296–7; Good Neighbor Policy of, 153–54; policies of, 32–33, 37, 38, 39, 151, 152, 294, 296; tropical medicine in, 35–36, 116–17, 153, 154, 250–53, 294

American Foundation of Tropical Medicine, 146–47, 153, 154, 157, 251, 253

American Institute of the Biological Sciences, 251

American Society of Parasitology, 250

American Society of Tropical Medicine, 43, 145–46, 153, 157, 170, 251; Committee on War and Postwar Problems of, 251, 255

American Society of Tropical Medicine and Hygiene, 251, 252

American South: diseases in, 33–34; hookworm in, 72–74; medical schools in, 33–34; as model for South Africa, 131–32

antimony tartrate. *See* drugs, antibilharzial

Ashford, Bailey, 39–40, 72, 73, 152

Aswan Dam, 51, 199, 267, 299

Atkinson, Lt. Edward, 66–67

Australia, troops of, in World War II, 158, 168

Azim, Abdel, 191

bacteriology: in Britain, 25–29; in United States, 35–36

Balfour, Marshall, 198

Bang, F. C., 161, 162, 250

Baring, Evelyn, 51

Barker, L. F., 42

Barlow, Claude, 102, 104f, 264, 267; in China, 102–3, 193; in Egypt, 105–6, 108–11, 112f, 113, 188–91, 193; self-infection of, 104, 258–59

Basch, Paul, 213–14

Bayer and Co., 99, 286, 289

Bayer 73 (Bayluscide), 272, 279, 281, 284

Bechuanaland, 145

beriberi, 42

Bevan, Ernest, 145, 265

Bilharz, Theodor, 5, 48f, 49, 50, 54, 55, 57, 60

bilharzia: academic research on, 124, 301, 324n23; acute form of, 165, 167, 247; "break point" of, 285–86, 303; diagnosis of, 167–68, 284; distribution of, 3, 6, 7f, 54, 264; early views about, 54; epidemiology of, 8–10; etiology of, 3, 5–6; importance of, 3, 115, 157–59, 169–70, 232, 249, 250, 255, 266t, 274, 275t, 294, 300–1; incidence of, 281, 283, 286, 303; irrigation and, 47, 51, 114–15, 121–24, 199, 244, 246, 261, 263t, 262–65, 274, 298; morbidity of, 299–300, 303; naming of, 5, 62; pathology of, 6, 8, 54, 165, 167, 244, 246–47, 278–79, 301; prevalence of, 6, 255, 256t; skin-infection theory of, 59–60, 61, 63, 64, 66, 67, 69; *see also* schistosomes

–campaigns against. *See* Brazil; British Empire; China; Cyprus; Egypt; Gambia; Ghana (Gold Coast); Japan; Mozambique; Nigeria; North America; Nyasaland; Philippines; Puerto Rico; St. Lucia; South Africa; Southern Rhodesia; Sudan; Tanganyika (Tanzania); Uganda; West Indies; World War I; World War II

–prevention of, 70–1, 269, 270, 296, 303; by canal clearance, 70, 109–10, 111, 112f, 113, 189, 191; by community participation, 303–4; by drying, 70, 109; by prophylactic drugs, 247, 288; by sanitation, 102, 106–8; by uniform impregnation, 164f, 165; *see also* molluscicides

–therapeutic for. *See* drugs, antibilharzial

Blackett, B., 145

Blackie, William, 135, 136

Blair, D. M., 264, 287

Boer War, bilharzia in, 4

Bradley, David, 277, 278f, 279, 302

Brazil, bilharzia in, 58

Brewer, Isaac, 125

British Army, diseases of, 13, 64, 158

–medical schools: Chatham, 21; Millbank, 21, 27, 68; Netley, 20, 21, 22f, 27, 308n23

British Empire, 15–16, 16f, 274; bilharzia in, 232t, 265–66, 266t, 274, 275t, 277; criticisms of, 147; educational commissions of, 224, 225–27; expenditure of, 141–2, 143, 145, 274, 275t; medical policies of, 17–18, 35, 145, 175–78, 219, 293–94, 296, 297; research in, 227–28, 230; *see also* Colonial Office; South Africa; Southern Rhodesia; *and individual countries*